I0813797

GOOD, BETTER, BEST

A **Three-Tiered Approach** to Weight Maintenance with **100 Low-Carb, Sugar-Free Recipes** for Lasting Success

BRENDA BENNETT

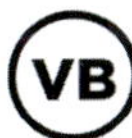

VICTORY BELT PUBLISHING INC.
LAS VEGAS

First published in 2025 by Victory Belt Publishing Inc.

Copyright © 2025 Brenda Bennett

No part of this publication may be reproduced or distributed in any form or by any means, electronic or mechanical, or stored in a database or retrieval system, without prior written permission from the publisher.

ISBN-13: 978-1-628605-45-7

The author is not a licensed practitioner, physician, or medical professional and offers no medical diagnoses, treatments, suggestions, or counseling. The information presented herein has not been evaluated by the U.S. Food and Drug Administration, and it is not intended to diagnose, treat, cure, or prevent any disease. Full medical clearance from a licensed physician should be obtained before beginning or modifying any diet, exercise, or lifestyle program, and physicians should be informed of all nutritional changes.

The author/owner claims no responsibility to any person or entity for any liability, loss, or damage caused or alleged to be caused directly or indirectly as a result of the use, application, or interpretation of the information presented herein.

Cover design by Kat Lannom

Interior design and illustrations by Elita San Juan

Cover photo and author photos by Shawon Davis

Printed in Canada

TC 0125

TABLE OF CONTENTS

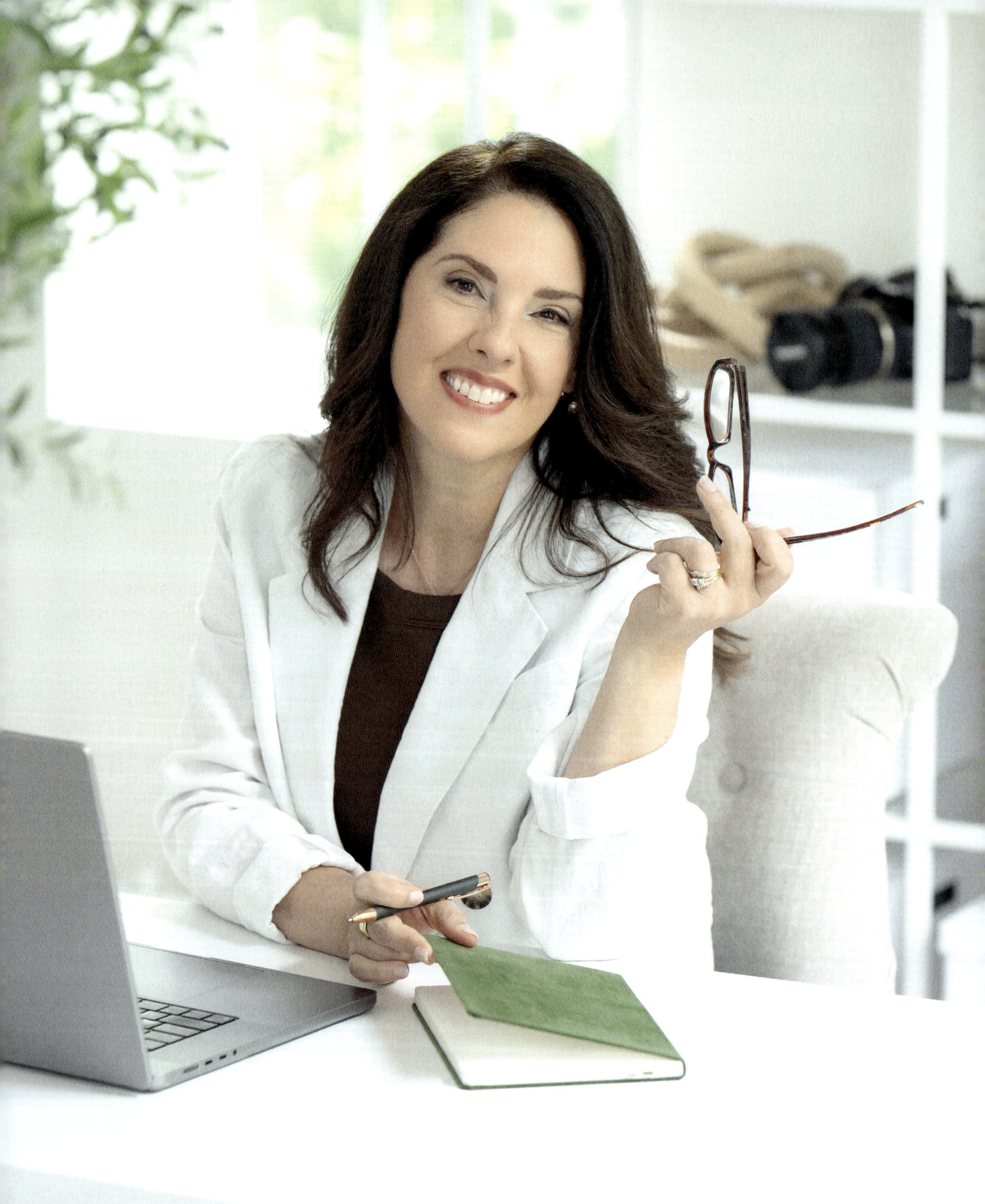

A LETTER TO THE READER

What if making healthy choices was simpler than you thought?

No elaborate plans, significant expense, or culinary expertise required. Just a willingness to prioritize your well-being.

Good, Better, Best offers a practical approach to stay on track so you can end the cycle of stopping and starting yet another "diet."

This book combats and conquers the all-or-nothing attitude that sabotages weight loss, triggers overeating, and hinders you from keeping weight off for good. It debunks the myths that eating whole-food, healthy meals takes too much time and effort and lacks sufficient variety, that you need more willpower, that you have too much stress to eat healthily, or that making healthy choices when eating out or at social events is too hard.

While I do love a good salad, I also love dessert. Maintaining weight shouldn't be a lifelong sentence to never indulge in foods you love! When you apply the *Good, Better, Best* mindset to your daily food decisions, keeping the weight off is simple and permanent, and you won't be required to eat salads for the rest of your life or never go out to eat again.

My goal with this book is to help you learn to make wise food choices more often than you make poor ones so that you can maintain weight loss. It's the sequel to my bestselling book *The 30-Day Sugar Elimination Diet,* which hundreds of people have successfully used to lose weight. That book explains how to detox from sugar and refined carbs, and this book teaches you to make better decisions about what you eat despite a food craving, an emotional trigger, or a generally bad day.

If you struggle with overeating—whether it's overeating sugar and refined carbs or overeating healthy keto foods—the answer is simple for everyone. The sole requirement is making better food choices and overcoming temptations that lead to overeating. Even if you don't have weight to lose or a desire to reduce or eliminate sugar and refined carbs, *Good, Better, Best* will help you.

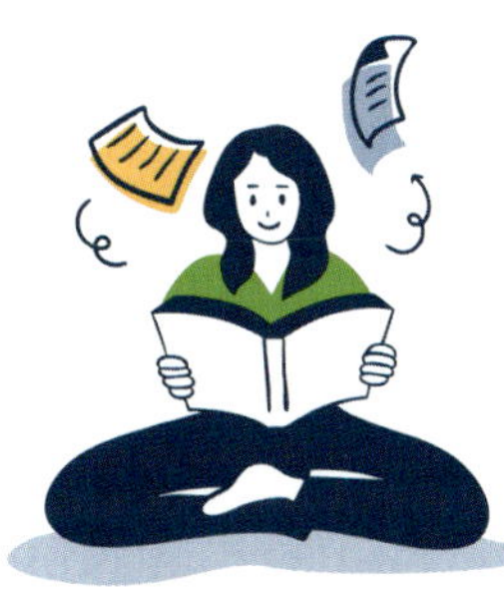

There are two parts to this book. Part 1 explains how to apply the Good, Better, Best mindset to every food decision you make, which will allow you to stay on track with your health goals and keep the weight off for good.

Part 2 provides meal plans and 100 delicious low-carb and mostly keto recipes categorized as Good (Enough), Better, and Best, with a back-to-basics whole-food approach and some simple planning and prepping that allows you to decide what you have time to make and how much effort you want to expend:

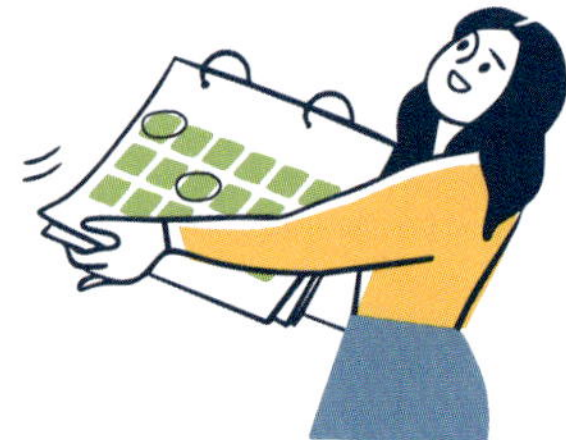

- Good (Enough) recipes take less than 20 minutes.
- Better recipes take 15 to 45 minutes, with much of the time for longer recipes being hands-off.
- Best recipes require more than 30 minutes. These recipes are for the days you have extra time to meal prep, cook, and enjoy your meals.

(You'll find a detailed discussion of the concept on pages 11 to 12, in the section titled "Good, Better, Best Defined.")

There's no one-size-fits-all plan that works for everyone to lose weight, but the one thing I am sure of is that no one ever intends to regain weight. Old habits have a way of creeping back in, one small decision at a time, until the number on the scale starts inching up. Maybe panic doesn't set in until you're up 10 or even 20 pounds, but the all-or-nothing attitude is the culprit that stalls and stops you from getting back on track in the moment. The all-or-nothing attitude starts with the thought, "I promise I will do better tomorrow."

Because let's face it: You know exactly how to lose weight. You may have done it successfully more than once in your life. You know all the things that help you achieve the right weight, yet you gradually slip with your food choices on a day-to-day basis when you're stressed, tired, bored, or anxious or when convenience foods win you over because of lack of planning.

This book is for anyone who feels they are a stress eater or lets good habits fall by the wayside on difficult days when the best intentions for a healthy meal fall apart.

Do any of these thoughts sound familiar?

- *It's almost lunchtime, and I didn't pack a healthy meal. I already blew it today with that pastry at the staff meeting this morning, so I will start over tomorrow.*
- *It's the weekend. I can't get back on track on the weekend when I have plans to go to a party, and there will be so much food. I'll have to start Monday.*
- *I really don't know what happened! I hit my goal weight, and now it's a month later, and I'm back up 10 pounds.*
- *I'm so stressed out and not motivated today to eat healthy, but I'll strategize and do better first thing in the morning.*

Before you dive into this book, begin to think about the common patterns you see in your life that cause you to steer off your healthy-eating food choices, which leads to weight gain:

- Are social events and FOMO (fear of missing out) your downfall?
- Is it a lack of planning healthy snacks that leads you to the vending machine or office breakroom for donuts?
- Is it a lack of time to make meals at home, so ordering takeout has become the norm?
- Is it stress from work, family, and other obligations that make you want to run to comfort foods like sugar and refined carbs?
- Could it be all of the above?

After coaching thousands of women (and some men) in my tribe membership, the most common themes are lack of planning for better options and lack of time. The easy route becomes takeout, drive-thru, or packaged convenience foods on the go.

You're not alone. It happens to the best of us.

The next common reasons for not being able to stick to healthy food plans are temptation, trying not to give in when everyone else is indulging, and a fear of missing out. The prevailing thought is "If I have one slip, it's over; I might as well just eat whatever I want and try again tomorrow." This all-or-nothing attitude comes about when you think perfection is necessary to keep weight off.

I'm here to tell you, it's not true. You can be imperfect *and* lose weight and keep it off. You can have slips without letting them ruin your day, so you throw in the towel and feel you should just wait and start again on Monday.

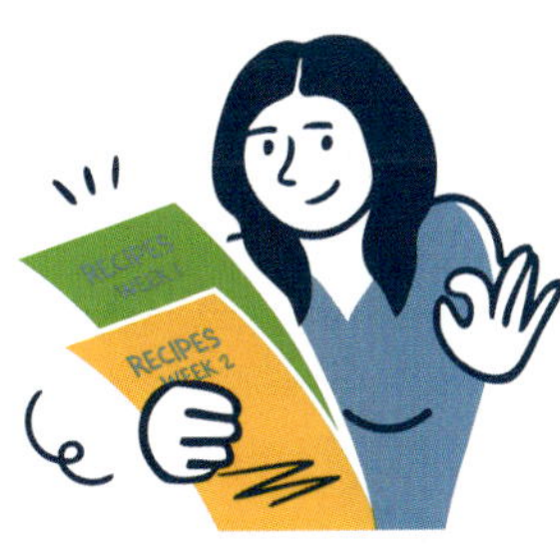

While I can't give you more time in your day, my prayer is that reading *Good, Better, Best* and applying this mindset strategy to your life will empower you to believe you can surely keep your weight off, no matter what life throws at you.

Wherever you are in your health journey—working on weight loss, maintaining your weight, or taking off some regained weight—you have the tools and habits to keep it off for good with the Good, Better, Best method.

With a little planning, some preparing, and an attitude of confidence, you will learn to make Good, Better, Best food choices daily. And when you make a choice that steers you off the path toward your goals, you'll realize why it happened and figure out how to get back on track quickly.

The days of delaying until after the weekend to start again on Monday are over. You'll live in the moment and make food choices based on Good, Better, or Best, and that will be enough.

You'll see how simple it truly is to lose weight successfully and stay at your happy weight for life—one choice at a time.

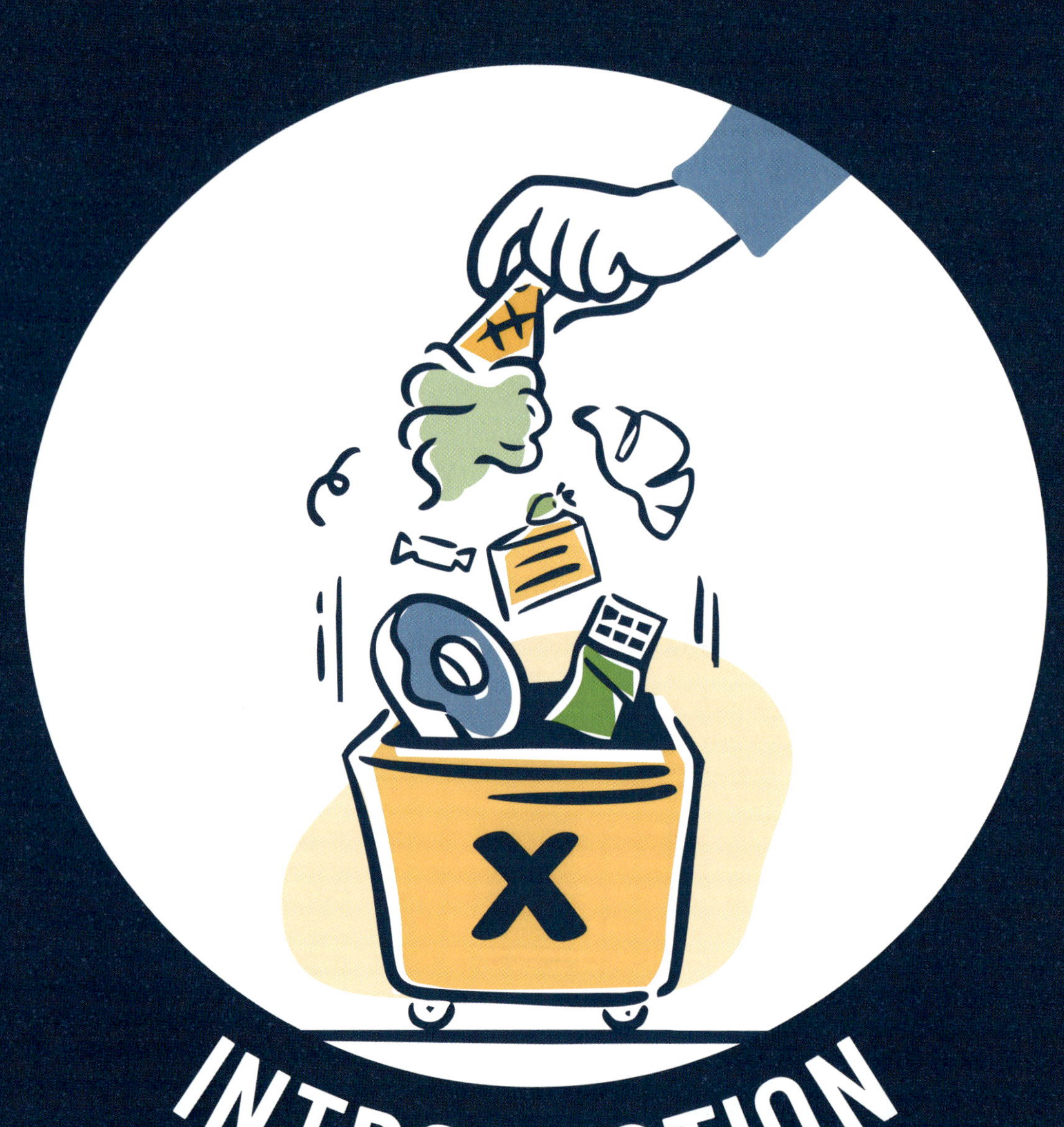

INTRODUCTION

Hi! I'm Brenda Bennett, aka Sugar Free Mom. Food blogger since 2011. Author of three cookbooks. Mom of three. Wife of twenty-eight years. Retired special education teacher. Sugar Free Course creator. Certified as a keto coach, Nutritional Therapy Practitioner, life coach, and the visionary behind the SFM Tribe weight-loss membership.

I started my health journey in 2004 when I first went sugar-free and discovered more freedom than I ever imagined. I was desperate to lose the extra baby weight from my second child, but to be honest, this wasn't the only time I had lost and regained weight.

I'd been the typical dieter since the age of twelve. Finding comfort in refined carbs like potato chips and sugary foods was the norm, and I quickly discovered and tried a dozen fad diets throughout my teens. By the time I was in my college years, my sugar addiction was the only way I knew how to cope with stress, anxiety, and relationships.

By the age of thirty-four, I had tried all the things to conquer my weight: Overeaters Anonymous, Jenny Craig, private nutritionists, Weight Watchers, excessive exercise, and on and on. Nothing lasted; nothing stuck for good. I just felt hopeless each time I tried once again to include sugar but moderate it.

It took me a very long time to simply say, "I don't have to be like everyone else. I don't have to include sugar in my life just because all the experts say I shouldn't deny myself because that will make me want it more."

That philosophy didn't work for me. Giving in to just one bite triggered intense cravings. I never experienced what they said would happen. They said that the craving would go away once I indulged. They were wrong. It was always worse.

When I decided that I was going to pave a new path for myself, my life changed forever.

I didn't want to be in any programs that said I could never again eat anything that resembled a dessert, even if it was sugar-free. They said it would only keep me addicted. I decided I could make a sugar-free dessert using natural sugar-free sweeteners without it triggering me to eat more, and I found out they were wrong.

I proved to myself what worked best for me. I proved to myself that I don't have to fit a norm. I didn't have to keep eating sugar just because others do.

In 2006, I gave up sugar for good. I can't tell you it was easy. I can't tell you I didn't struggle. But I can tell you that I never quit on myself. I can tell you that I haven't chosen to put sugar in my mouth intentionally since then.

My food choices have changed from gluten-free to low-carb to keto. I spent a short time on carnivore, went back to keto, switched back to low-carb, and then went keto once again. The one constant has been my sugar freedom.

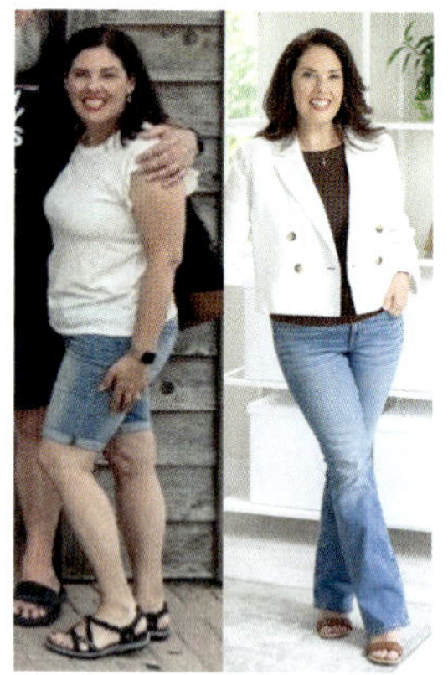

Life hasn't been easy just because I stopped eating sugar. I was diagnosed with hypothyroid in 2019 after suffering for years, and in 2021, we had toxic mold in our home, which caused both weight gain and horrific symptoms, but with my keto lifestyle and thyroid medication, the extra weight came off. But when I turned fifty-two in 2023, a multitude of uncomfortable symptoms—like thinning hair, brain fog, histamine intolerance, insomnia, body temperature fluctuations, fluttering heart palpitations, and inevitable weight gain—started coming back, despite no change in my diet, intermittent fasting routines, or weekly strength training. I thought it was hormones, but I was still menstruating, so I assumed it was perimenopause.

My hormones were tested twice in one year, and I discovered they were perfect, but my cholesterol went through the roof as it had back in 2018 when I was undiagnosed with hypothyroid, and I finally realized my thyroid must be the issue. I talked with my endocrinologist to adjust my thyroid medication. At the time of writing, I'm now eight months into the change in dosage and a switch to natural NP thyroid, and I can feel an improvement in fluctuations in temperature; less hair loss in my head, eyebrows, and lashes; improved sex drive; no more fluttering heart palpitations; and better sleep. I would love to tell you that the 10 or 15 pounds I had gained in 2024 all came off easily once the thyroid medication was correctly dosed, but that was not the case this time around. I had to tweak my keto diet to see results, and in Chapter 3, I share all the things I did to get back to my happy weight.

If you'd like to stay in the know about my health and life, I regularly update my email list on SugarFreeMom.com.

Through all this struggle, I remain steadfast in my self-care practices and commitment to my sugar-free lifestyle. I do not desire sugar and refined carbs and have no thoughts or cravings for any of it.

I don't do cheat days or cheat meals because I don't need to get a break from my diet. I don't eat for my emotions. I don't eat when I'm stressed, sad, angry, lonely, tired, or bored. Food comfort is not my first choice to feel better anymore.

I make a Good, Better, or Best decision in the moment, and that's enough. I don't negotiate with my toddler brain or compromise on my non-negotiables when faced with challenges.

I've learned how to create a sustainable sugar-free lifestyle for myself and paved the way for others who believe as I do. My chosen path may be quite different than some addiction experts recommend or believe is possible, but it's worked for me for almost two decades, and I plan to continue this way for the years to come.

I've come to learn that every small decision is just a daily choice. It's not good or bad; it's just a plain old choice. Making that one decision back in 2006 to leave sugar behind for good has given me incredible freedom, and I'm grateful every day to be able to help others find their own definition of food freedom.

GOOD, BETTER, BEST DEFINED

The Good, Better, Best method is a mindset shift. It's a way of allowing yourself to be imperfect while keeping weight off. It's about making decisions with one goal in mind: "What can I confidently choose to eat in this moment that still aligns with my goals and keeps me on track? Even if it's not the very best choice, it's still a good enough choice."

This method can be applied not only to how you eat to maintain weight loss but to how you take care of yourself daily. It can be applied to self-care, mindfulness, exercise, and meal planning. Once you learn this method, your life will forever change, and you will stop quitting on yourself when the going gets tough.

Instead of throwing in the towel on your healthy habits, you will learn how to apply the Good (Enough) rule to life so you don't say, "Screw it," and eat all the things while waiting for Monday to come around so you can start the cycle all over again.

The Good, Better, Best method gives you control of your choices and empowers you to choose each day how you can roll with the punches and still move toward your health goals.

I define Good, Better, and Best like this:

- A Good food option is something you have 100 percent confidence that you can choose and still stick to your non-negotiable food plan.
- A Better food option is an improvement on your Good option, but you may only feel about 75 percent confident that you can make that choice in a moment of weakness.

- The Best food option is a great choice and better than the others, but you are only about 50 percent confident you'd make that choice when you've had a stressful day.

The Good, Better, Best options are realistic and manageable stepping stones for where you are in a given moment. These options mean your brain doesn't try to resist the change; instead, you can get out of that all-or-nothing mindset.

Here's an example: When my kids were babies, every night at 9 p.m. I wanted a snack. My stomach was truly growling. My brain had a habit of desiring a snack—usually sugar and refined carbs—exactly at 9 p.m. as I arrived at my only relaxation time all day, once the kids were in bed.

This habit created false hunger pangs. When I started asking myself if I was hungry enough to eat a hard-boiled egg, the answer was always, "No way!" I wanted chips or chocolate to soothe my stress away. I was dealing with habit hunger, and here's how I conquered it:

- A Good food option instead of eating a whole bag of chips, which is what I wanted to do, was being 100 percent confident that I could put chips in a bowl and not eat from the bag.
- My Better option, about which I was 75 percent confident, was choosing pork rinds or nuts in a bowl instead of potato chips.
- And my Best option, about which I was 50 percent confident, was to have a cup of tea or decaf coffee or just go to bed.

The Good, Better, Best method is a great way to bridge the gap to get you closer to the place where you feel like you're making better choices even if you're not quite where you want to be in choosing the best options. Even if you make a good or better food decision only 50 percent of the time, you're still winning and not quitting on yourself, bringing you closer to your goals.

The Good, Better, Best mindset can be used for any habit you're trying to make stick or any health goal you desire.

To make the content in this book super accessible and easy to use, I've broken it into two parts. Here's a snapshot of what you can expect to find in this book.

Part 1 gives the foundation for understanding how to use the effective Good (Enough), Better, Best philosophy as a practical tool in your life, enabling you to maintain your weight and health goals.

Chapter 1 is about understanding why you make certain decisions regarding what, how much, and when to eat. This chapter explains the science behind decision-making; why hunger is elevated; why overeating happens with certain foods; how to tame the toddler in you to get control back; how sleep, sunlight, and stress impact your decisions; and why protein is so important as you age.

Chapter 2 helps you define your non-negotiables, teaches you how to incorporate indulgences without going overboard, explains how to apply the GBB mindset when eating out, helps you redefine your why to maintain your weight, and gives you my 1-1-1 method to successfully tackle any social event with tempting food.

Chapter 3 provides you with a regain action plan to get back on track, explains protein-only days for weight loss and maintenance, and outlines the lifestyle interventions needed for successful maintenance.

Part 2 includes a meal prepping guide, three 7-day meal plans with shopping lists, and 100 recipes to choose from to get back on track with your goals. There's also an "About the Recipes" section that highlights recipe features and gives several ingredient substitution options; I suggest you review that section before delving into the recipes.

All the recipes in this book are sugar free, gluten free, and low carb, and the great majority are ketogenic as well. For the sake of clarity, recipes with 10 grams or less of total carbs per serving are considered keto friendly. Recipes with 11 to 19 grams of total carbs per serving are considered low carb. The carb counts are in the nutritional information below the recipes. That said, you can make most of the recipes keto friendly simply by using ingredient substitutions. For example, swapping in shirataki noodles or egg white noodles for higher-carb spaghetti squash or zucchini noodles will lower the total carbs per serving. Recipes requiring modification to be keto friendly are flagged with a keto-friendly icon; required ingredient substitutions are noted below each of these recipes.

To help with meal prepping, you'll find a sampling of super simple freezer-prep recipes in the Good (Enough) chapter, while more time-intensive freezer-prep recipes are in the other two chapters. The batch-cooking recipes in the Best chapter are ideal options for when you have more time to devote to meal prepping. Freezer-prep meals have you prepare a recipe up to the point of cooking it. You put the prepped ingredients in a freezer bag; all you need do is thaw the frozen ingredients in the refrigerator the night before, then the day of cooking, you simply put the thawed contents of the bag in a slow cooker, Instant Pot, or Dutch oven and cook the meal! Batch-cooked meals are, as you probably guessed, recipes with a large yield that can be divided into serving portions and refrigerated or frozen for later.

Hands-off time, such as for marinating or chilling, is not factored into the recipe prep times. For example, though the Quick Berry Chia Jam (page 93) in the Good (Enough) chapter takes just a couple of minutes to prepare, but it requires 1 hour to chill. All passive prep times are listed in the prep time field at the top of each recipe so that you can plan accordingly. Also note that the time needed to prepare recipe components, such as batch-cooked bacon or hard-cooked eggs, is not factored into the total prep time assigned to each recipe category. To help you plan your efforts in the kitchen, these prep times are noted in the information at the top of the recipes.

Chapter 5 includes basic recipes for sauces and other staples that are used in multiple recipes throughout the book or that can be used to make a quick plan B meal.

Chapter 6 contains Good (Enough) recipes that require no more than 20 minutes, with many recipes taking much less time than that. A couple of them can even be made as simplified freezer-prep meals, which is great for meal planning. Some take advantage of convenience foods, such as packaged egg white wraps or fully cooked meats, to allow you to prepare a meal quickly. Most of these recipes make only one or two servings. The dessert choices in this chapter are very simple, created to give you a fast way to satisfy a sweet tooth and keep you from going off the rails. (More elaborate dessert options are in Chapters 7 and 8.) At the end of this chapter, I suggest some quick, throw-it-together-in-a-pinch meals you can fall back on when you need a plan B. By using prepared ingredients you're likely to have in your pantry, fridge, and freezer, you can whip up a satisfying meal that meets your needs with little effort.

Chapter 7 contains Better recipes that require anywhere from 15 to 45 minutes to prepare, though much of the time for the longer-to-prepare recipes is hands-off. These are made from scratch and do not use convenience ingredients. Some even work as freezer meals or are designed as meal prep options for busy weekday mornings. Many of these recipes are suitable for larger family meals or entertaining.

Chapter 8 contains Best recipes that mostly require 30 minutes or more of your time. Like the Better recipes, they are made from scratch and do not use convenience ingredients. Freezer prepping and batch-cooking instructions are included! These recipes are for the days when you have extra time to prepare, cook, and enjoy your meals. Many of these recipes are suitable for larger family meals or for entertaining.

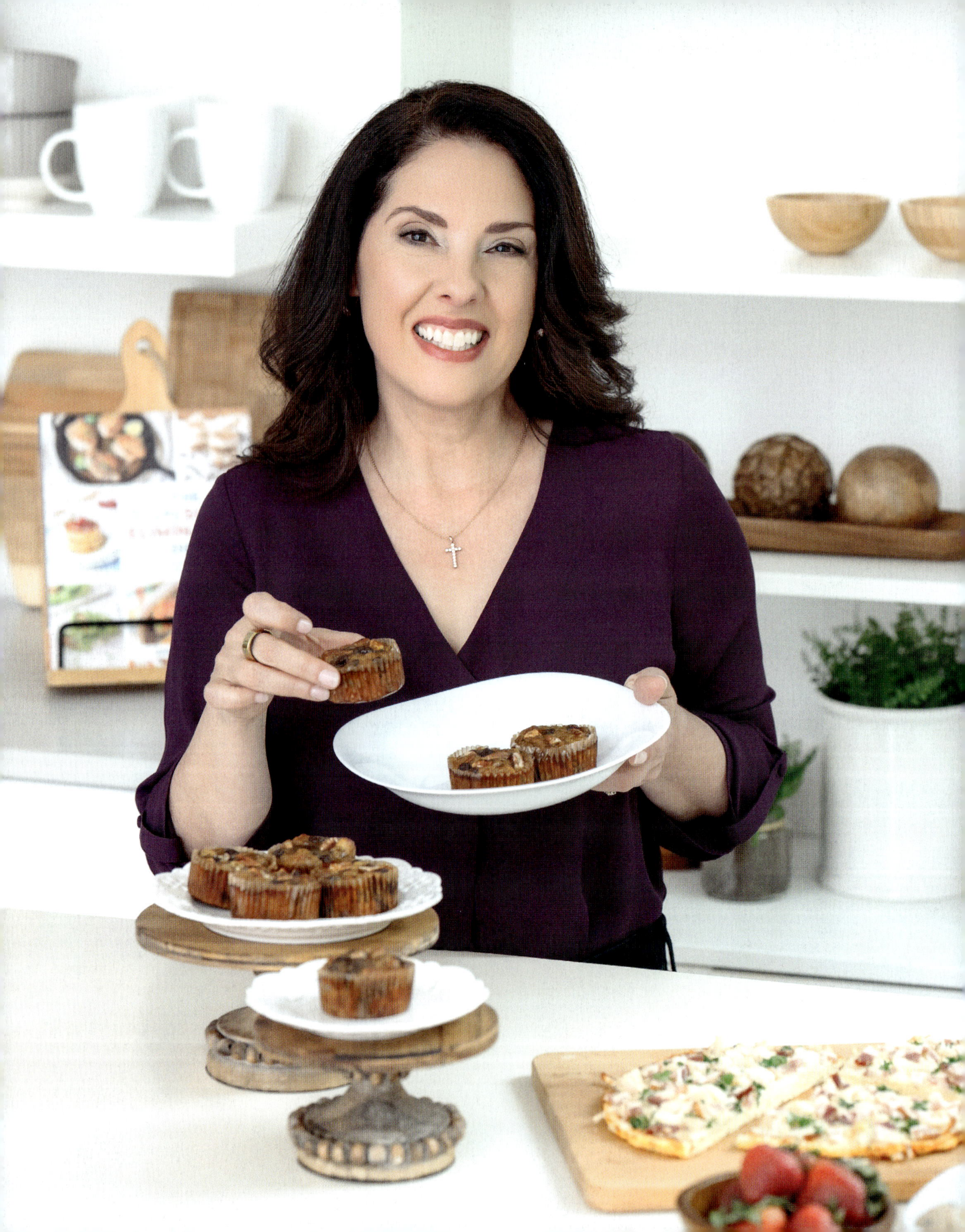

PART 1

THE DECISION-MAKING PROCESS

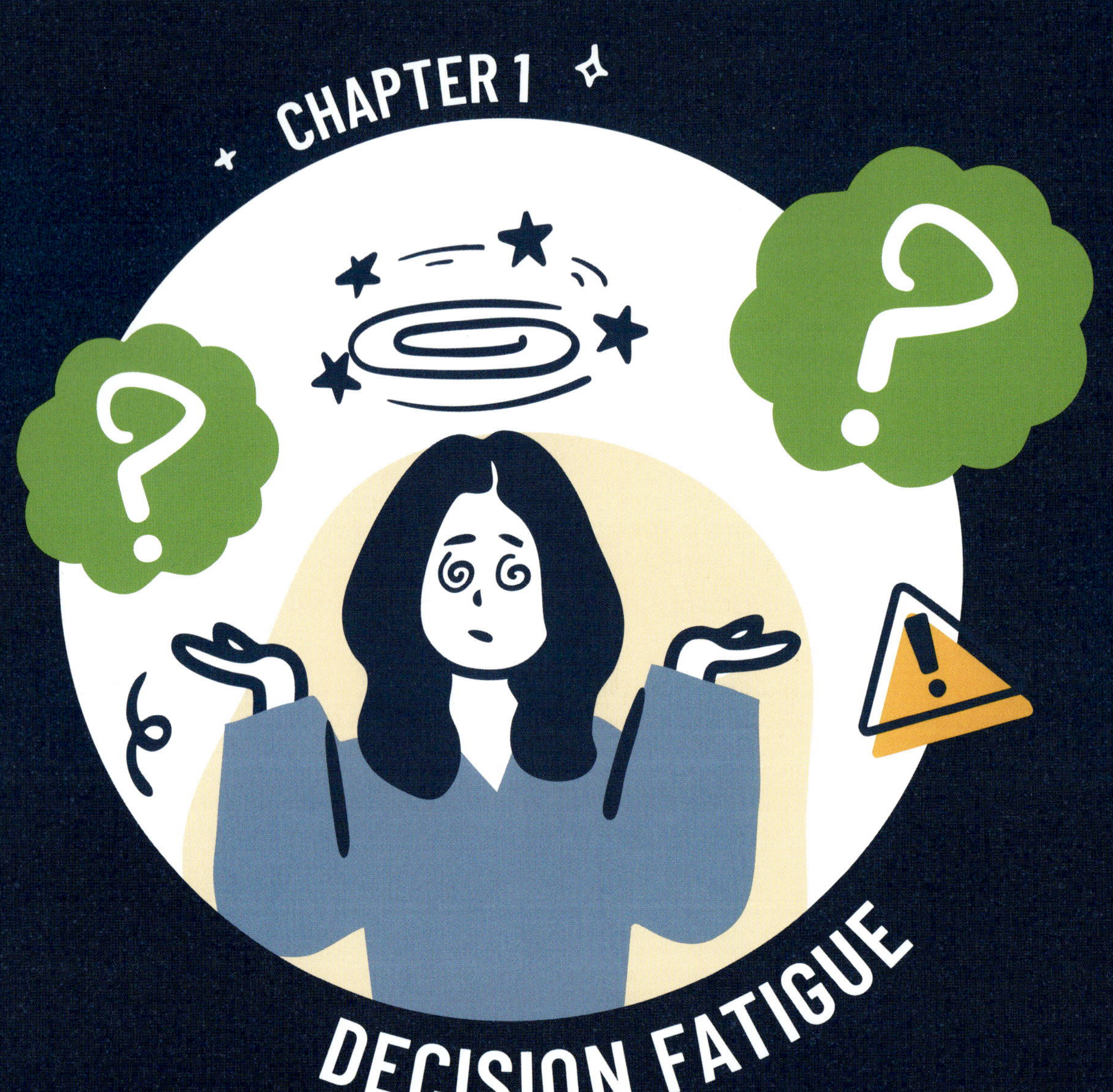
CHAPTER 1
DECISION FATIGUE

You make a lot of decisions in the course of a day. One study suggests the average American adult makes 35,000 decisions daily![1]

Just as your muscles can get fatigued by exercise, your brain can become less efficient when it's overloaded with too many decisions. That state is called *decision fatigue*, and it can impair your ability to make rational decisions and maintain self-control. Basically, when your brain needs to make any decision, regardless of whether it's minor or major, decision fatigue can set in, and it can impact your ability to regulate and experience emotions.[2]

A person experiencing decision fatigue may make impulsive decisions that have negative consequences, delay or procrastinate, completely stop all activity, or experience a lot more frustration than other people.

If you've successfully lost weight in the past, it's most likely because you planned exactly what you would eat to be in a calorie deficit and lose weight. You probably didn't guess or wing it. You calculated and tracked everything. So, when you're in weight-loss mode, most of your decisions are planned—because, you know, without a plan, things fall apart, and it's too easy to give in to temptations.

When you get to maintenance mode or complete a program or diet, impulse decisions often become more the norm because of the simple thought, "I should be able to relax now, so I can stop meal planning and tracking." Planning doesn't seem as important or necessary as it was when you were in weight-loss mode.

This chapter shares the science behind impulses and planned decisions and offers a happy balance of both using the Good, Better, Best method to stay on track.

IMPULSE EATING

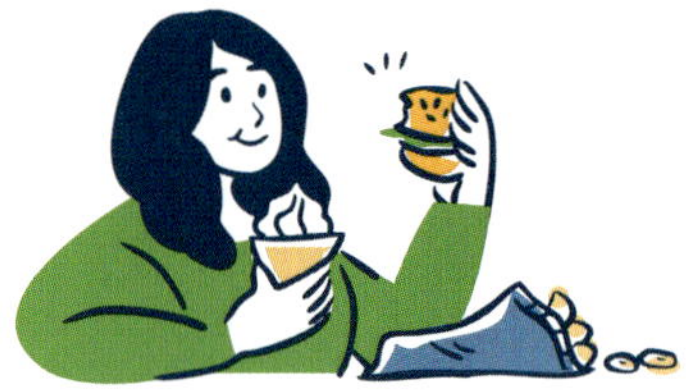

A lot of us make decisions we struggle to follow through on—not because deciding is difficult but because commitment requires more effort.

To support the big decision to lose weight or stop eating sugar and refined carbs, you have to do small things each day to follow through and honor that decision.

The primal human brain is wired for reward and wants to avoid pain at all costs. This animal instinct part of your brain is what's working to keep you alive, flee or fight, run from a dog, and so on. That part of your brain also seeks to find the pleasure in things. Refined carbs and sugar are hyperpalatable and designed to make you want more of them, which gives you that trigger of dopamine and a high reward each time you indulge.[3]

One reason for overeating is that many people soothe themselves with food, stuffing negative, uncomfortable feelings down without learning how to process them. Food becomes a comfort and reward because eating is so much easier than processing feelings.

Here's what happens when you stop overeating or cut out certain foods, especially foods that brought you great comfort. When you know you need to stay away from them and stop eating them, you start truly feeling your emotions, like stress, exhaustion, boredom, anger, sadness, worry, and hunger. You also have to face the impulses to eat the very things you said you wouldn't.

Your brain goes into fight-or-flight mode because all the emotions you start feeling are new to you. For years, you'd avoided them and chose to eat instead. Now, there's no reward from food, and you feel pain.

The primal part of your brain doesn't care about the future. It's like a three-year-old toddler who just wants what they want when they want it. Toddlers are only interested in instant pleasure and don't think about the pain. (Read more on taming the toddler later in this chapter.)

The good news is you have another part of your brain. The sensible, adult part of your brain that handles reasoning (the prefrontal cortex) looks into your future, understands delayed gratification, and has your best interest at heart. It's your conscious thinker. If you were using this part of your brain all the time, you wouldn't give in to impulse eating! Instead, your toddler has been winning, right?!

So, how do you use the adult part of your brain more than you let your primal/toddler brain control you?

In *The 30-Day Sugar Elimination Diet,* I spoke a lot about daily habits and rewiring your brain so that the old habits of turning to food stopped being automatic and were replaced with new habits. You use your prefrontal cortex to do that. You think ahead of time of how you can avoid temptations and distract yourself with something else.

Your toddler brain only makes decisions in the moment, but you can't rely on it because it wants instant gratification all the time. It always chooses the easiest path. Deciding what you're going to eat ahead of time requires use of your prefrontal cortex, which instructs your toddler brain to follow along.

When you make an advance decision rather than waiting to decide as your day unfolds, you reduce your chances that decision fatigue will set in, and you regain control because the choice has been made, end of story. You won't be relying on how you feel in that moment, so you won't impulsively choose foods that don't serve your health goals.[4]

You've probably already experienced this and can attest to the fact that when you've planned your food before the day begins, you've been able to stop reacting to the issues of the day and give in to temptations. Is that true? I hope so!

Perhaps in the past when you've lost weight and gotten to your goal, you stopped planning. You might have started to succumb to the problems of the day and eat whatever looked really good in the fridge and pantry, thinking, *Well, I'm at my goal weight, so this indulgence won't matter too much.*

This happened because of decision fatigue. You didn't plan a healthy food option for yourself and had to think about what to eat, and the healthy option that would maybe take more time is your last choice. The easier choice would be a convenient packaged or store-bought food because your brain doesn't want to make another decision, so it switches to automatic responses in the face of discomfort. If you've followed this pattern for years when stressful days happen, the easy choice has become automatic.

If you want to stop giving in to those unhealthy food choices in the moment, you've got to make your decision on what you will eat before the moment comes so you have one less decision to make, and decision fatigue won't set in.

When you do this regularly, you take back control of your choices by not giving in to your toddler brain.

TAMING THE TODDLER

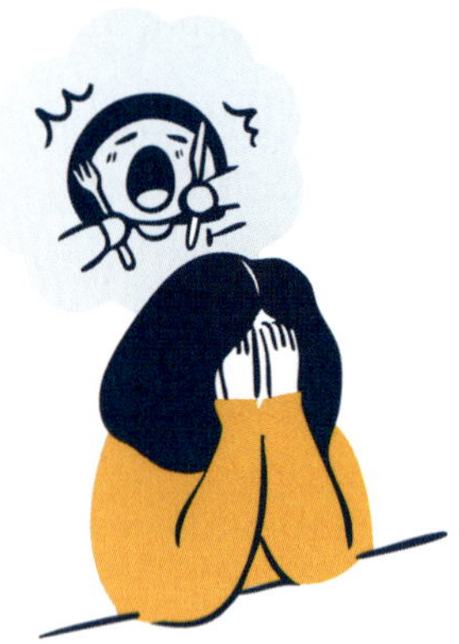

Every person's brain has thousands of thoughts each day—some positive, some negative—and we all have what I call the "toddler" in us. The three-year-old who wants what they want, when they want it. This toddler is your impulse decision-maker. They come out to play every time decision fatigue happens.

The toddler is the one who acts quickly in the face of danger. Fight or flight is their way of life, and they seek to always comfort you. The toddler doesn't understand or care about future goals; they only live in the moment, and they're strong and quite the rebel. When someone tells them no, they fight hard and negotiate with the sensible part of your brain, who I have coined the "adult" in the relationship.

I'm sure you've seen this scenario (or lived it): Imagine a toddler in the grocery line screaming at their parent because they want a candy bar. What happens when the parent tries to stop the toddler and get them to be quiet? The toddler gets worse and has a hissy fit tantrum. Then what?

The parent gives the child the candy bar to stop the fit, and the toddler wins! They learn that screaming and having a tantrum will get them exactly what they desire. If this pattern continues and the toddler gets a treat every time, the automatic habit has been created.

Have you been the parent who let the toddler have the fit without giving in to it? I have. I didn't care. That's what it's like not to give in to the impulse feeling. You want something, but you don't obey your inner toddler's demands.

When you don't plan your meals of healthy food ahead of time, you have to negotiate with your toddler all day long. Here's how it often plays out:

Late for work, didn't make a lunch the night before. No plan B for when this happens. Coffee will have to do for breakfast. No problem, I can run to the deli and grab a healthy chicken salad on my lunch break.

Emails, deadlines, meetings, and now my one-hour lunch is shortened to 20 minutes. I won't make it to the deli for that healthy chicken salad, but I have to eat something. I'm starving and didn't eat breakfast. Crackers. I'll get some crackers from the break room that will hold me over until I get home.

It's now 3 p.m. and those crackers didn't help at all. I'm so hungry, I can't concentrate. I'm also sleepy, and I know I need a pick-me-up, but I am committed to my ______ diet, and there's nothing here to eat! Screw it, I'm eating this candy bar, and I'll get back on track tomorrow!

This is the worst commute in the worst traffic, and I have no idea what to make for dinner, plus I haven't gone shopping, so there's nothing healthy to eat anyway. Ordering pizza is a good idea since I already ate that candy bar, and I'm going to start back on track tomorrow. I deserve pizza, but also ice cream since I won't be able to have that once I start back on my ______ diet. While waiting for the delivery of the pizza, the cookies in the cupboard are too tempting to resist; after all, it's been a stressful day.

This is how decision fatigue, constant mind chatter, and your toddler convince you to comfort yourself every time you have a stressful day! Automatic habit formed!

Taming the toddler in you requires some daily, deliberate discipline to avoid sabotaging your future health goals by demanding satisfaction in the moment. When these skills become a daily practice, your toddler voice will only be a quiet whisper, and you will be back in the driver's seat.

Being aware that you're negotiating with yourself is a good start to building the discipline to keep your toddler in check. You'll know your toddler is talking to you when you're struggling with the Better food choice. For example, when you have a choice between a chicken salad or pizza, the toddler says, "Eat the pizza; you've had a difficult day."

This is why making a food plan ahead of time is so important. When decisions are already planned, you can talk to yourself as if you're the parent speaking to your toddler: "It's okay, Honey. I know you really want that pizza because you're feeling stressed, but no, not today. We can plan for it tomorrow."

There are a few actions you can take to help tame your toddler.

NOTE: My "Tame the Toddler" five-session video workshop will help you control your impulse decisions when you're faced with temptation. The workshop tells you exactly what to do to conquer self-sabotage. Use the QR code for free access.

Writing Your Meal Plan

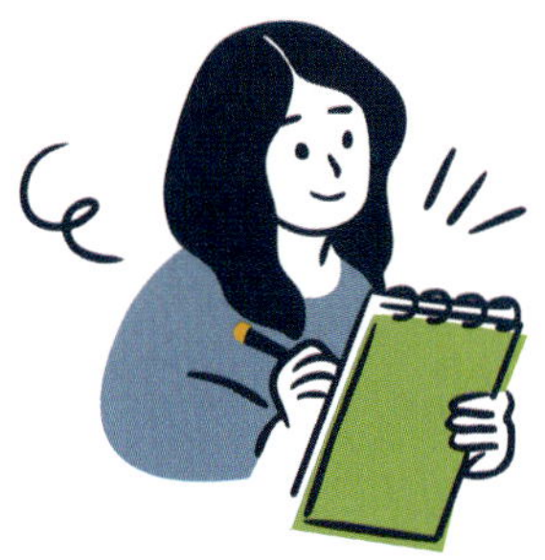

If you've had some weight gain after getting to your goal weight, it's time to get back on track by taming the toddler. Writing down *exactly* what you will eat each day is one tool you can use to do that.

No one plans to overeat when they're trying to lose weight, but in maintenance, it's easy to become somewhat lax with eating, and that's why weight gain creeps up a little at a time.

Getting back on track with writing down your food plan each day might upset your toddler brain because they're a little rebel who doesn't like to be told what to do. Despite that, it's worth the effort. You will always make a better choice twenty-four hours ahead of time than you will in the moment.

You must practice this new habit. Eat only exactly what you plan. If the broccoli you have planned has gone bad, you can swap it with another green vegetable. The only reason to eat something other than what you planned is if you thought you plugged in the slow cooker in the morning when you left for work, but you didn't.

That said, you also need a backup plan B meal for times when you absolutely cannot eat what you had planned. Eggs and bacon are a good backup, if you always have those items in the house. (Chapter 5 includes easy store-bought items to have in your fridge, pantry, and freezer as your plan B.)

But otherwise, eat only what you planned. This helps you maintain integrity with yourself, because once you open the door to your "right" to change your plan, you're giving an inch to your toddler brain. And that side of you is going to go for the mile and take advantage. Stick to eating only what was planned.

Accepting Discomfort

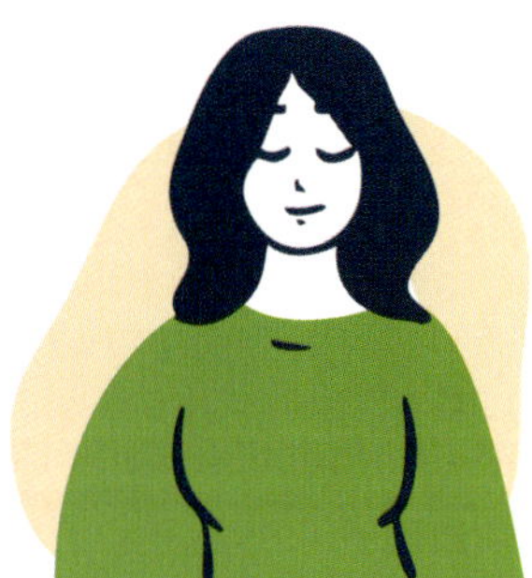

You must override your toddler brain, which is determined to be comforted. It wants to be safe and comfortable and to avoid overwhelming emotions. Your toddler brain may say, "Eat the donut. It's going to comfort us and make us happy, and we will *die* if we don't eat that donut!" But this is just a thought; it has no control.

Because I'm willing to be uncomfortable even when I'm stressed, as well as willing not to eat the tempting thing, I have amazing confidence. No food controls me, and no feelings control me. I hold every thought captive, and they are powerless without my consent to act.

When you're confronted by an impulse to eat something, know it's powerless over you if you don't give it consent. The toddler brain can't force you to do anything. You have the final decision of whether to obey that impulse or just allow it to be there. You become powerless only when you give in to a moment of unconscious eating.

Applying the Good, Better, Best Strategy

Every single time you overeat, it's because of a thought coming from your primal brain—the toddler in you. Every time you don't overeat, it's because of a thought coming from your future self who wants to reach your goals; that's your prefrontal cortex. You need to increase the thoughts that help you not to overeat and decrease the thoughts that cause overeating so you can start changing those automatic habits and make new habits form.

Learning to recognize the sabotaging thoughts from your toddler voice is a great start, but if you're not at the point where you can ignore the voice and not eat the donut, you have an opportunity to apply the Good, Better, Best strategy. Consider these things:

- The best option is not eating the donut. How confident am I to make this choice?
- The better option is to choose something else to eat that won't spike blood sugar and continue cravings for more. How confident am I to make this choice?
- The good option is to own the decision to eat the donut but commit to just one rather than bingeing and eating three. Another good option is eating the donut but walking away from the rest of the donuts in the breakroom. Or eating the donut but confiding in a friend who's supporting me so I can come up with a plan for next time I'm in this situation.

The whole point of using the Good, Better, Best strategy is to end the all-or-nothing attitude that would cause you to give in to the temptation of the donut, learn nothing from why it happened, and throw your hands up and say, "Forget it; I failed today. I'll eat whatever I want for the rest of the day because it's ruined. I'll start again tomorrow."

Using the Good, Better, Best mindset reminds you that you have choices. You didn't fail; you decided. You had control not to eat the donut. It's not the end of the world. You are not a lost cause; you simply decided to eat the donut. Good, Better, Best enables you to look more objectively at why you ate the donut. It helps you start discovering areas in your environments where you're vulnerable to temptation so you can set up a strategy to conquer the donut the next time.

Remember, if you do give in to your toddler thoughts, dust yourself off, remind yourself you're human, forgive yourself, and move on. Own the decision you made and stop judging it but also examine why it happened and how you can overcome that challenge the next time.

Removing shame and guilt creates an opportunity to simply learn from your past mistakes without judgment. Instead of wallowing in guilt, your brain can start coming up with strategies to reduce and decrease self-sabotage in the future.

PROCESSED PACKAGED FOODS INCREASE HUNGER

Besides learning to ignore the toddler in you by planning your food ahead of time to avoid decision fatigue, learning which type of foods trigger hunger and cravings is important.

High-calorie foods full of sugar and refined processed carbs and deficient in quality nutrients will cause you to overeat simply because of the ghrelin hormone being stimulated. Ghrelin is your hunger hormone—the one that gives your body the we-need-to-eat-right-now signal.

Unfortunately, ghrelin can be dysregulated by sugary, processed, and packaged foods that have little to no quality nutrients. Overprocessed, sweet, and refined packaged foods are the biggest culprits because they contain so many additives to maintain freshness while they sit on the shelves. Also, they're specifically engineered to be addictive. Even packaged snacks labeled as keto can ignite your ghrelin hormone to want more.

If you've ever eaten a pastry, snack bar, or donut from your local coffee shop and felt hungry again within an hour, that's ghrelin at work.[5]

The standard American diet is full of convenient, processed "foods" that often lack protein and are high in sugar, fat, and inflammatory seed oils. They might provide quick energy, but they lack long-lasting fuel and nutrients your body seeks to function optimally, so you need to eat every two to three hours for energy.

In a study on protein leverage, David Raubenheimer and Stephen Simpson state that a low protein intake is the main driver of overconsuming calories from carbs and fats: "A preference by consumers for foods rich in carbohydrates and fats has incentivized the processed food industry to mass-produce food products rich in energetic carbohydrates and fats, which have resulted in a proportional reduction of the protein content of human diets, causing energy overconsumption."[6]

Think of an outdoor fire. You use kindling to get the fire started quickly, but you need some big logs once it's lit to keep the fire going for a longer period. Otherwise, you will have to keep adding sticks constantly to keep it going. Similarly, when you're constantly burning glucose for your energy, you need to eat more frequently.

After you eat, food is either used for fuel or stored as fat for later use. Insulin is your fat-storage hormone, and its main job is to balance your blood sugar. When insulin is high, you can't burn fat. Eating processed foods with sugar and carbs, eating too frequently (think meal, snack, meal, snack, and so on), or just overeating leads to insulin spikes, and you can't tap into your body fat for fuel.[7]

Your body always chooses the first available fuel source, so when glucose is always present in your bloodstream, your pancreas must continue to produce insulin to keep your blood sugar down. This is a problem if you want to lose weight and keep it off because you'll constantly be in fat-storing mode rather than using your stored fat for fuel.

If you do need a snack, avoid sugar and processed foods that feed ghrelin and cause cravings.[8] Instead eat a protein-rich food that will help balance blood sugar and reduce your chance of ghrelin screaming at you that you're hungry when you most likely aren't.[9]

Check out some high-protein quick snacks in the Good category of the recipe section that take just a few minutes of time to prep!

SLEEP, SUN, STRESS, AND OVEREATING

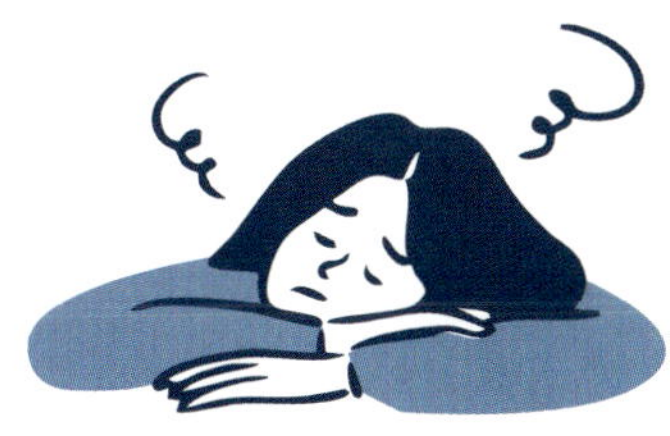

When it comes to our hunger signals and giving in to cravings and overeating, sleep is a huge factor. You can't make good decisions when you're sleep deprived. The toddler in you will be cranky and try to bully you to eat whatever looks the most appealing in the moment. In this section, I talk about ways disrupted sleep can make it harder for you to ignore your inner toddler.

Imbalanced Leptin and Ghrelin

A lack of sleep results in less leptin, your satiety hormone, and more ghrelin, which you know tells you how hungry you are. Because leptin is a hormone that tells your brain you've eaten enough, if you're sleep deprived and producing less of it, you're going to feel hungrier. In addition, that feeling of satisfaction and satiety can be greatly decreased for several other reasons besides lack of good-quality sleep.

Low leptin can be a result of a diet high in inflammatory foods, especially sugar and refined carbs; having consistently high spikes in blood sugar and insulin levels; chronic disease; inflammation; and undereating. Even certain medications can hinder or reduce your ability to detect the signaling from leptin to stop eating.

Taking steps to reduce overeating and having the ability to make better food decisions throughout the day starts with prioritizing a good night's sleep. Research has shown repeatedly that poor sleep or inadequate sleep is linked to weight gain. In experimental sleep deprivation studies, researchers have found that the reward centers of the brain are *more* stimulated by food when you're sleep deprived. Poor sleep can increase the brain's pleasurable response to food and decrease your self-control and decision-making abilities.[10]

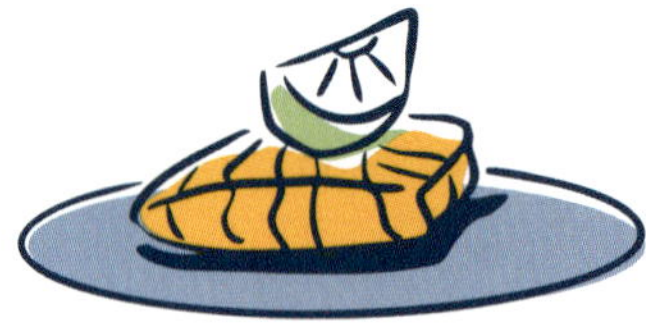

Also, eliminating snacking between meals is a great way to reduce spikes in your blood sugar and insulin, allowing you to become more sensitive to leptin signaling. And if you've been on a weight-loss protocol with a calorie deficit for some time, having a higher-calorie day once a week can allow your body to believe it's safe and not think it's starving and has a need to preserve body fat.

Eating nutrient-dense animal protein from red meat, pasture-raised eggs, chicken, turkey, pork, and seafood rich in omega-3s (like wild-caught salmon, sardines, tuna, herring, and mackerel) is another great way to increase leptin sensitivity.

Another easy way to increase leptin sensitivity is to get sun exposure. In fact, if you want to improve your overall mood, daily sun exposure will increase the production of serotonin. Getting little breaks outside will improve mental and emotional fatigue.

Reducing Exposure to Artificial Light

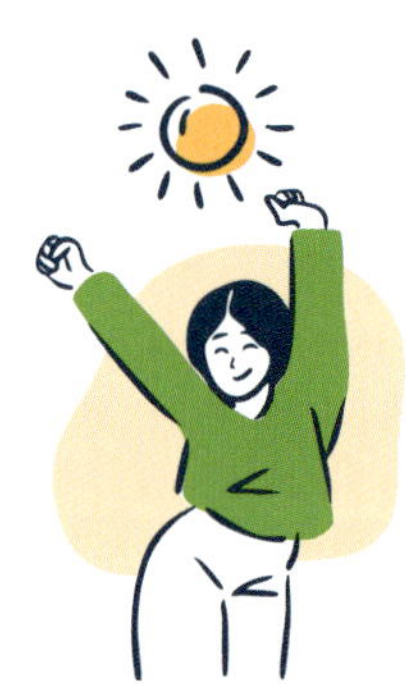

When you're overexposed to artificial light all day long and are on computers while working in an office (or even at home), watching TV, or being on a phone, the blue light exposure can cause an imbalance in your natural circadian rhythm. Taking breaks throughout the day to see natural light is especially important if you work inside for many hours because glass windows block the beneficial rays of the sun. I try to bring my laptop outside during the day, weather permitting. If it's too chilly to be outside, I have a place in my home to open a window so I can still receive the beneficial rays through the window screen.

Getting up for the sunrise or early morning light as well as watching the sunset are very beneficial to regulate your circadian rhythm. The beneficial rays in your eyes can help set your internal clock, so to speak, which makes you more naturally ready to go to bed at a reasonable time and wake with the sunrise.

If you live where it's too early to wake for sunrise without negatively affecting how much sleep you can get, just create a routine to get up between 6:00 and 6:30 a.m. to get that first light in your eyes. It's OK to wear glasses, but contacts block some of the beneficial rays, so try to take them out for sunrise and sunset.[11]

A small 2015 study found that when people are exposed to blue light in the evening hours, their bodies don't release as much melatonin, and their sleep cycles are delayed or disrupted.[12] Wearing blue light blocking glasses after sunset while you watch TV or use your device is another helpful way to enable you to fall asleep easily and stay asleep. (My husband doesn't like wearing blue light blocking glasses, so I purchased a TV screen cover instead.)

Grounding

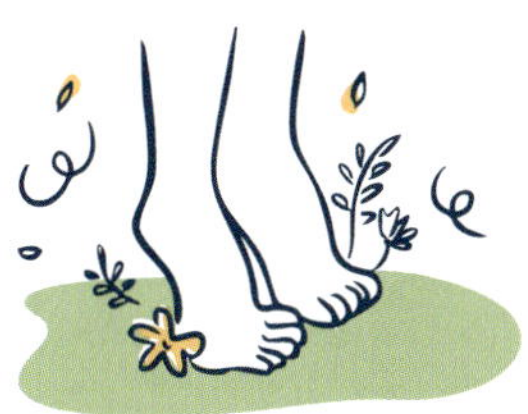

You can also improve sleep by practicing grounding.[13] Our ancestors worked outdoors and walked barefoot, but today, we rarely do that. We're often in our homes or work environment with shoes on while being bombarded with electromagnetic fields from all our lights, computers, TV, and so on. We're exposed to unnatural electric pollution.[14]

To offset some of this pollution, get grounded daily by walking barefoot outside and connecting to the ground so the earth's surface electrons can transfer energy into your body. It can be a profound effective strategy against chronic stress, inflammation, and poor sleep.

Grounding is free and effective. Of course, the weather doesn't always make it possible to go barefoot during the winter season, so there are earthing products for in-home use while you sleep, sit, and even use your computer.[15]

Supporting Good Sleep

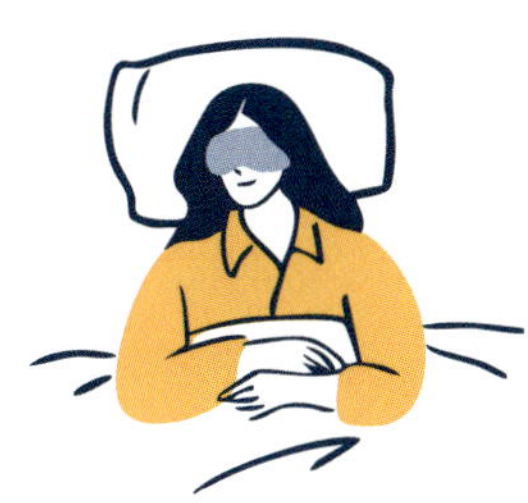

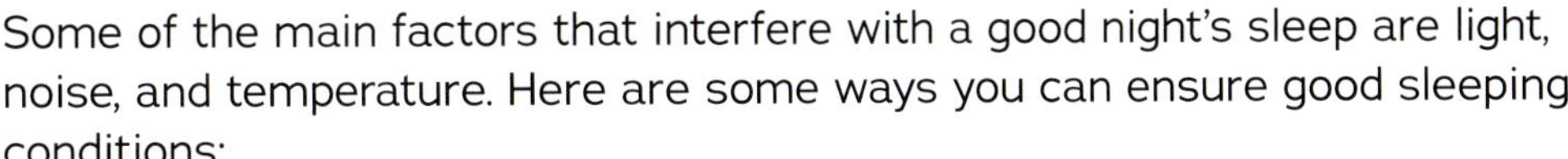

Some of the main factors that interfere with a good night's sleep are light, noise, and temperature. Here are some ways you can ensure good sleeping conditions:

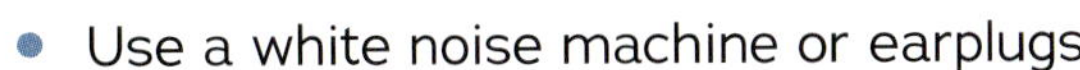

- Use a white noise machine or earplugs.
- Keep your bedroom as cool as possible—between 65°F and 68°F is best.
- Darken your bedroom as much as possible so no light comes in through your windows or through devices in your bedroom. Use an eye mask or blackout curtains.
- Put your phone charger in the bathroom to block any notifications from waking you.
- Try to avoid eating shortly before your typical bedtime. Snacking or a late meal interferes with your body's natural ability to wind down to sleep because it's working to digest the food you've eaten instead. Aim to stop eating at least two or three hours prior to your bedtime.

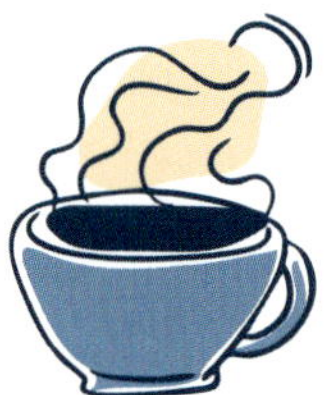

Beyond those simple modifications, you can also try limiting caffeine to just the morning. Some people are slower metabolizers of caffeine than others; I'm one of them. My husband, on the other hand, is a fast metabolizer of caffeine and can enjoy an espresso at 6 p.m. but still fall right to sleep by 9 p.m. Caffeine sensitivity is genetic for the most part, and you probably know how much caffeine you can tolerate. Typically, caffeine has a half-life of five to seven hours.[16] If you have issues falling asleep, avoid caffeine after 2 p.m.[17]

If you embark on all these changes for better sleep and you still have difficulty getting quality sleep, consider whether your mind and thoughts won't quit when you lay your head on your pillow.

You can also try using a magnesium supplement. I've recommended and used magnesium for years now. It helps with bowel regularity and also promotes stress and anxiety relief. However, all forms of magnesium are not created equal.

Cheaper forms pass through the body and do not get absorbed well. For instance, magnesium bisglycinate is superior in both absorption and function serving to replete magnesium status.[18] In a magnesium glycinate comparison study reported by Graff et al. at Weber State University, it had

- 8.8 times greater absorption than magnesium oxide
- 5.6 times greater absorption than magnesium sulfate
- 2.3 times greater absorption than magnesium carbonate[19]

Evidence supports the use of magnesium in the prevention and treatment of many common health conditions, including migraine headache, metabolic syndrome, diabetes, hyperlipidemia (high cholesterol), asthma, premenstrual syndrome, preeclampsia, and various cardiac arrhythmias.[20]

When I started using a supplement called Relax & Regulate, which is part of the Naturally Nourished line created by functional registered dietitian Ali Miller, I noticed I was better able to fall asleep and stay asleep. Her product includes inositol, and that seems to have been the game changer for me.

Although inositol is referred to as vitamin B8, it isn't a vitamin. It's a compound found naturally in the human body. One benefit is its ability to help balance blood sugar. Myo-inositol has been shown in clinical studies to promote healthy blood sugar levels and to support healthy glucose metabolism. It also supports receptors in the brain that bind to neurotransmitters like serotonin, dopamine, and norepinephrine, which helps with improving mood.[21] Inositol has been successfully used to support balanced hormones, mostly in women,[22] and support a healthy body weight.[23] Various double-blind controlled trials demonstrate positive clinical outcomes of inositol on depression, panic attacks, OCD, and ADHD.[24]

Another game-changing supplement in my life has been gamma-aminobutyric acid (GABA). Specifically, I use GABACalm from the Naturally Nourished line. GABA is an amino acid that serves as a major inhibitory neurotransmitter in the brain and spinal cord. It helps balance an overstressed nervous system. It's best used as needed in stressful situations.

For my coaching clients who always feel stress in certain situations and then want to turn to food for comfort, I recommend they try GABA. An uncomfortable family party, anxiety with flying, road trips, holidays, getting home from work after a stressful day—whenever you feel some stress, GABA gets depleted in your brain.[25] In a study on humans, prefrontal brain GABA levels decreased by 18 percent after acute psychological stress.[26]

If you've been someone who falls asleep yet wakes in the early morning hours with constant thoughts of anxiety, overwhelm, or stress, GABA could be helpful for getting back to sleep. In my experience, a chewable form of GABA has been the most helpful to quickly get back to sleep.[27]

MOOD, MOVEMENT, STRESS EATING & SELF-CALMING TOOLS

If you want to reduce the urges to give in to food temptations when stress hits and improve your ability to make a good decision that aligns with your non-negotiable health goals, you have to make a commitment to improve your mood. In this section, I cover some suggestions for doing that.

Daily Movement

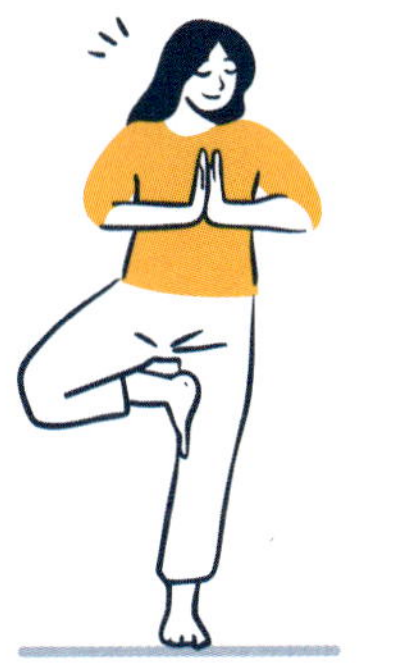

The first thing to try is some daily movement.

Now I know what you're thinking: *I don't have time to exercise.* I'm not saying you need to head to the gym every day. I'm asking you to consider small movements throughout your day to relieve stress. When you can calm your nervous system in a moment of heightened stress, you will be better equipped to make food decisions that honor your health goals.

There are many ways to find stress relief, but the best one is the one you will easily do without having to negotiate with your toddler brain. When you can find the one you need no motivation to do, you've hit the jackpot! That's the best fit for you.

Studies show that just going from a sedentary sitting position to getting up for a quick stretch—basically moving to any degree—has an immediate effect for feeling more hopeful, optimistic, and energized with improved mood because endorphins are released.[28] For example, if you're sitting at your desk feeling overwhelmed, just standing up can immediately release endorphins and help you feel a sense of improvement.

If you've been a person who runs to the cookies or chocolate to regulate your nervous system when emotions are intense, you'll be happy to know that movement has been proven to help your brain's ability to experience and amplify natural pleasure.

This is exactly what you want rather than getting your reward dopamine hit from food. Your brain also becomes better able to handle and navigate difficult or challenging situations. Again, it's a win-win.

If you've been a person who has had a habit of snacking at night as a way to feel better from a crappy day, adopting some type of body movement will be a key strategy for you to better handle emotional processing because movement activates the parasympathetic nervous system. Regular body movement boosts serotonin and dopamine, enhancing mood and reducing anxiety, boosting overall energy levels, reducing cortisol levels, improving sleep, and promoting neuroplasticity, which enhances your brain's ability to adapt and process emotions.

I noticed this effect long ago when I first participated in Overeaters Anonymous (OA) and experienced the no-snacking between meals guideline. I had to learn to adopt other ways to destress, and walking was one of them. It became a need and deep desire. On days I couldn't do it, I noticed my mood suffered drastically.

Self-Calming Tools

When you start feeling emotions from any circumstance—restlessness, overwhelm, sadness, boredom, or any other emotion—that causes you to run to food for self-comfort, to take the edge off, or temporarily distract yourself, this pattern of emotional eating is reinforcing your toddler brain behavior, and it's more likely to repeat.

I wrote my master's thesis in 1999 on a natural treatment option for middle school children with hyperactivity, and self-calming tools were key in my research. My research confirmed that long-lasting gains and the most significant success long term were a combined behavior therapy, emotional counsel, and practical support, which may be more effective than drugs alone. The thesis also shared studies on how food additives, artificial flavors, dyes, sugar, and wheat all contributed to an adrenaline reaction.

(Little did I know back in 1999 that I would become sugar-free just five years later and then write cookbooks and be a coach!)

One of the things I discussed in my thesis was something called Brain Gym, which is basically a series of simple movements that encourage and access the whole brain, right and left hemisphere, which can help reduce adrenaline reactions. The left side of your brain deals with language, sequences, analysis, math, science, facts, and logic, and the right side is involved with imagination, art, images, symbols, creativity, intuition, and feelings.

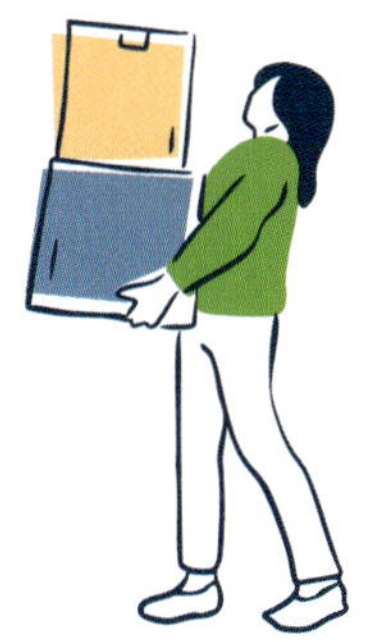

Certain movements can help send positive messages to your brain. For example, if someone is sad but makes a smile, that act can encourage a temporary lift in their feelings.

Here are some physical activities that can promote this integration:

- Pushing, pulling (I love pulling weeds), carrying objects, bringing your knees to your chest, curling up your body, swinging, sliding, and sitting on some kind of air cushion.

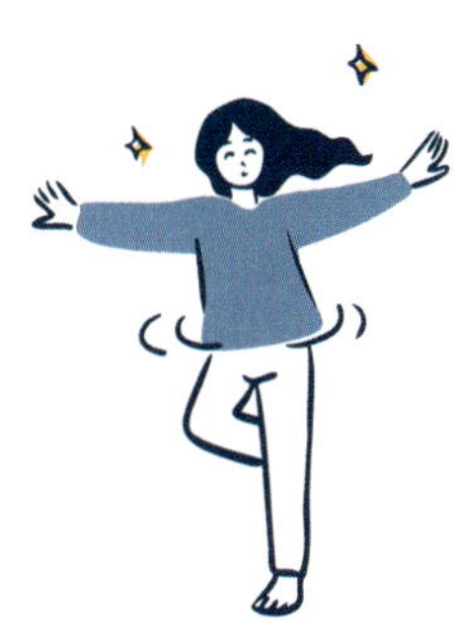

- Spinning is very effective. You find a focal point to look at and stretch your arms out to your sides while you spin around in place. Keep your eye on the focal point and count or set a timer for 15 to 30 seconds. This activity replicates what ADHD medication would do for my students but without the side effects. It was very calming and centering.

So, you're probably thinking *Those ideas are great, but what if I can't do something like that in the moment or don't have the space for that much movement?* Here are some other ideas:

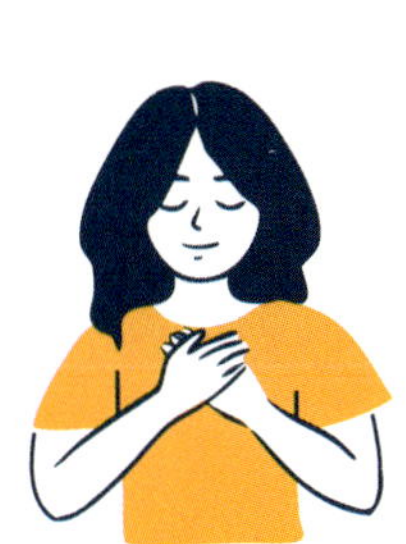

- **Hand on heart and breathe:** When you're feeling overwhelmed by fear, uncertainty, worry, anger, or stress, and you'd normally grab something to eat to cope with that feeling, try this activity. Bring both hands (or just one) over your heart, close your eyes, breathe in deeply, and then exhale twice as long. I like to close my eyes, but you don't have to. I'm a fast talker, and when I was teaching my Tribe membership, I noticed my speed of talking even slowed down!

  This exercise could take you just 3 seconds or however long you like. Placing your hands over your heart helps release oxytocin, which is fantastic for combating stress. Your heart rate also slows. The breathing technique signals to your brain that there is no threat, you're not in flight-or-fight response, and you're not being chased by a tiger.

- **Bilateral stimulation:** When it comes to fear, worry, or stress, which is just an overactivation on one side of the brain, bilateral stimulation crosses the midline to activate the whole brain and create new pathways or patterns and bring balance. (*Bilateral* just means accessing both sides.) Bilateral stimulation is simple and very powerful. Grab something in your left hand—a rock, your phone, a ring, whatever you

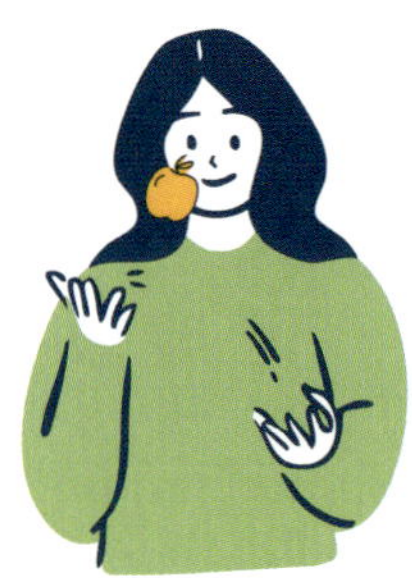

have handy—and move it from left to right, swapping the object to your right hand as it passes the midline of your body (in line with your nose). Then do it again in reverse, going from right to left. You don't have to do it for a long time—30 seconds or so. And to be honest, you don't need anything in your hand. The idea is that you're crossing your midline to bring symmetry to both sides and activate both sides of your brain.

If you're out and about or at a restaurant with friends and trying to calm yourself when everyone is ordering dessert, you can be as discreet as you want. For example, you can do this under the table on your lap. I love crossing my arms and tapping each shoulder. Whatever you choose to do for bilateral stimulation, the idea is that you're interrupting the habit of emotional eating with this activity instead of eating to comfort yourself.

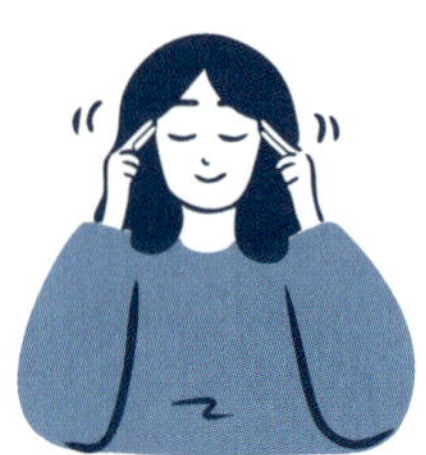

- **Emotional freedom tapping (EFT):** This is a fast, accessible, powerful tool. It's convenient and simple. It's just as easy to do as walking to the pantry or fridge to get something to eat. EFT focuses on acupuncture points in your head, eyebrow, side of your eye, under your eye, chest, and wrist. Tap the index and middle fingers of your dominant hand on the top of your head with short quick taps for as long as you like; then tap to the side of your eyebrow, on your temple, under your eye, and on your chest. Repeat this as many times as you like until you feel a sense of calm or diminished cravings. You can do it for as little or as much time as you want. Some research supports EFT's ability to help with cognition, relieve stress, and to help with emotion processing, so this method can be a great way to interrupt that habit of making a poor food decision that doesn't support your goals.[29]

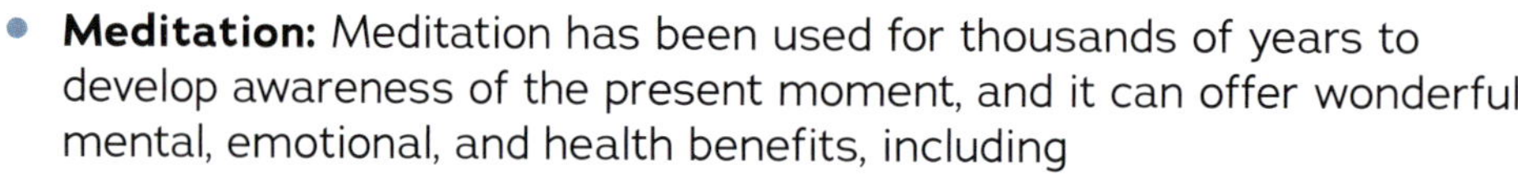

- **Meditation:** Meditation has been used for thousands of years to develop awareness of the present moment, and it can offer wonderful mental, emotional, and health benefits, including

  - Lowering blood pressure
  - Reducing stress
  - Improving sleep
  - Improving emotional regulation
  - Increasing focus
  - Enhancing mood

  A 2019 review found that mindfulness-based interventions reduced levels of the stress hormone cortisol in employees participating in workplace mindfulness programs, and a 2018 review suggests that meditation may contribute to healthy aging.[30] Meditation may also help with symptoms of specific conditions, including

  - Depression and anxiety disorders
  - Cardiovascular disease, such as arterial hypertension[31]
  - Dementia, Alzheimer's disease, and Parkinson's disease[32]

- Insomnia[33]
- Attention deficit hyperactivity disorder (ADHD)[34]
- Chronic pain

Meditation can involve practices to sharpen focus and attention, connect to the body and breath, and develop acceptance of difficult emotions. My favorite type of meditation is movement meditation, which incorporates my love of nature. Although most people think of yoga when they think of meditation practice, meditation can also be simply walking, bike riding, gardening, or hiking in nature. Movement meditation is an active form of meditation where the movement guides you into a deeper connection with your body and the present moment. It's especially good for people who find peace in action. I don't need any motivation to go for a walk with my dogs. It's something I seek each day, and I've done it for years now.

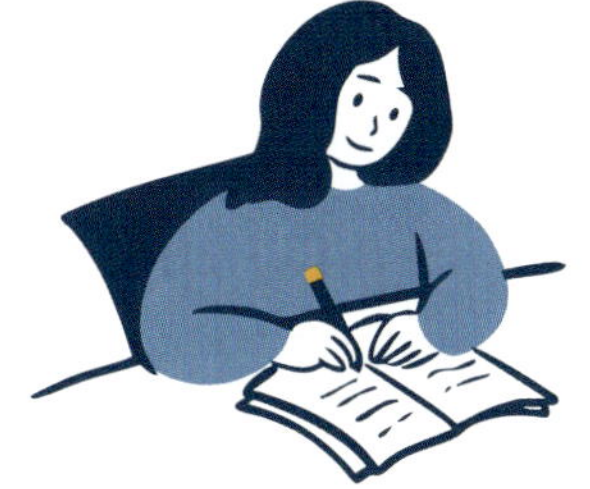

- **Writing:** Writing provides a structured way to process feelings and emotion. I've practiced writing for years, basically starting when I began my journey with OA back at the age of 22. My weight went from 159 pounds to 124 in six months, and I needed to learn to do something other than eat my emotions.

  The action of writing allows you to release energy by physically moving. When I was angry, I'd almost tear through the pages as I held the pen to write! It was and is very therapeutic! The act of writing helps you move through any emotions you feel in your body, and it releases some of the adrenaline you might feel when you're amped up. It stimulates the release of dopamine and decreases the levels of stress hormones (like cortisol), and that's exactly what you want if you're trying to fight an urge to eat and make a Good, Better, Best decision.

  Writing helps engage your prefrontal cortex, which you know is the sensible, decision-making center of your brain. This activation helps organize your thoughts and regulate emotions, bringing you a clearer understanding of how you're feeling. Amazing, (write!!) right?

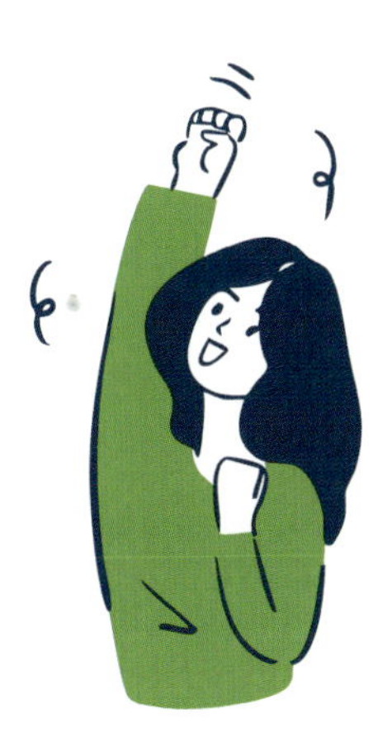

- **1, 2, 3, Yes!** This practice is a physical way to let go of the day's mistakes or upsets. You're saying to yourself, "I am letting this go." Open your hands in front of you, close your eyes, and think about the last twenty-four to forty-eight hours. Think about the people who may have hurt your feelings, things that happened that upset you, or things you did that you regret. Count to three, scream "YES," and toss your hands over your shoulders. Or you can write names or situations on paper, count to three, and wad up the paper and toss it over your shoulder while you scream "YES." You can use this technique at the end of the day or first thing in the morning. The idea is to use a simple action that can bring relief to process emotions and release stress.

Using any of these quick self-calming tools before you take the action to put something in your mouth for comfort or stress is a great step in the right direction. It allows you to pause for a moment so you can get back in control of your emotions and let your sensible prefrontal cortex make a Good, Better, or Best decision. You can even combine the techniques, as I've done in these examples:

- It's the middle of the day at work, and you feel stressed and emotionally tired. Normally, you might go to the office breakroom for a snack. Now, you want to change that habit, so you step outside, use some self-calming tools, take some deep breaths, get some sunlight, take your shoes off, and ground if possible.
- It's after dinner, and you feel a need to unwind with a snack. Try stepping outside, looking at the moon and stars, taking some deep breaths, and doing some hand-over-heart or tapping. You've just started a great new pattern to interrupt and rewire your brain from those old habits of eating to unwind.

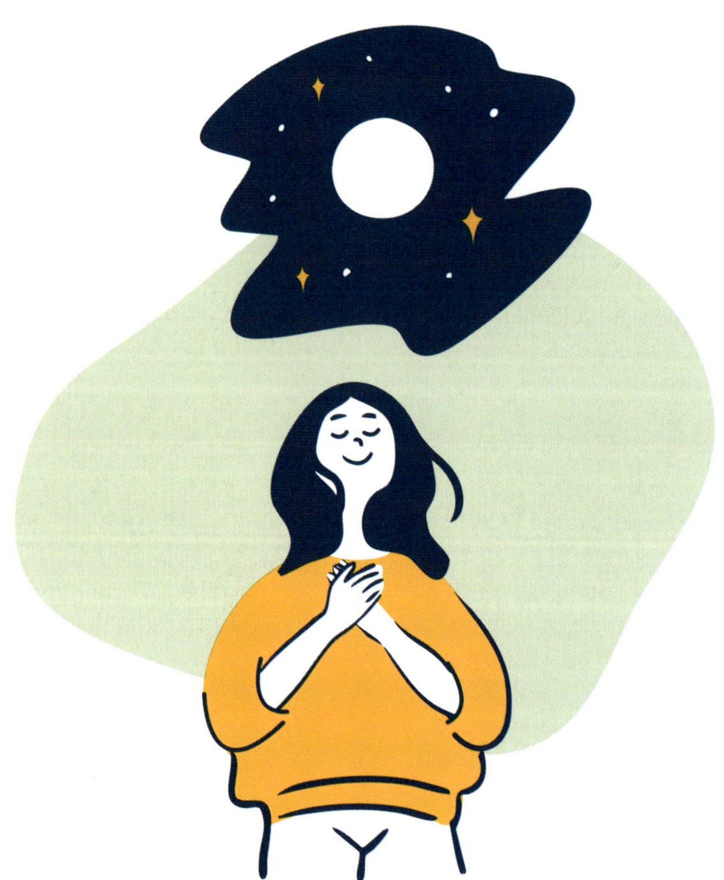

CHAPTER 2

WHAT KEEPS THE WEIGHT OFF

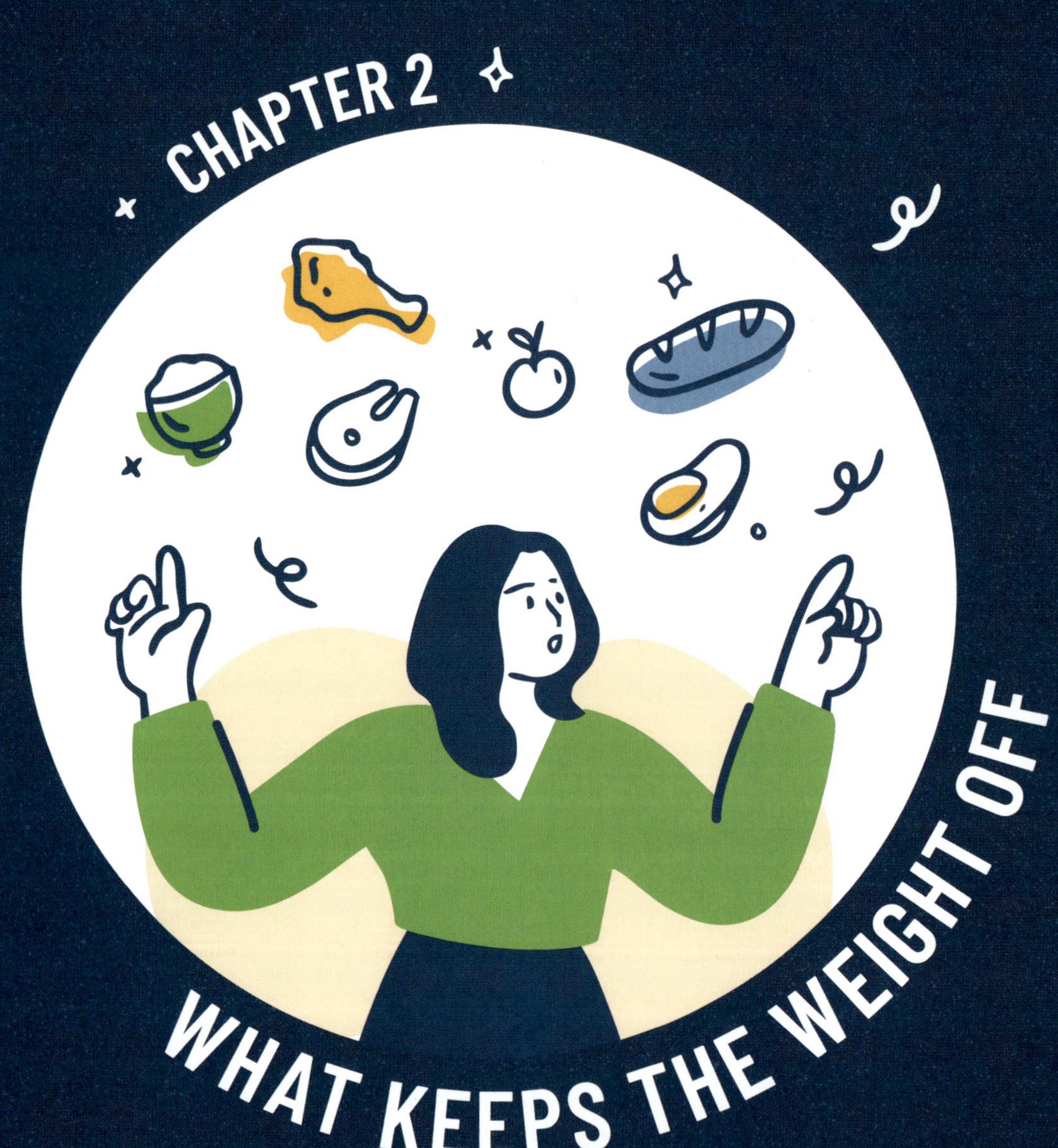

Once you've reduced processed foods in your diet, worked on improving your sleep, started planning food ahead of time to avoid decision fatigue, and practiced some self-calming techniques, you should notice it gets easier not to give in to your toddler voice. You'll be making better food decisions.

Non-negotiables are the foods and ingredients you can commit to never consuming—no matter what. You create a boundary for yourself. Even if your toddler brain tends to give in to temptations, you won't cross the line of eating anything on your non-negotiable list.

When you're in weight-loss mode, your non-negotiable foods are clear, concise, and consistent. Then, after you've hit your weight-loss goal, mastering maintenance for continued success requires a new perspective. You may want to include foods you didn't include while you were actively losing weight. You're now maintaining weight rather than losing it, but the facts remain the same: You should avoid certain ingredients and foods—or at least eat them only occasionally—if you're looking to achieve a good-quality life without health issues as you age.

My non-negotiables involve staying away from inflammatory vegetable seed oils, sugar, grains, and gluten and prioritizing protein daily. I describe these things in the following sections. You will need to decide whether you'll have similar non-negotiables or need different ones specific to your situation.

Inflammatory Vegetable Seed Oils

I don't purchase any store-bought item that contains canola, corn, cottonseed, grapeseed, soybean, sesame, safflower, sunflower, or peanut oil. Aside from being used for cooking, these types of oils are found in salad dressings, frozen meals, and processed, packaged foods. Learning to read labels of all packaged products that aren't single-ingredient foods will be an empowering lifelong skill for better health.

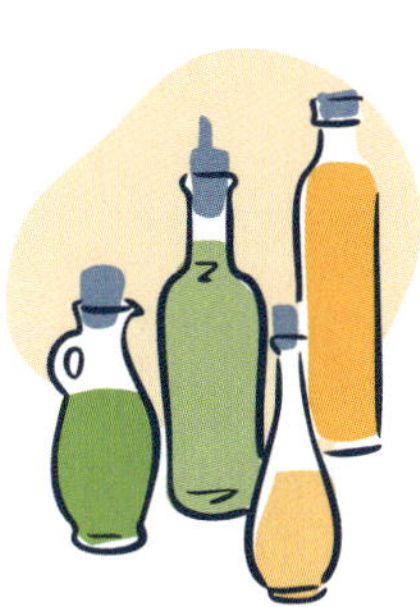

All these vegetable seed oils are high in omega-6. This is important to understand because a diet high in grains, vegetable seed oils, meat from grain-fed animals, and processed foods contain an abundance of omega-6, which will cause inflammation in the body. Omega-3s have anti-inflammatory properties, so it's important to be diligent in including more in your diet. And although you need both omega-6 and omega-3 fatty acids, the standard American diet has an excess of omega-6 but not enough omega-3. I've written extensively about oils in my book *The 30-Day Sugar Elimination Diet*.[35]

Chronic inflammation in the body leads to serious health issues. Eliminating inflammation in your body starts with changing your food choices and being adamant about your non-negotiables. I cook with butter, olive oil, lard, bacon grease, avocado oil, and coconut oil.

Sugar

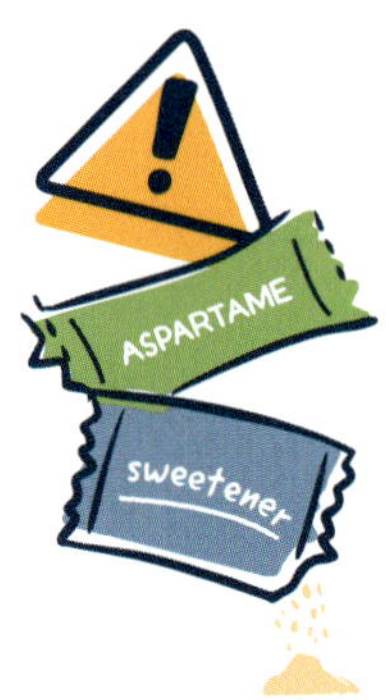

When I'm looking for a convenient store-bought item for my family, if there is any form of sugar listed within the first five ingredients, I won't buy it. Often a product has both inflammatory seed oils and sugar, which gives it two strikes.

Remember that ghrelin, your hunger hormone, gets amped up, and your appetite and cravings increase when you eat sugar and refined carbs. (See page 26 in Chapter 1.) I also avoid artificial sweeteners like Splenda, aspartame, and saccharin because studies have shown them to spike blood sugar and cause cravings.

If you choose to have a dessert with sugar on occasion, that's totally up to you. I suggest you plan for it ahead of time and be prepared for a spike in blood sugar. You may also possibly find that strong cravings return, but at least you will know to expect it. Eating on an impulse decision will give your toddler brain a chance to get a leg up and gain control again.

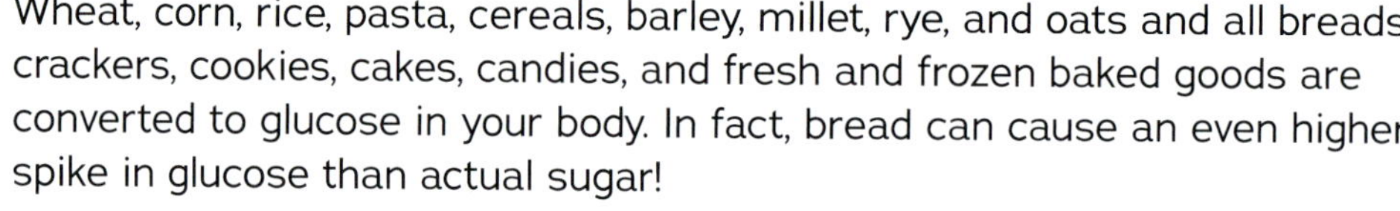

NOTE: I've created a handy downloadable cheat sheet of all the sneaky sugar types. Get the "Hidden Names of Sugar & Artificial Sugar" list with this QR code.

Grains and Gluten

Wheat, corn, rice, pasta, cereals, barley, millet, rye, and oats and all breads, crackers, cookies, cakes, candies, and fresh and frozen baked goods are converted to glucose in your body. In fact, bread can cause an even higher spike in glucose than actual sugar!

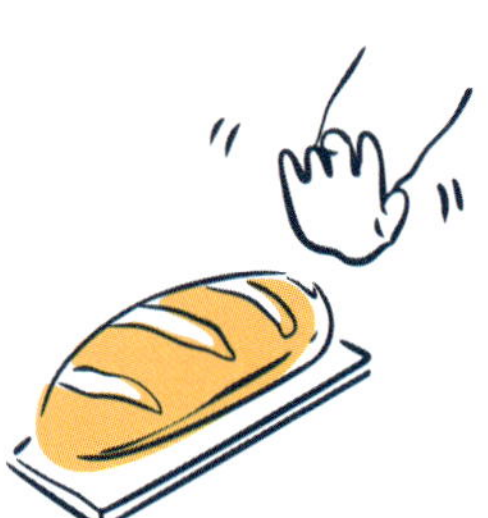

You'll notice your blood sugar spiking shortly after eating something with grains. It increases your hunger, and you crave more of that food.

Whole grains block the absorption of many nutrients you need and increase appetite because of the high carbohydrate load increasing blood sugar and insulin. In addition, grains have minimal nutritional value and decrease absorption of vitamins and minerals, compromising your digestion and immune function and leading to inflammation in the body.

Protein

The last item on my non-negotiables list is protein, but it's here for a different reason than the others. I believe protein is the most important macronutrient as we age. One study confirmed that daily protein intake is usually 0.8 to 1.5 grams per kilogram of ideal body weight to preserve lean body mass.[36]

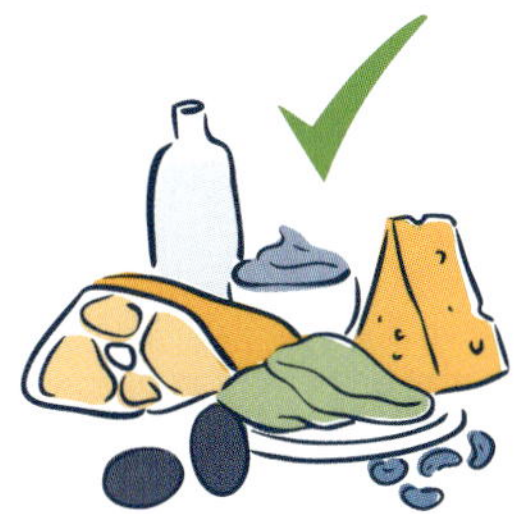

Every meal I eat has a good amount of protein in it, and that's a non-negotiable for me. I aim for 100 grams a day or more. Here are some reasons you need ample protein:

- You must eat an adequate amount of protein each day to manage ghrelin. (See page 26 in Chapter 1 for more information about ghrelin.)
- Eating enough protein is satiating and improves leptin sensitivity, which is what you need for long-term weight maintenance. When you prioritize protein, enjoy healthy fats, and eat low carb, you should be able to go from eating every two to three hours to not feeling hunger for four to six hours or more.
- Protein helps you maintain your muscle mass and function for strength and function; in turn, that will make you able to maintain your independence in your later years.[37]
- Eating an insufficient amount of protein will lead you to overeat until your body meets its nutrient needs. This is called the protein leverage hypothesis.

In 1995, Australian researcher Susanna Holt created the satiety value, which measures how much of a specific food will satisfy hunger. She found high-protein foods have the highest satiety value. How much protein you need to eat depends on your activity level, age, and goals. Every day, you experience a certain amount of muscle breakdown and muscle protein synthesis, which means you're gaining muscle, maintaining it, or losing it. You have to eat a certain amount of protein to gain or maintain muscle.

In the past, studies on protein stated a cap of 20 to 25 grams per meal for muscle protein synthesis. Eating any protein beyond that amount wouldn't be beneficial because it would be oxidized. However, a recent study found there is *no* upper limit to how much protein your body can use. This is exciting for those of us who like to eat a lot of protein.[38] My goal for the recipes in *Good, Better, Best* is that each has at least 20 grams of protein per serving.

HANDLING SOCIAL EVENTS

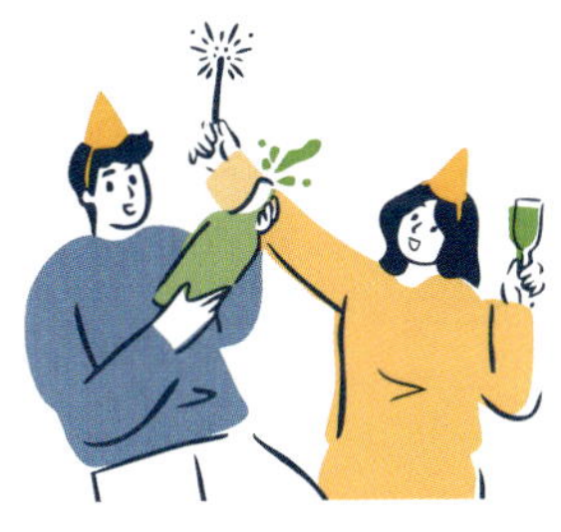

I know what you're thinking. It's probably something like, *Sure, fine, I can plan my food when I'm at home or work to avoid decision fatigue. I can reduce my processed foods intake. I can work on improving my sleep and reducing my artificial light exposure. I can work on taking measures to reduce my stress. But there is no way I can make better food decisions when I'm at a party, and everyone else is eating tempting foods!*

Yes, you can. I have a method that calms down your toddler voice when you experience FOMO (fear of missing out). This method gives you a plan for any social event because you can do it anywhere. It's easy, it's free, and it puts you in control of your choices.

In my coaching practice and in my own life experience, I see many people struggle with grazing and snacking throughout the day. It also happens at parties because the food is always out, and it's easy to walk by and grab something, so you're essentially eating the whole time you're there. If you work from home, you may also have an issue with snacks from the pantry when you need a break from the work.

The 1-1-1 method is something I've used for years when I'm at a party or celebrating a holiday. Even though I always make sure to be prepared with keto-friendly options for myself, I have to have a plan, so I don't give in to the tendency to get swept up in the constant eating at my Italian family's gatherings. Eat the appetizers. Then have the big meal, have coffee, have dessert, have another meal, snack after dinner. Next thing you know, you're up a few pounds, and it takes a week or more to lose it. It's frustrating, especially if you didn't eat anything with sugar or refined carbs and you still gained.

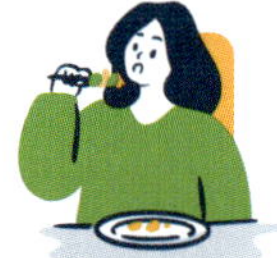

Here's the concept of the 1-1-1 method. The first 1 is for one plate. If you want appetizers, you can have them, but you must put them on a plate and sit down to eat what you've selected. No standing and grazing and adding more to the plate. Take a plate, add the food you want, sit down, and eat. Once the food on the plate is gone, you're done.

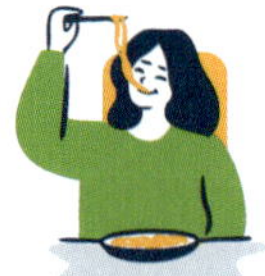

You then do this same thing with the main meal and desserts. You allow yourself to pick the foods that are available to you and align with your non-negotiables.

The second 1 is for one portion of what you want. You do not go back for seconds.

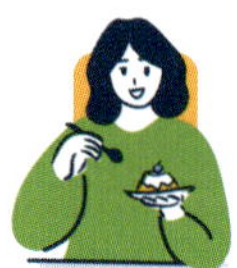

Pretty simple concept, right? One plate, one portion of the foods you want. No second plate or helpings.

The final 1 means you have a start and finish to your meal with a firm time limit. Remember, I was a teacher, and I like giving rules.

You have a clear beginning and end of your meal. For appetizers at a party, I recommend 30 minutes. Once the food on your plate is gone, grab a drink and mingle. For the main meal, I recommend 1 hour. Dessert, 30 minutes.

What does this do? Your brain likes rules, just like teachers do. It really does! There's comfort in habits and boundaries. The sensible part of your brain, the adult in the prefrontal cortex, loves routines and consistency. Only your toddler brain, the impulse part of your brain, will always choose immediate gratification.

The time limit for your meal is one way to control the impulsive toddler brain. You decided to begin and end your meal within one hour. When that hour is done, you won't be negotiating with the toddler brain. You don't have any more food; your meal is done. As you practice this habit, you will find the toddler brain will become quieter and stop asking.

As you practice this method, you will also find that you'll start making better choices of what to put on the plate to stay in alignment with your goals.

Implementing this method will stop you from constantly snacking, grazing, and gaining when you attend social events. It's how I maintain my weight and don't have to track anymore.

Instead of thinking, "I'm at a party, and I will never get to eat this food again, so I'd better eat everything. I'll have to start my diet on Monday," simply allow yourself the one plate. It provides more freedom and less of the all-or-nothing attitude.

Here's a tip to increase your success with the 1-1-1 method. It'll work better for you if you plan your food ahead. Taking a low-carb dessert to a party is helpful if you get FOMO every time you see desserts. It helps you to be on the defense. I offer plenty of delicious sugar-free, low-carb desserts in the recipe section. Try one and watch that FOMO disappear!

APPLYING THE GOOD, BETTER, BEST MINDSET TO EATING OUT

I may be a mind reader. I totally know what you're thinking about eating out because I've coached so many people with these same thoughts:

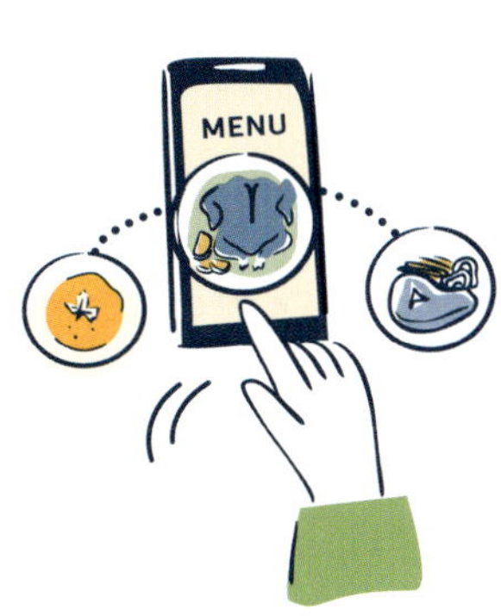

- *It's impossible to eat healthy when going out to eat.*
- *I can't make a healthy choice when everyone else isn't eating healthy.*
- *There's nothing good to choose from—just boring salads—when going out to eat.*
- *I can't say no to dessert.*
- *There's no way I can avoid sugar and refined carbs when eating out.*
- *I can't go out to eat because I won't enjoy sticking to my food plan.*

Instead of going into a restaurant with uncertainty about what you will find to eat, be prepared. Look at the menu online prior to going to the restaurant and make a Good, Better, Best decision about what you'll order. This habit will help you avoid decision fatigue because of the many menu choices. Tell a friend or family member what you plan to order. This will offer some accountability.

One of the tools I teach in my coaching practice is avoiding decision fatigue, keeping choices simple, and challenging the thoughts that seem true. For example, thinking it's impossible to eat healthily when eating out is just a thought. Does it empower you to feel confident or make you feel hopeless?

When you challenge the thought that it's impossible to eat healthily, ask yourself why you think that way. Could it be true that other people make healthy choices when going out to eat? Yes, many people have no trouble making healthy choices when eating out. Why does it seem impossible for *you* to make healthy choices in a restaurant? Keep asking yourself why until you can get to the core reason.

Learning to recognize the thoughts that don't serve you and challenging them is a great skill. As you practice it, you'll uncover a lot more about yourself.

Of course, you could instead continue to think it's too hard to make healthy choices when going out to eat and believe it. What will that do? Keep you isolated and believing that you can never go out to eat when you're on a "diet" and trying to be healthier. But isn't it preferable to choose to reframe this all-or-nothing thought and allow your prefrontal cortex to get to work in coming up with solutions to make better choices when you eat out?

Here's an example: *It's possible to eat healthy when going out to eat if I keep it simple and look for a protein and vegetable.*

How does that thought make you feel? Discouraged or encouraged that you can follow through with making a healthy choice?

Once you've uncovered your own sabotaging thought (or thoughts) that makes eating out feel hard for you and then challenge and reframe it, you've opened the door for solutions.

I teach all my coaching clients a simple strategy to be able to eat at any restaurant:

1. Look for naked proteins and vegetables. Naked proteins don't have breading on them. If you can't find any, ask the waiter if a menu item can be customized to be made without breading or sauce. Same with vegetables. Search the menu for any entrees that include simple low-carb vegetables like asparagus, broccoli, zucchini, and cauliflower. If they come with an added sauce, ask the waiter what's

in it and request that it can be put on the side. If it's not on your non-negotiables list, choose that option.

2. If the entrée choices all come with a high-carb starch like rice, pasta, or potato, ask to replace the starch with additional vegetables or salad.

Here's another example, which uses the thought *I can't say no to dessert.*

Is it true you *can't* say no to dessert or just that you *don't want to*? It's likely that you go into a restaurant with the intention of not getting dessert and then your toddler brain starts making demands. The next thing you know, you're diving into the very thing you said you wouldn't indulge in. This happens most easily when you head into a restaurant experience without a plan of what you will allow yourself to have. Whether it's dessert, alcohol, or French fries, planning beforehand is the best gift you can give yourself.

I'll say it again, planning your food *before* you get to the restaurant is the key to avoiding decision fatigue because you can use the sensible, adult part of your brain—the part that wants you to reach your goals.

Now that I've covered the logistics, what happens if you plan, commit to a friend what and how much you'll eat, and then your little toddler brain offers you all the sabotaging thoughts? Thoughts like these:

- *You never get to go out to eat. You can enjoy all the things and get right back on track tomorrow.*

  Challenge it with this thought: *That excuse has tripped me up and made me overeat for too long. I will not wait for tomorrow; I'm sticking to my plan.*

- *You can live a little because you've been good all week.*

  Challenge it with this thought: *It's not about being good or bad. If I want anything, I can plan for it tomorrow.*

- *It's just one. One bite won't matter.*

  Challenge it with this thought: *Not true! Every time I try one bite, it makes me want more. Not today, toddler!*

Being able to stand firm against those toddler thoughts is a skill that takes practice. I've been developing it over many years.

Many of my clients have had a difficult time not listening to sabotaging thoughts. They end up giving in to them. Realizing this made me understand that I needed to develop some steps that would allow clients to work toward the goal of not giving in while developing their ability and confidence at their own pace and on their own terms. That realization was what led to the Good, Better, Best process.

Since your toddler brain is ruled by instant gratification and impulse, when you make a Good, Better, or Best choice, you are still in control. There's an amazing feeling of empowerment as you start practicing this method.

I recommend using some self-calming tools (pages 32 to 36) to regulate your nervous system before making a Good, Better, Best food decision.

A Best decision is to stick to your planned food choice for the restaurant. How confident do you feel to make this choice? 100 percent, 75 percent, 50 percent?

A Better decision is if you really want a starch, ask for a sweet potato or baked potato instead of fries. How confident do you feel to make this choice? 100 percent, 75 percent, 50 percent?

A Good decision is if you really want french fries, ask if you can have only half the amount that they typically serve. How confident do you feel to make this choice? 100 percent, 75 percent, 50 percent?

Any of these choices will create strength that you have made a better choice than you would have prior to learning this strategy. If you can walk away from any restaurant experience feeling pretty good about your choices instead of being angry at yourself and regretful, that's a win.

REDEFINING YOUR WHY IN MAINTENANCE

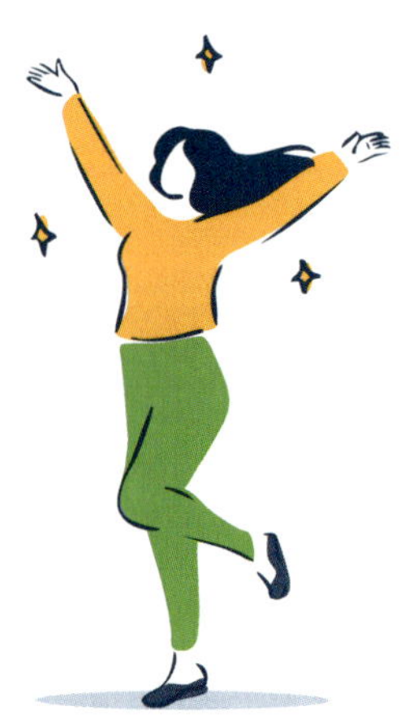

Once you lose your weight and you hit maintenance, you must create new, purposeful thoughts about your habits that make doing them important for maintenance. Hitting your goal weight often changes how your brain automatically thinks about the habits that got you here. Your brain might make the habits seem less important because there's no scale goal or immediate reward attached to them anymore.

The bottom line is that if the thoughts you're having aren't useful, you need to replace them with something *you* can believe about your habits. Don't let your brain turn your habits into enemies that prevent you from having fun or living. It's on *you* to turn your habits into allies for being able to maintain your weight loss. The best gift you'll give yourself in maintenance is teaching yourself deliberately and purposefully how you'll think about the things you do to keep to the weight off.

Maintenance won't be perfect, so planning for how you handle each day and correcting when things get off track is part of the ups and downs of this phase. I really think redefining your why is important in maintenance. You had whys for weight loss, so now you have to figure out your whys for maintaining.

Start by writing the story of all the things you did to get into maintenance. What changes did you have to make? What were the "whys" that drove you to act? How did you get through the hard parts? Which "whys" for losing weight have come true for you (for example, being able to sit in an airplane seat without an extender, getting off meds, fitting into a certain size of clothes)? One of the whys that came true for me is that I no longer had that constant chafing of my inner thighs. I hated that so much.

Imagine ten years into the future and see yourself still maintaining your weight. Which of the whys are still important to you? Here are some examples:

- I'm still off my meds.
- I'll be able to travel without a seatbelt extender after I retire.
- I wear all the cute clothes I want.
- I enjoy shopping.
- My thighs don't rub together.

Which habits do you think you need to start, stop, or redefine now that you're in maintenance so that you stay there long term? For example, I need to make food planning easy for myself, or I want to make sure I manage emotional eating.

Now put it all together. Redefine your maintenance habits by combining them with your maintenance whys: I want to keep fitting into my size 8 clothing by learning to love meal planning and make it easy.

What I found is that my habits and food choices didn't stop after I got to my goal weight. My top priorities stayed the same and were not just the things I did to lose weight. They became part of my lifestyle. I see freedom and find joy in my habits, my sugar-free, low-carb food choices, and my self-care practices because I know I am worth it. Why would I give up those things when I'm at my happy weight? Why would I think of them as a burden or too time-consuming to continue?

I started my first website with sugar-free, low-carb recipes in 2011. I wrote my first course for detoxing from sugar in 2012. In 2019, I went to nutrition school, became a keto coach, and then became a life coach. I've written three books on sugar-free eating, and I share my lifestyle with all who will listen. Just imagine what could happen for you when you have space to think about other things besides your weight. When weight loss isn't something you have to spend so much mental energy on, you can figure out what new and wonderful things you want to do next. Your weight isn't a problem to solve anymore!

INCORPORATING INDULGENCES

If you've read *The 30-Day Sugar Elimination Diet* and followed the meal plan in that book, you were willing to give up sugar and refined carbs for 30 days. What happened at the end of that month?

You may have started listening to your toddler brain saying that it was time to treat yourself. Or maybe you simply decided to bring sugar and refined carbs back into your life. Maybe one decision was an impulse decision, and it snowballed from there.

That's why I wanted to write this book, my friends! You can get back on track with the Good, Better, Best method—one decision at a time.

If you want to make exceptions for certain foods occasionally, how do you do that and keep your weight off without ending up in a roller coaster of emotional eating, spiking glucose, and ignited cravings?

Eating off your food plan is simple: You just plan for it. Plan exactly what and how much of said food you will indulge in. Tell someone in your life that you commit to that amount so they can hold you accountable and help you stick to it.

I don't want you to be afraid of any food. I'm not afraid of sugar or refined carbs; I just have absolutely no desire for them. My life is so much better than I ever could have dreamed because I gave it up a long time ago and don't keep giving in to it, even a little.

Don't misunderstand me here. I'm not telling you to be like me and choose to never eat sugar again, but I'm also not advocating eating sugar and refined carbs.

I know I was addicted. I know that many other people are also addicted to sugar and refined carbs and have yet to admit that, so I will never be the coach that says, "Yes, you should indulge in your wants and desires." I don't see a need for sugar and refined carbs. I had enough in my lifetime, and I choose to never touch them again. They serve me no purpose. I am not missing out, and I am not deprived.

However, I do understand that your personal food plan may include exceptions on occasion. I'm here to help you make those exceptions (or "off plan" food) less detrimental if you choose to indulge. You have to own your decision.

Never make exceptions for food indulgences as an *impulse* decision. I hope by now you realize that doing so will only strengthen the primal toddler brain.

You can incorporate an indulgent meal or dessert into your maintenance lifestyle without causing weight gain. I suggest you do this only once you get to maintenance, though. Plan your food of choice ahead of time and then commit it to your support person, who will hold you accountable to the amount you committed to.

But if you start listening to your toddler brain and give in to cravings and temptations—a few here and there—after a month of making poor decisions, you may notice you've put 10 pounds back on. Then it's time to sound the alarm and make a game plan.

My action plan in the next chapter can help you get right back on track if that happens.

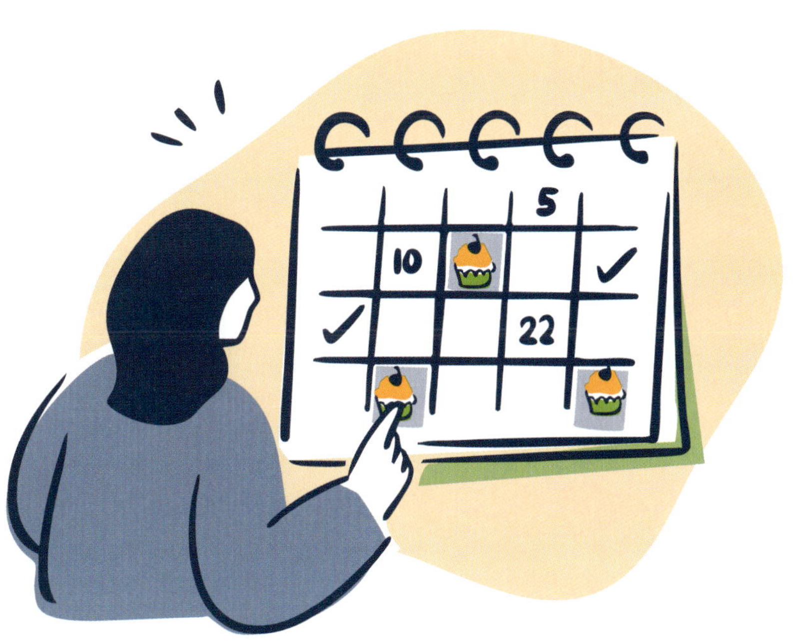

CHAPTER 3

REGAIN ACTION PLAN

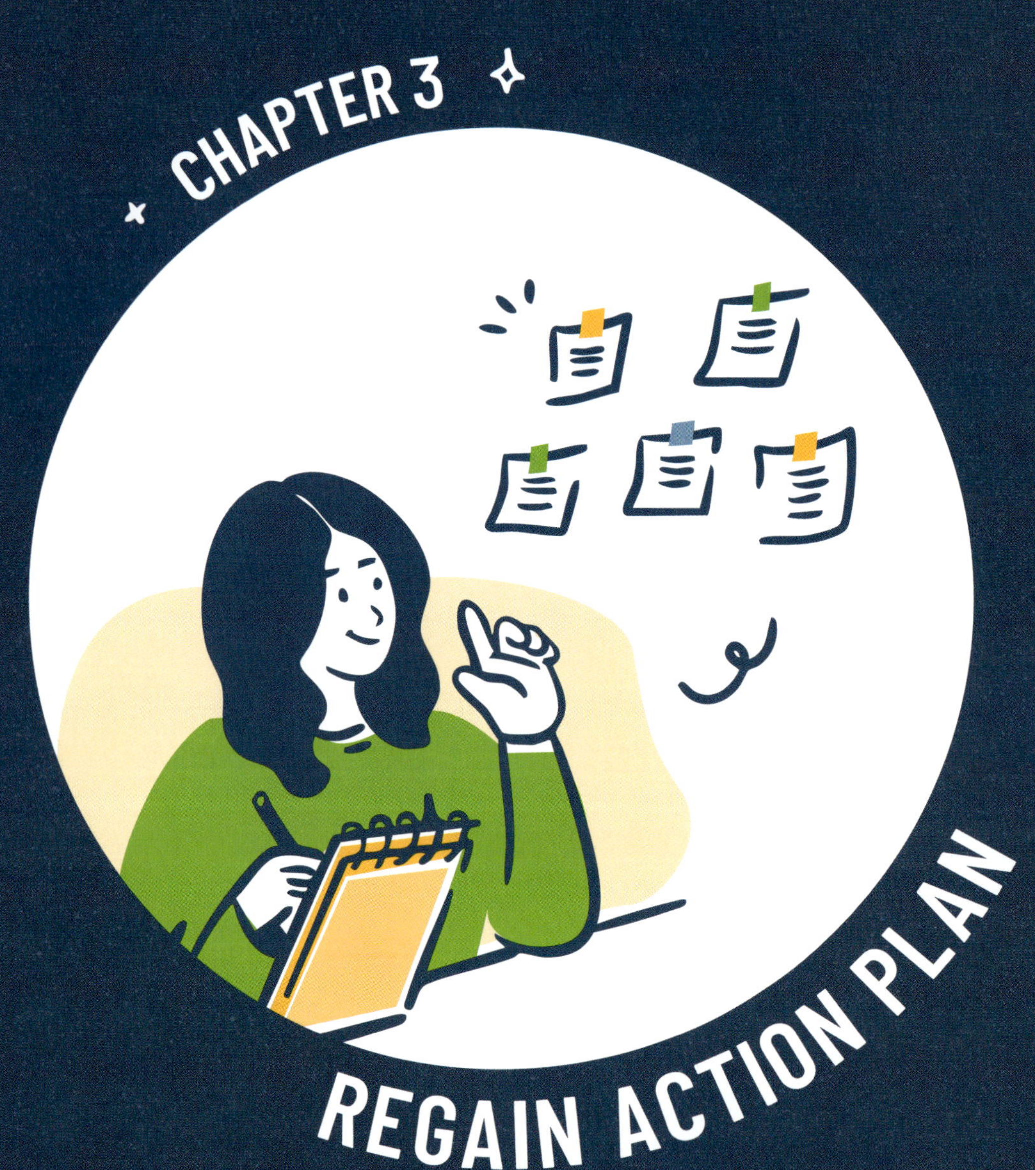

Maintenance is the act of repairing, correcting problems, pivoting when needed, and preventing damage to maintain a good condition. Sometimes, when you're in a maintenance phase, you regain some weight—for whatever reason. You're still a weight-loss success; you just need to figure out why you regained so you can learn from it and move on from it.

The process you use to work through regained weight is simple, whether you regained 5 pounds, 10 pounds, or more: Remove the guilt, accept that it happened, own it, and work on why it happened. In this chapter, I talk about reasons you might regain some weight and how to handle it when you do.

UNDERSTANDING WHY YOU REGAIN

Here are some common reasons for a regain:

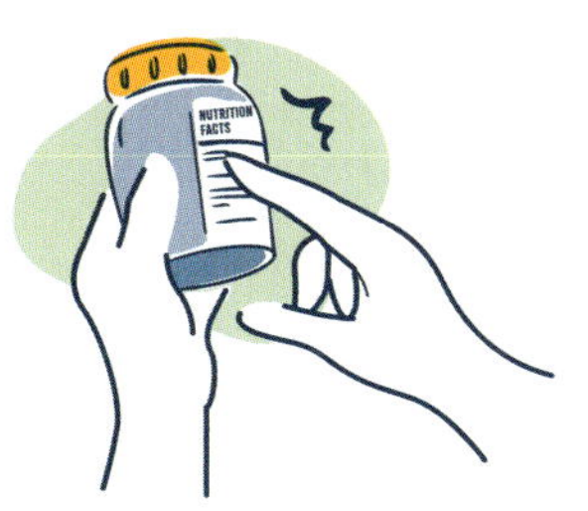

- **Too many calories and fat:** Even on a low-carb plan, calories matter. While low-carb eating can naturally reduce hunger, it's possible to overeat, especially high-fat foods like nuts, cheese, and keto treats.
- **Too many hidden carbs:** Certain processed foods labeled as "low carb" or "keto friendly" may contain hidden sugars or starches. Ingredients like maltitol, dextrose, and hidden sugars in processed foods can slow progress.
- **Dairy sensitivity:** Some people experience stalls due to dairy products, which can cause inflammation, bloating, or insulin spikes.
- **Not enough protein or too much fat:** Protein is essential for maintaining muscle and metabolism. Too little protein can slow weight loss, while excessive fat intake can lead to a calorie surplus.
- **Not enough sleep or high stress levels:** Poor sleep and chronic stress increase cortisol levels, which can slow weight loss and increase cravings.
- **Hormonal fluctuations:** Menstrual cycles, menopause, thyroid imbalances, and other hormonal shifts can temporarily affect weight.
- **Body composition changes:** If you're working out or building muscle, the scale may not reflect fat loss accurately. Measuring nonscale victories like measurements, clothing fit, and energy levels is key.

How Intermittent Fasting Can Help You Get Back into Your Maintenance Range

Intermittent fasting (IF) is a powerful tool that can help break through a weight loss stall or regain. By limiting when you eat, IF allows your body to

- Lower insulin levels, making fat-burning more efficient
- Improve metabolic flexibility, allowing your body to use stored fat for energy
- Reduce overall calorie intake naturally without strict tracking
- Enhance autophagy, the body's cellular repair process, which can reduce inflammation and improve metabolism

Experimenting with different fasting windows—such as 16:8 (fast for sixteen hours, eat within eight hours) or 18:6—can provide metabolic benefits. Additionally, longer fasts like twenty-four-hour fasting once or twice a week can be helpful for breaking through a stall or regain.

Become a scientist: Check the data and look at the facts. How often are you overeating? Do you only overeat certain foods? Processed snacks? Too many salty snacks like nuts? Too much alcohol? Get the data so you can plan to conquer it. You know how to lose weight, so you can easily make a reentry plan.

Choose one or more of these ideas to get back on track:

- Go back to tracking everything you eat.
- Skip dessert.
- Consider removing dairy and nuts temporarily.
- Include a few protein-only days each week.
- Lower your fat intake three to five days per week.
- Try moving your big meal from the end of the day to the start of the day.
- Follow any of the meal plans in this book.
- Rally a buddy or an accountability group for support. Share what you're committing to regarding your food and eat only that.

I give more details about protein-only days, changing the timing of your high-calorie meals, lowering the fat, and finding your tribe in the following sections.

TRYING SOME PROTEIN-ONLY DAYS

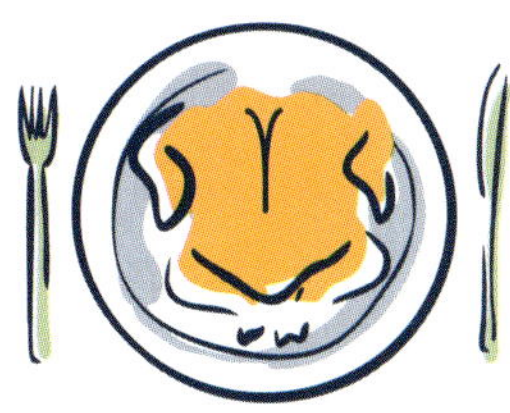

If you've been following a low-carb or keto lifestyle for any length of time, I'm sure you're aware of the carnivore and protein-sparing modified fast diets. Both adhere to a strict protein-with-minimal-carbs approach. Both can help with weight-loss stalls, but many people have difficulty sticking to them.

I tried carnivore because I had chronic hives. I'm not talking one or two; they covered my entire jawline, and they were horribly itchy. Carnivore is a great idea for anyone who's dealing with gut issues or undiagnosed symptoms. It certainly helped me, but I wasn't doing it for weight loss. I was lean and felt great, but I missed my veggies for sure.

I've also tried protein-sparing modified fasts when my weight wouldn't budge and I hadn't yet been diagnosed with hypothyroid. It helped move the needle a little but was my least favorite weight-loss method because of how low in calories and fat it was.

In my opinion, protein-only days, whether they are higher-protein keto or lower in fat like a protein-sparing modified fast, do support weight loss. The minimal carb intake in either strategy is the key to weight loss.

If you've never tried doing one to three days in a week of eating only protein, I highly recommend it, especially if you're in a stall or regain. A strict carnivore approach usually consists of just beef and water, but I think protein-only days are easier when you include dairy (if you can digest it well) and other sources like whey protein powder, collagen peptides, and egg white protein powder. I also opt for sauces and dips when doing protein-only days. To avoid palate exhaustion, I find it super helpful to combine two or three different proteins at each meal.

Include all the protein sources you like, and don't worry too much about calories. The goal is to eat minimal carbs but achieve satiety on the days you eat only protein. Here are some good sources of protein to help you get started:

- Beef
- Chicken
- Clams
- Cod
- Cottage cheese
- Crab
- Eggs
- Egg white protein powder

- Herring
- Lamb
- Liver
- Oysters
- Pork
- Ricotta cheese
- Salmon
- Sardines
- Scallops
- Tuna
- Turkey
- Whey protein powder

Turn to page 66 for a seven-day meal plan that incorporates three protein-only days. If this helps move the needle, do more than three days.

EATING YOUR HIGHER-CALORIE MEAL EARLIER

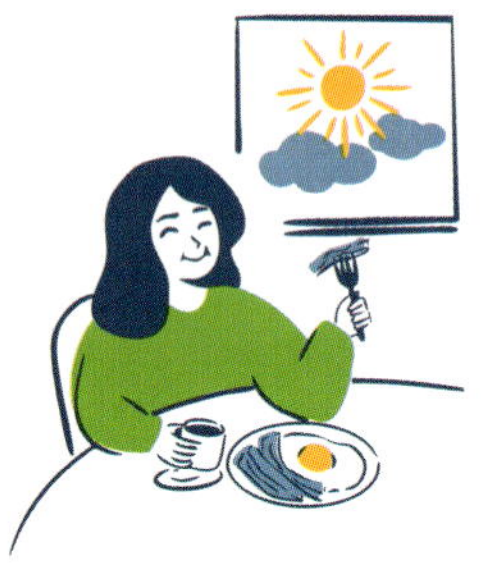

Having a larger meal at breakfast rather than dinner has also shown benefits as an effective tool for decreasing the hunger hormone ghrelin and improving weight management long term.

One study found that the amount of food eaten, type of food eaten (macronutrient composition), and timing of meals are the key components of weight-management strategies.[39] Another study tested overweight women for twelve weeks.[40] Half were in the higher calories at breakfast group, and the other half ate the same number of calories at dinner. The two groups had the same macronutrients for the entire day. The only difference was a simple swap of the timing for the higher-calorie meal.

The findings were quite interesting. The group with higher calories at breakfast had more weight loss and less hunger—so a decrease in ghrelin—than the dinner group. The high-calorie dinner group also had a higher glucose and insulin response. This is consistent with previous studies that have shown that insulin sensitivity and glucose tolerance decrease progressively throughout the day, a factor that may explain why nighttime meals and snacking cause weight gain.

Trying this change even for just one week may move the needle in the right direction. See the seven-day meal plan on page 68. It includes three days of swapping a higher-calorie breakfast and a lighter dinner.

LOWERING YOUR FAT INTAKE

I've been on a ketogenic diet since 2015, and through the years, even with my struggles with hypothyroid, I have felt amazing and still do. But since turning fifty-three (and being at the beginning of my hormone journey with low estrogen), I need to change my macros to see weight loss again. For years, I've been accustomed to a higher fat intake for maintaining my weight, but recently I've needed to have a more moderate fat intake to move the needle.

A popular method for anyone in a stall or weight regain is to incorporate two or three days a week of a protein-sparing modified fast (PSMF), which drastically lowers fat intake to about 30 grams daily. It's a temporary means to see changes on the scale. In a *Clinical Nutrition* study, researchers found that diets higher in protein and moderate in fat, combined with regular physical activity, were more effective for preserving lean mass and promoting fat loss in overweight individuals, including women approaching menopause.[41] The method works well for many people. The key is to be compliant.

Some people love PSMF, and I wanted to see if I needed to reduce my fat by much to see results. My goal was fat loss without muscle loss. My month of testing proved that a moderate fat intake of between 50 and 70 grams per day was the right amount for me, and I lost 8 pounds in one month. I continued my high protein, moderate fat intake for another month and saw another 7-pound loss, getting me back to my optimal happy weight.

Both the 7-day Minimal Time meal plan and the 7-day Protein Only meal plan use this high-protein, moderate-fat-intake approach five days per week.

FINDING YOUR TRIBE

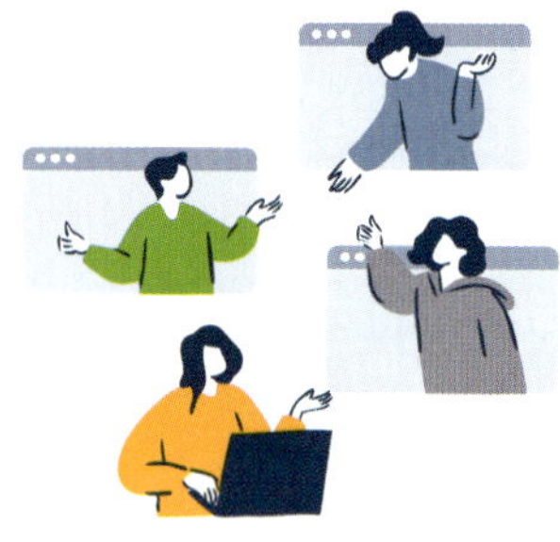

Strength in numbers: It's not just a cliché.

Courage, hope, power, unity, and accountability are things you can get from a group of people who support you. Finding people in your life who bring you encouragement is a blessing and gift that keeps on giving.

When you find a group of people who have a common goal, belief comes, hope increases, camaraderie develops, and you can truly know you're not alone. It can inspire you to dream big when you know others are rooting for you.

Studies show that being in some type of support with others, whether in person or online is the key for lasting results. Having community increases weight-loss success rates for keeping the weight off long term.[42]

A study considered three types of online programs: Some just offered info and self-tracking tools, others had a group chat feature where people could check in with each other and build friendships, and then there were programs with a professional coach available to answer questions. Researchers found that the ones with community support or coaching were just as effective as in-person weight-loss programs.[43]

In my experience, a successful weight-loss maintenance program includes the following things:

- Monitoring food intake and physical activity. What you monitor, you manage.
- Scheduling weekly contact with a supportive group of people who support your goals and don't sabotage you.
- Having problem-solving tools in place to resolve and prevent old habits from resurfacing.
- Managing stress if you overeat and/or comfort eat in response to stress.

Finding your tribe takes time and requires vulnerability but can be the most rewarding pleasure of your life. Allowing yourself to let others build you up when you feel weak, offer an encouraging word, vent with you, and listen to you will help you keep going even when you struggle. If you don't have people in your life, even just one, it can be harder to reach that goal. You can do it through pure determination and diligence, but it can be a lonely way to go.

I hope this book encourages you to find support to make the road ahead easier and more enjoyable as you continue your health journey and find your tribe. As a thank-you for purchasing this book, you can use this QR code to receive a free fourteen-day trial for the Sugar Free Mom Tribe, access to the five-session "Tame the Toddler" video workshop, and a download of "Hidden Names of Sugar & Artificial Sugar."

Going Alone or Together: My Experience

I've done it both ways—with support and without—and I can tell you with certainty that it's far better when you're not alone. That's why I've shared my story, my recipes, and my strategies with you in this book. My hope is that you feel like you finally have someone in your corner who truly understands what it's like to crave change but fear you'll fail again.

You don't have to prove anything to anyone. You don't need to do this perfectly. You simply need to be willing to try a new way—your way—with a little more compassion, a little more curiosity, and a lot less comparison.

Freedom from sugar isn't about isolation or deprivation. It's about discovering how good you can feel when you finally stop trying to fit into someone else's rules. It's about reclaiming your joy, your health, and your life—one good, better, best choice at a time.

You are not alone anymore.

Just keep going and find your tribe. .

Now, let's get to the delicious part: the recipes.

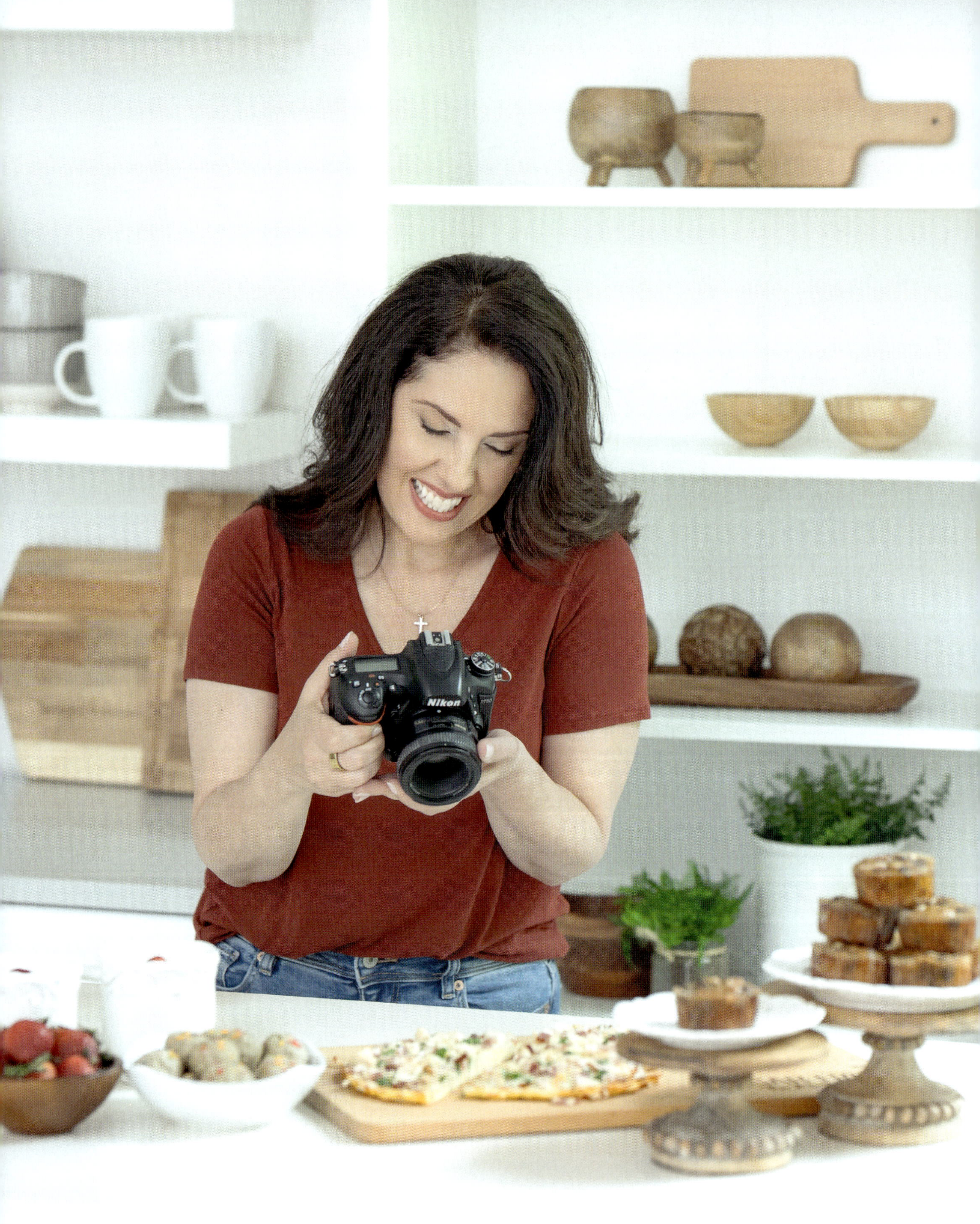
Nikon

PART 2

LET'S GET COOKING

CHAPTER 4 MEAL PREPPING GUIDE

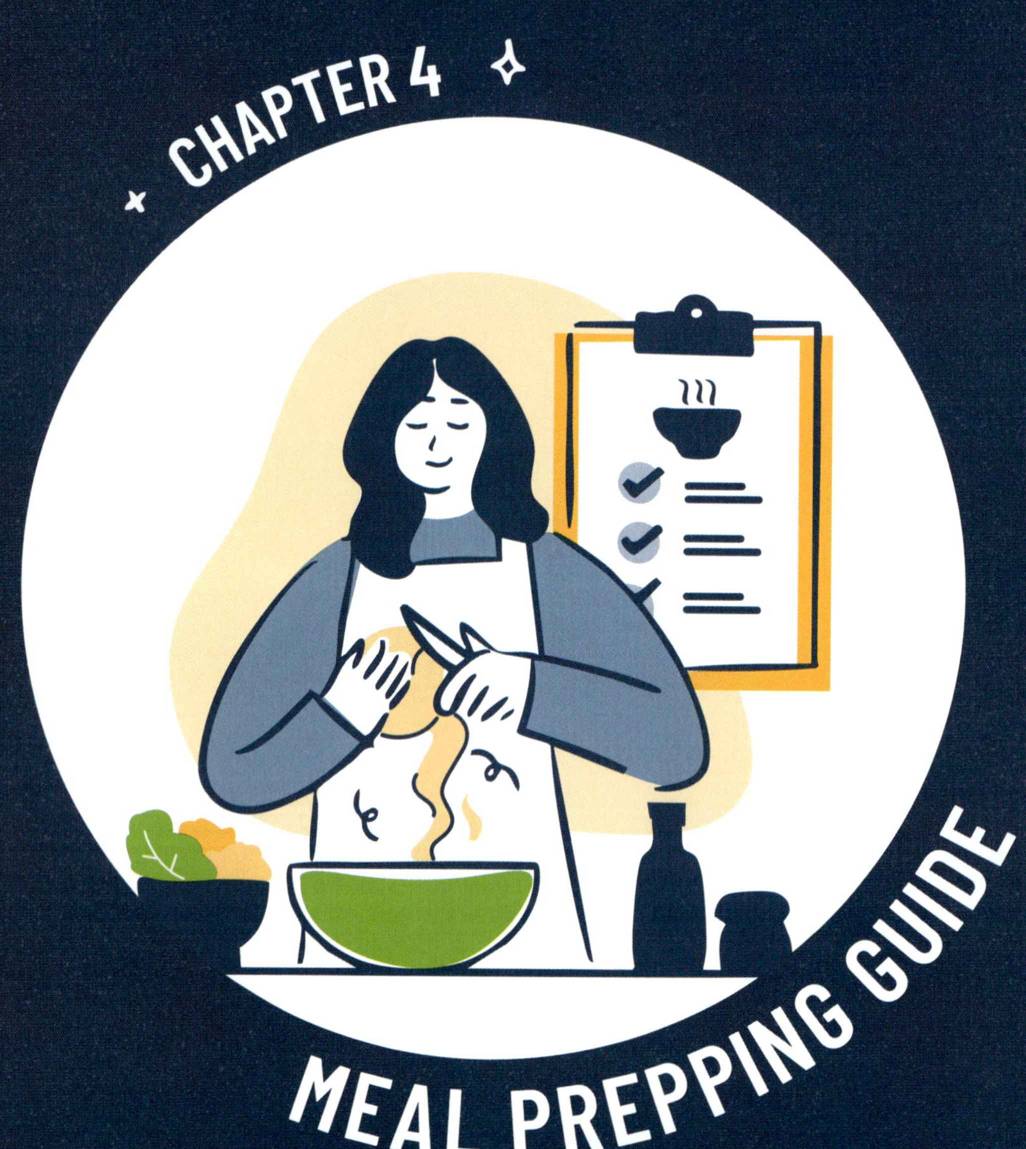

As someone who has had to work hard to maintain her weight, I can tell you wholeheartedly that planning ahead and doing some simple meal prepping can make a big difference in your actions and choices throughout the day.

Remember decision fatigue? Meal prepping is how to avoid it. Having simple options planned for breakfast, lunch, dinner, or snacks makes it a lot easier to make the better choice rather than succumb to ordering takeout, hitting the drive-thru, or raiding the vending machine. Applying the Good, Better, Best method to meal prepping each week is a win for long-term maintenance of your weight.

Throughout the recipes in this book, you'll find several practical meal-prep strategies you can use to help you stay on track. They include batch cooking, freezer prep, and single-serving meal prep. Using the kitchen strategies presented in this book will make your life easier while allowing you to stick to your non-negotiables.

Here's an example of what you can prep when you have at most 15 minutes, 30 minutes, or 1 hour:

- **In 10 minutes,** you can make my Tiramisu Overnight "Oats" (page 105) and my 90-Second Protein English Muffin (page 100) to have for breakfasts during the week.
- **In 15 minutes,** you can chop lettuce, cucumbers, peppers, and rotisserie-cooked chicken and put them in individual containers so you can pull them out for lunch any day of the week. Don't forget dressing and a fork, and you're set to go!
- **In 20 minutes,** you can hard-boil eggs—just skip the peeling until you are ready to eat them—or measure out slices of deli ham and cheese to wrap in lettuce or egg white wraps for roll-ups. Put some pickles in baggies, and you're done. Even better, make my Hard-Baked Eggs (page 166) so you don't need to peel the shells at all!
- **In 30 minutes,** you can easily prepare my Cottage Cheese Protein Waffles (page 94) or meal-prepped lunch bowls or containers for easy breakfasts and lunches during the week ahead.
- **In 1 hour,** you can freezer prep any of the following easy meals, freezing them raw, ready to be thawed and cooked in a slow cooker, Instant Pot, oven, or air fryer when you need them. (And yes, I did time myself making them.)
    - Italian Sausage & Peppers (page 257)
    - Sheet Pan Ranch Burgers (page 124)
    - Chicken Spinach Alfredo (page 205)

- Bacon-Wrapped Chicken Tenders (page 128)
- Ricotta Meatballs in Marinara Sauce (page 206)

If you have a larger window of time, you can do some batch-cooking to prepare recipes with larger yields (8 or more servings); then you refrigerate or freeze portions for wonderful dinners for yourself or the family. Batch-cooking multiple meals at once is an amazing use of your time (it pays dividends later). Making use of multiple appliances—such as an oven, Instant Pot, and slow cooker—allows you to cook several recipes simultaneously. I timed myself prepping four recipes in the Best chapter: three batch-cook meals plus the roasted vegetables. It took 1 hour 15 minutes of active prep time to get them all prepped and cooking away.

Here is how I did it:

I started with the Braised Brisket Dinner (page 263) because we wanted to eat it for dinner, and it takes the longest to slow-cook in the oven (about 3 hours). After I got that in the oven, I prepped the BBQ Pulled Chicken (page 260) for the slow cooker. Since we weren't having that for dinner, using the faster Instant Pot method wasn't critical. I set the slow cooker to cook on high for 3 hours so that it would be completed that evening with time left to cool and package it for freezing. Next on the list was preparing the Beef Stew using my Instant Pot. Once that finished cooking, in about 45 minutes, I let it cool to be packaged into 1-cup servings.

Once I had the three meat dishes cooking, I realized I had time to prep Roasted Vegetables (page 264), which I got into the oven as soon as the brisket came out. Thirty minutes later, the vegetables were roasted and ready to be cooled and packaged into servings of 1 cup for freezing.

MEAL PLANS & SHOPPING LISTS

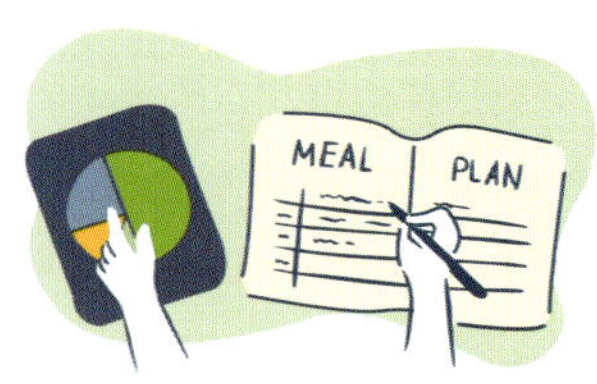

In this section, you will find the following three meal plans along with accompanying shopping lists:

- A 7-Day Minimal Time meal plan
- A 7-Day Protein-Only Days meal plan
- A 7-Day Higher-Calorie Breakfasts and Lighter Dinners Days meal plan

Each of these meal plans was designed with a different focus. The first is for when you have limited time but want to stay on track with your macros and address weight regain by lowering fat. The week includes six days with moderate fat intake and one day of higher fat. The second plan features three protein-only days for dropping weight quickly (the protein-only days are in green). The third features days with higher-calorie breakfasts and lower-calorie dinners, a way of eating that has been shown to improve long-term weight maintenance.

Bear in mind that all three meal plans are a guide. You can modify a day's meal plan if you determine you should have more servings, more protein, or more total carbs per day based on your nutritional needs for your age, height, and current weight. The best way to determine the appropriate number of calories for weight maintenance or weight loss is to use an online macro calculator or app like Carb Manager or Cronomete

Please note that the shopping lists for these meal plans do not include optional ingredients, such as garnishes or toppings, or secondary ingredient choices (just as the nutritional information for the recipes doesn't factor in these ingredients). Do a quick read of the recipes you'll be making before heading to the store to decide whether you want to include optional ingredients or prefer to use alternative ingredients.

I assume you have the following basic pantry items on hand, so I haven't included them in the shopping lists. Check the ingredient lists in the recipes you plan to make to verify that you have the quantities needed before you head to the store:

- Cooking oils: Extra-virgin olive oil, avocado oil, and coconut oil
- Cooking spray(s): Olive oil, avocado oil, and/or coconut oil
- Low-carb sweeteners: Confectioners' style, granular, and liquid
- Fine sea salt and ground black pepper

The meal plans assume you're feeding yourself breakfast and lunch and then feeding a family of four dinner, with dinner leftovers sometimes used for lunches the next day. Recipes that make more than one serving for breakfast or lunch or more than four servings for dinner can be refrigerated or frozen for later. You will find storage instructions with the recipes. If a larger recipe doesn't keep or reheat well, then the plan may suggest making a smaller batch to avoid waste.

In addition to sometimes eating an extra portion of a recipe as a leftover, occasionally components from one or two meals are repurposed later in the week, such as a couple of leftover waffles and an egg muffin being used to construct a breakfast sandwich or leftover barbecued pulled chicken from dinner going into a BBQ chicken bowl for lunch. For this reason, before freezing extra portions, be sure to skim the rest of the meals planned for the week to be sure the same recipe (or part of it) isn't used later on.

7-DAY MINIMAL TIME

DAY	BREAKFAST	LUNCH	DINNER	NUTRITION INFO	
1	1/2 batch **Quick Creamed Eggs** 97	**Hot Cottage Cheese Pizza Bowl** 117	**Sheet Pan Double Smash Cheeseburgers with Secret Sauce** 134	Calories Fat Protein Total Carbs Fiber Net Carbs	1,671 146g 78g 12g 1.5g 10.5g
2	**90-Second Protein English Muffin** 100	2/3 batch **Dill Pickle Egg Salad** 182	**General Tso's Chicken Meatballs** 210	Calories Fat Protein Total Carbs Fiber Net Carbs	719 52g 51g 14g 3.4g 10.6g
3	**Sheet Pan Omelet** 174	**General Tso's Chicken Meatballs** leftovers	**Pork Ragu** 209	Calories Fat Protein Total Carbs Fiber Net Carbs	755 51g 55g 14g 2.4g 11.6g
4	**Sheet Pan Omelet** leftovers	**Pork Ragu** leftovers	**Chicken Tacos** 131	Calories Fat Protein Total Carbs Fiber Net Carbs	705 45g 62g 8g 2.4g 5.6g
5	**Vanilla Protein Power Smoothie** 106	**Dill Pickle Egg Salad** leftovers	**Turkey Sausage Pepper Zucchini Skillet** 132	Calories Fat Protein Total Carbs Fiber Net Carbs	921 60g 79g 19g 5g 14g
6	**Strawberry Protein Mug Muffins** 102	**Pork Ragu** leftovers	Double batch **Buttery Filet Mignon** 213	Calories Fat Protein Total Carbs Fiber Net Carbs	943 61g 81g 13.3g 4.1g 9.2g
7	**Parmesan Eggs** 98	**Salmon Patties** 119	**Bacon-Wrapped Chicken Tenders** 128	Calories Fat Protein Total Carbs Fiber Net Carbs	777 38g 9g 7g 2.01g 4.99g

Shopping List for 7-Day Minimal Time Meal Plan

PRODUCE

bell peppers, red, 2 large

garlic cloves, 7

ginger (grated), 3 tablespoons

lemon, 1

onion, red, 1 small

onions, yellow, 3 medium

parsley, 1 bunch

scallions, 3

strawberries, 2 large

zucchini, 1 large

DAIRY

butter, salted, 1 stick

cheddar cheese, shredded, 1¼ cups

cheddar cheese, 4 slices

cottage cheese (4% milkfat), 11 ounces

eggs, large, 23

heavy cream, 7 ounces

milk, unsweetened almond, ½ cup

mozzarella cheese (part skim), shredded, ¼ cup

Parmesan cheese, grated, 2 tablespoons

PROTEIN

bacon, 12 slices

beef, filet mignons, 1½ inches thick, 4 (8-ounce)

beef, ground, 80/20, 2 pounds

chicken breast, boneless, skinless, 2 pounds

chicken breast strips, grilled, ready-to-eat, 2 pounds

chicken, ground, 2 pounds

pepperoni, ½ ounce

pork, ground, 1 pound

salmon, 1 (5-ounce) can

sausage, turkey links, 1 pound

PANTRY

allulose, granular, 2 tablespoons

baking powder, 1 teaspoon

bone broth, chicken, 2 cups

coconut aminos, ½ cup

collagen peptides, vanilla flavored, ⅓ cup

dill pickle, 1 medium

dill pickle juice, 2 teaspoons

flour, blanched almond, 7 tablespoons

gelatin powder, unflavored, 10 grams

ketchup, sugar-free, 1 tablespoon

marinara sauce, low-carb, 1 tablespoon

mayonnaise, avocado oil, 1¼ cups

mustard, Dijon, 1 teaspoon

mustard, prepared yellow, 2 tablespoons

peanut butter, powdered, 2 tablespoons

peanut butter, unsweetened, 1 tablespoon

pork rind panko, ¾ cup

red wine, ½ cup

stevia, liquid, vanilla flavored, ½ teaspoon

taco shells, low-carb, 8

tomato paste, 2 tablespoons

tomato puree, unsweetened, 2 tablespoons

tomatoes, crushed, 1 (14-ounce) can

vinegar, apple cider, 2 tablespoons

vinegar, distilled white, ¼ cup

whey protein powder, vanilla flavored, ½ cup

DRIED HERBS/SPICES

cayenne pepper

chili powder

cumin, ground

fennel seeds

garlic powder

Italian seasoning

onion powder

paprika

red pepper flakes

sesame seeds

smoked paprika

7-DAY PROTEIN-ONLY DAYS

DAY	BREAKFAST	LUNCH	DINNER	NUTRITION INFO
1	**Caramel Apple Scones** 230	**Hot Cheeseburger Cottage Cheese Bowl** 114	**Beef Stew** 258	Calories 937; Fat 67g; Protein 67g; Total Carbs 21g; Fiber 6.5g; Net Carbs 14.5g
2	**Basic Egg Muffins*** and 2 slices thick-cut bacon 232	⅓ batch **On-the-Go Cottage Cheese Egg Salads** 181	**Baked Breaded Pork Chops** 190	Calories 994; Fat 59g; Protein 101g; Total Carbs 11g; Fiber 2.32g; Net Carbs 8.68g
3	Leftover **Caramel Apple Scone**	**Salmon Poke Bowl** 186	**Sheet Pan Ranch Burgers** and **Cottage Cheese Cloud Bread Rolls** with **Crispy Smashed Cauliflower** 124 88 271	Calories 1,183; Fat 92g; Protein 69g; Total Carbs 28g; Fiber 7.2g; Net Carbs 20.7g
4	**Savory Cottage Cheese Protein Waffles**** 94	Leftover **Ranch Burger** (burger only)	**Mississippi Pot Roast** 267	Calories 950; Fat 67g; Protein 81g; Total Carbs 7g; Fiber 1.2g; Net Carbs 5.8g
5	**Chocolate Protein Granola Bars** 168	Leftover **Mississippi Pot Roast**	**BBQ Pulled Chicken***** 260	Calories 909; Fat 60g; Protein 81g; Total Carbs 13g; Fiber 4g; Net Carbs 9g
6	**Prep-Ahead Breakfast Sandwich** (using 2 leftover waffles, 1 leftover egg muffin, and 2 slices thick-cut bacon) 237	**Hot BBQ Chicken Cottage Cheese Bowl** (using leftover BBQ Pulled Chicken) 113	Double batch **Air Fryer Salmon** 127	Calories 1,268; Fat 81g; Protein 116g; Total Carbs 14g; Fiber 0.4g; Net Carbs 13.6g
7	Leftover **Chocolate Protein Granola Bars**	**Shrimp Escabeche****** 185	**Cheeseburger Pie** with **Garlic Parmesan Broccoli** 198 137	Calories 1295; Fat 100g; Protein 71g; Total Carbs 23g; Fiber 6.4g; Net Carbs 16.6g

Shopping List for Protein-Only Days Meal Plan

PRODUCE

apple, 1 small

avocado, Hass, 1 small

broccoli florets, 1 pound

carrots, 2 medium

cauliflower florets, 1 pound

cucumber, 1 medium

daikon radish, 1 medium

garlic cloves, 5

lettuce, romaine, 1 medium head

lime, 1

onion, red, 1 large

onions, yellow 2 large

parsley, 3 sprigs

tomato, 1 medium

DAIRY

butter, salted, 1 stick

butter, unsalted, ½ stick

cheddar cheese, shredded, 1¾ cups

cottage cheese (4% milkfat), 24 ounces

eggs, large, 31

heavy cream, 18 ounces

mozzarella cheese (part skim), shredded, ¼ cup

Parmesan cheese, grated, ¼ cup

PROTEIN

bacon, regular cut, 2 slices

bacon, thick cut, 4 slices

beef chuck roast, boneless, 6 pounds

beef, ground, 80/20, 4 pounds

beef, ground, 90/10, 1 (3-ounce) patty

chicken thighs, boneless, skinless, 2 pounds

pork chops, bone in (½ inch thick), 4 (5-ounce)

salmon fillets, skin on, 4 (6-ounce)

salmon, raw, sushi grade, 4 ounces

shrimp, large, peeled and deveined, 1 pound

PANTRY

allulose, liquid, ⅓ cup

apple extract, 1 teaspoon

baking powder, 2 teaspoons

BBQ sauce, sugar-free, ½ cup

bone broth, beef, 4 cups

bone broth, chicken, ½ cup

chocolate chips, sugar-free, ¼ cup

coconut aminos, 4 tablespoons

collagen peptides, chocolate flavored, ⅓ cup

dill pickle, 1 small

egg white protein powder, ¼ cup

flour, coconut, 7 tablespoons

glucomannan, ½ teaspoon

ketchup, sugar-free, 1 tablespoon

low-carb brown sugar–style sweetener, ¼ cup plus 1 teaspoon

macadamia nuts, raw, ½ cup

mayonnaise, ⅓ cup

mayonnaise, avocado oil, 3 tablespoons

mustard, Dijon, 2 teaspoons

peanut butter, natural, ⅓ cup

pepperoncini slices, 1 cup

pork rind panko, 1 cup

pumpkin seeds, hulled ½ cup

shirataki rice, ½ cup

Sriracha, 1 teaspoon

sunflower seed meal, 1 cup

sunflower seeds, hulled, ½ cup

tomato paste, 2 tablespoons

vanilla extract, ½ teaspoon

vinegar, distilled white, 2½ teaspoons

vinegar, white wine, ½ cup

whey protein powder, 1¼ cups

DRIED HERBS & SPICES

apple pie spice

cumin, ground

dill weed, dried

garlic powder

Italian seasoning

onion, dried minced

onion powder

parsley, dried

sea salt, flaked

smoked paprika

thyme, ground

*Save one egg muffin for the Prep-Ahead Breakfast Sandwich on Day 6. Freeze the rest for later.

**Reserve two waffles for the Prep-Ahead Breakfast Sandwich on Day 6. Freeze the rest for later.

***Set aside one serving of pulled chicken for the BBQ Chicken Cottage Cheese Bowl on Day 6. Freeze the rest for later.

****Shrimp Escabeche leftovers should be eaten by the next day.

7-DAY HIGHER-CALORIE BREAKFASTS AND LIGHTER DINNERS DAYS

DAY	BREAKFAST	LUNCH	DINNER	NUTRITION INFO
1	**Chocolate Protein Granola Bars,** 2 scrambled eggs, and 2 slices thick-cut bacon 168	**Tuna Cabbage Patties** 122	**Hot Shrimp Dip** with sliced cucumbers 120	Calories 1,482 Fat 114g Protein 95g Total Carbs 21g Fiber 6g Net Carbs 15g
2	**Lemon Poppyseed Muffins** 234	½ batch **Better BLT Salad** 178	**Ricotta Meatballs in Marinara Sauce** 206	Calories 1,273 Fat 101g Protein 68g Total Carbs 24g Fiber 9g Net Carbs 15g
3	½ batch **On-the-Go High-Protein Breakfasts** and ⅓ cup mixed fresh berries 173	Leftover **Ricotta Meatballs in Marinara Sauce**	**Bourbon Chicken Lettuce Wraps** 193	Calories 1,433 Fat 95.2g Protein 105.4g Total Carbs 30.8g Fiber 5.6g Net Carbs 25.2g
4	Leftover **Lemon Poppyseed Muffin**	Leftover **Better BLT Salad**	**Crustless Pepperoni Pizza Bake** 197	Calories 971 Fat 89g Protein 55g Total Carbs 18g Fiber 9g Net Carbs 9g
5	Leftover **On-the-Go High-Protein Breakfast** and ⅓ cup mixed fresh berries	Leftover **Crustless Pepperoni Pizza Bake**	**Garlic Butter Chicken Thighs** 268	Calories 1,190 Fat 92.2g Protein 100.4g Total Carbs 15.8g Fiber 4.7g Net Carbs 11.1g
6	**Cinnamon Roll Protein Pancakes** 170	Leftover **Garlic Butter Chicken Thighs**	**Italian Meatloaf** 249	Calories 949 Fat 66g Protein 78g Total Carbs 10g Fiber 3.1g Net Carbs 6.9g
7	**Breakfast Frittata** 177	Leftover **Italian Meatloaf**	**Chicken Caprese Casserole** 194	Calories 1,482 Fat 118g Protein 91g Total Carbs 14.5g Fiber 8g Net Carbs 6.4g

Shopping List for Higher-Calorie Breakfasts and Lighter Dinners Days Meal Plan

PRODUCE

basil, 3/4 bunch

bell pepper, red, 1 small

berries, mixed, 2/3 cup

cucumber, 1 medium

daikon radish, 1

garlic cloves, 16

green cabbage, 8 ounces

lemons, 4 medium

lettuce, Boston, 8 large leaves

lettuce, romaine, 1 heart

onions, red, 2 small

onions, yellow, 2 large

parsley, 1/2 bunch

scallions, 1 bunch

tomato, Roma, 1 large

tomatoes, grape, 1 cup

DAIRY

butter, salted, 2 tablespoons

butter, unsalted, 1 1/2 sticks

cheddar cheese, shredded, 3 cups

cottage cheese (4% milkfat), 7 ounces

cream cheese, 1 (8-ounce) package

eggs, large, 38

Folios cheddar cheese wraps, 6

heavy cream, 11 ounces

mozzarella cheese (part skim), shredded, 4 1/3 cups

Parmesan cheese, grated, 1 3/4 cups

ricotta cheese (part skim), 2 cups

sour cream, 5 ounces

PROTEIN

bacon, regular cut, 8 slices

bacon, thick cut, 6 slices

beef, ground, 80/20, 2 pounds

beef, ground, 85/15, 2 pounds

chicken breasts, boneless, skinless, 1 pound

chicken, rotisserie (2 to 2 1/4 pounds), 1

chicken thighs, boneless, skinless, 3 pounds (8 thighs)

pepperoni, 25 slices

pork, ground, 3 pounds

sausage, chicken links, fully cooked, 4 links

shrimp, frozen (any size), cooked and peeled, 1 pound

tuna packed in water, 2 (5-ounce) cans

PANTRY

allulose, liquid, 1/3 cup

baking powder, 2 1/2 teaspoons

bone broth, chicken, 2 cups

bourbon, 1 tablespoon

chocolate chips, sugar-free, 1/4 cup

coconut aminos, 1/3 cup

collagen peptides, chocolate flavored, 1/3 cup

flour, blanched almond, 1/2 cup

flour, coconut, 1 cup

glucomannan, 2 teaspoons

low-carb sweetener, brown sugar–style, 1/4 cup plus 1 tablespoon

low-carb sweetener, granular or confectioners' style, 1/2 cup

macadamia nuts, raw, 1/2 cup

marinara sauce, low-carb, 5 1/2 cups

mayonnaise, avocado oil, 1/2 cup plus 2 tablespoons

peanut butter, natural, 1/3 cup

pesto sauce, 1/2 cup

pork rind panko, 2 cups

pumpkin seeds, hulled, 1/2 cup

Sriracha, 2 teaspoons

stevia, liquid, cinnamon flavored 1 teaspoon

stevia, liquid, lemon flavored, 1/2 teaspoon

sunflower seeds, hulled, 1/2 cup

vanilla extract, 1 teaspoon

whey protein powder, vanilla flavored, 1/2 cup

DRIED HERBS & SPICES

cinnamon, ground

garlic powder

Italian seasoning

onion powder

poppyseeds

red pepper flakes

sea salt, flaked

seasoning blend (such as Bell's)

ABOUT THE RECIPES

The recipes are divided into four chapters: Basics, Good (Enough), Better, and Best.

BASICS

The Basics chapter contains recipes for sauces and other staples that are used in multiple recipes throughout the book or that can be used to make a quick "plan B" meal on the fly (like using a cloud bread roll to make a sandwich with deli meats).

GOOD (ENOUGH)

The Good (Enough) chapter provides easy recipes that can be prepped quickly and cooked in 20 minutes or less. Some require no cooking at all, and some take advantage of convenience foods, such as packaged egg white wraps or fully cooked meats, to allow you to prepare a fast meal. In addition to the recipes, you'll find a helpful list of plan B meals tucked at the end of the chapter. These meals give you options for staying on track with your macros even when finding time to make one of the Good (Enough) recipes becomes impossible.

BETTER

The Better chapter features recipes that take 15 to 45 minutes to prepare, with much of the time for the longer recipes being hands-off. These are made from scratch and do not use convenience ingredients.

BEST

Recipes in the Best chapter require more than 30 minutes of your time to prepare. Many have larger yields, making them great batch-cook options. These recipes are for the days when you have extra time to meal prep, cook, and enjoy your meals.

For a more detailed description of the three key recipe chapters and their concepts, see the section "Good, Better, Best Defined" on pages 11 to 12.

All the recipes are sugar-free, gluten-free, and low-carb, and the great majority are ketogenic as well.

Recipe Icons

The recipes feature quick reference icons to help you navigate them easily and discover at a glance which ones suit your dietary needs or are made with a cooking appliance you'd like to use. When possible, I provide multiple cooking methods so that you can make all the recipes regardless of whether you own a pressure cooker (such as an Instant Pot), a slow cooker, or an air fryer. When an ingredient substitution can be made to make a recipe dairy-free, egg-free, or nut-free, those options are noted. If you have a peanut allergy, look for the icon that indicates peanuts are an ingredient.

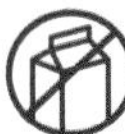 Dairy-Free

 Egg-Free

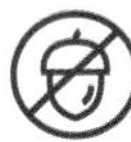 Nut-Free

 Includes Peanuts

 Vegetarian

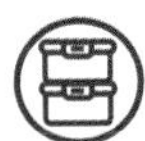 Meal Prep

 Freezer Prep

 Batch Cook

 Single Serving

 Microwave

 Pressure Cooker

 Slow Cooker

 Air Fryer

Ingredient Swaps

Use these ingredient swaps to customize the recipes to your needs. Keep in mind that substituting ingredients may alter the nutritional information for the recipe.

- Cottage cheese should be 4% milkfat. It can be swapped for plain Greek yogurt or part-skim ricotta cheese.
- Chicken can be swapped for salmon, tuna, or shrimp.
- Ground beef, ground turkey, or ground chicken can be swapped for bulk (ground) sausage.
- Almond flour or sunflower seed meal can be swapped for pork rind panko.
- Sunflower seed meal can be swapped for blanched almond flour.
- Canned full-fat coconut milk can be swapped for heavy cream.
- Avocado oil can be swapped for olive oil. I use extra-virgin olive oil in all recipes.
- I do not recommend swapping whey protein powder for anything else in baking recipes, such as for rolls or bread; you won't get the same result.
- For the low-carb sweeteners used in the recipes, I have specified only the basic form: liquid, granular, confectioners' style, or brown sugar style. Personally, I prefer to use liquid stevia, liquid monk fruit, and a blend of monk fruit and allulose in granular, confectioners' style, and brown sugar style. However, feel free to use any low-carb sweetener you like, just so it is liquid, granular, confectioners' style, or brown sugar style as specified in the recipe you are making.
- For cooking spray, you can use avocado oil, olive oil, or coconut oil cooking spray, according to your preference.

Miscellaneous Tips

The total prep and cook times are given for each recipe. Remember that when cooking food using an Instant Pot or other pressure cooker, the pressure must build up before the actual cooking can begin. The longer the cook time, the longer it takes for the needed amount of pressure to build. For example, if you are setting the cooker to cook a meal for 35 minutes, it will take 10 to 15 minutes for it to come to pressure. Knowing this will help you plan for when dinner will be ready.

Each recipe also features nutritional information, including both total carbohydrates and net carbs. Optional ingredients as well as secondary ingredient choices have not been factored into the nutritional information. If you'd like to include optional ingredients or use a secondary ingredient choice, keep in mind that doing so will alter the nutrition numbers.

CHAPTER 5

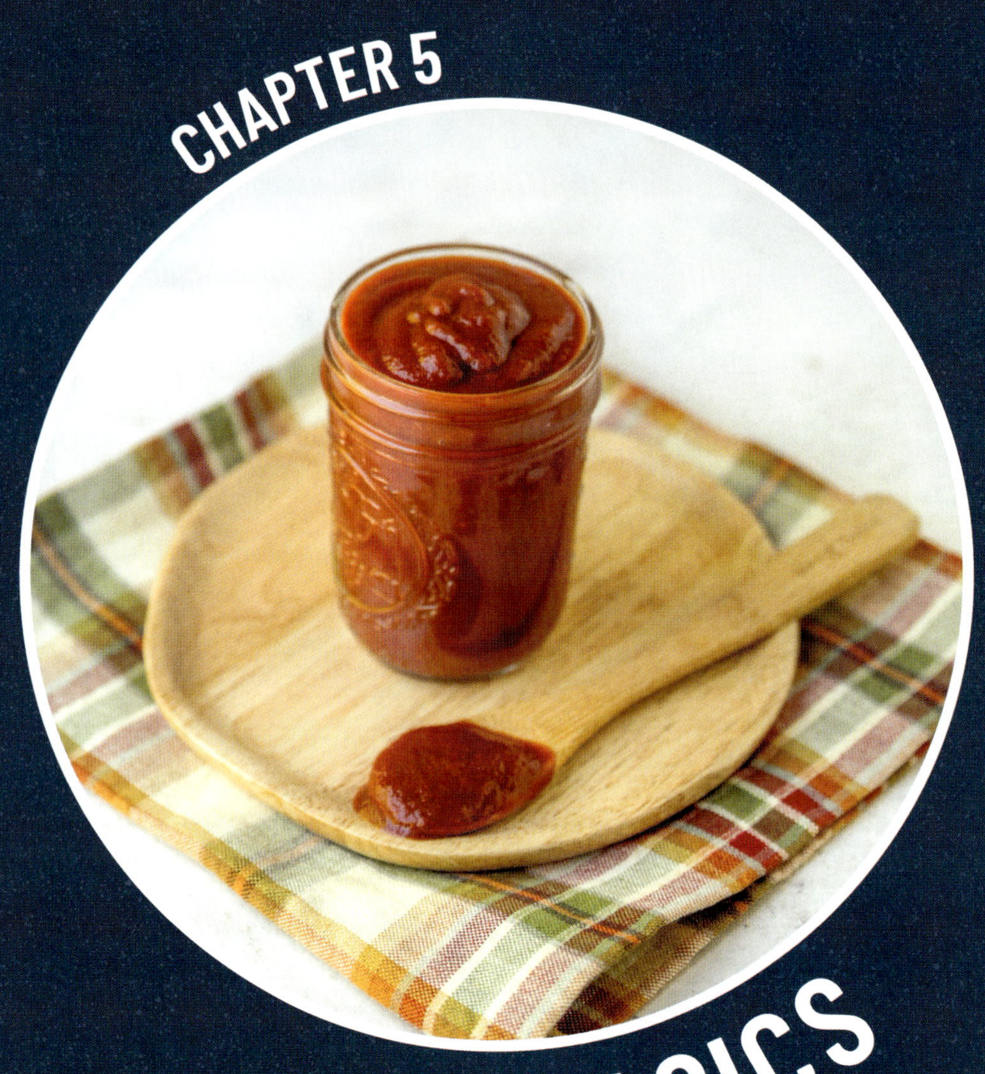

BASICS

YIELD: variable (two ½-ounce cooked slices per serving)

PREP TIME: 1 minute

COOK TIME: 8 to 20 minutes per batch (depending on cooking method and preferred doneness)

BATCH-COOKED BACON

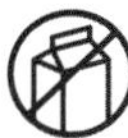  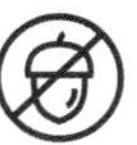 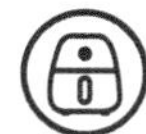
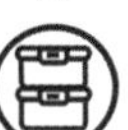 

Learning how to make bacon perfectly in my oven and air fryer was a game changer! I use this method often to cook a week's worth of bacon, which means I have it ready to be crumbled on salads or reheated and enjoyed alongside an egg for a fast and easy breakfast. Of course, you can also cook bacon as needed—1 slice here, 2 slices there. But I suggest you take advantage of meal prepping and cook, at a minimum, what you'll need for 5 days at a time, freezing any extra for later. Note that a 1-pound package of thick-cut bacon contains an average of 8 to 12 slices; it depends on the exact thickness of the cut. You can comfortably fit about 12 slices on an 18 by 13-inch rimmed baking sheet.

Thick-cut slices uncured bacon

OVEN DIRECTIONS:

1. Place an oven rack in the bottom position. Preheat the oven to 400°F.
2. Lay the bacon slices on a rimmed baking sheet, with no overlap.
3. Place the pan on the lower rack of the oven. Bake for 15 minutes for soft, chewy bacon or 20 minutes for crispy bacon.
4. Drain the slices on a paper towel–lined plate.

AIR FRYER DIRECTIONS:

1. Preheat an air fryer to 350°F.
2. Lay the bacon in a single layer in the air fryer basket. Cut the strips in half crosswise if needed to fit; cook in multiple batches if needed.
3. Air-fry for 8 to 9 minutes for chewy bacon or 12 to 14 minutes for crispy bacon. If cooking in batches, remove the grease from the drip pan between batches.

   Store the bacon in the refrigerator for up to 5 days or in the freezer for up to 1 month. I prefer to reheat cooked bacon in the air fryer at 350°F for 1 to 2 minutes, but you can also reheat slices in a skillet over medium-high heat.

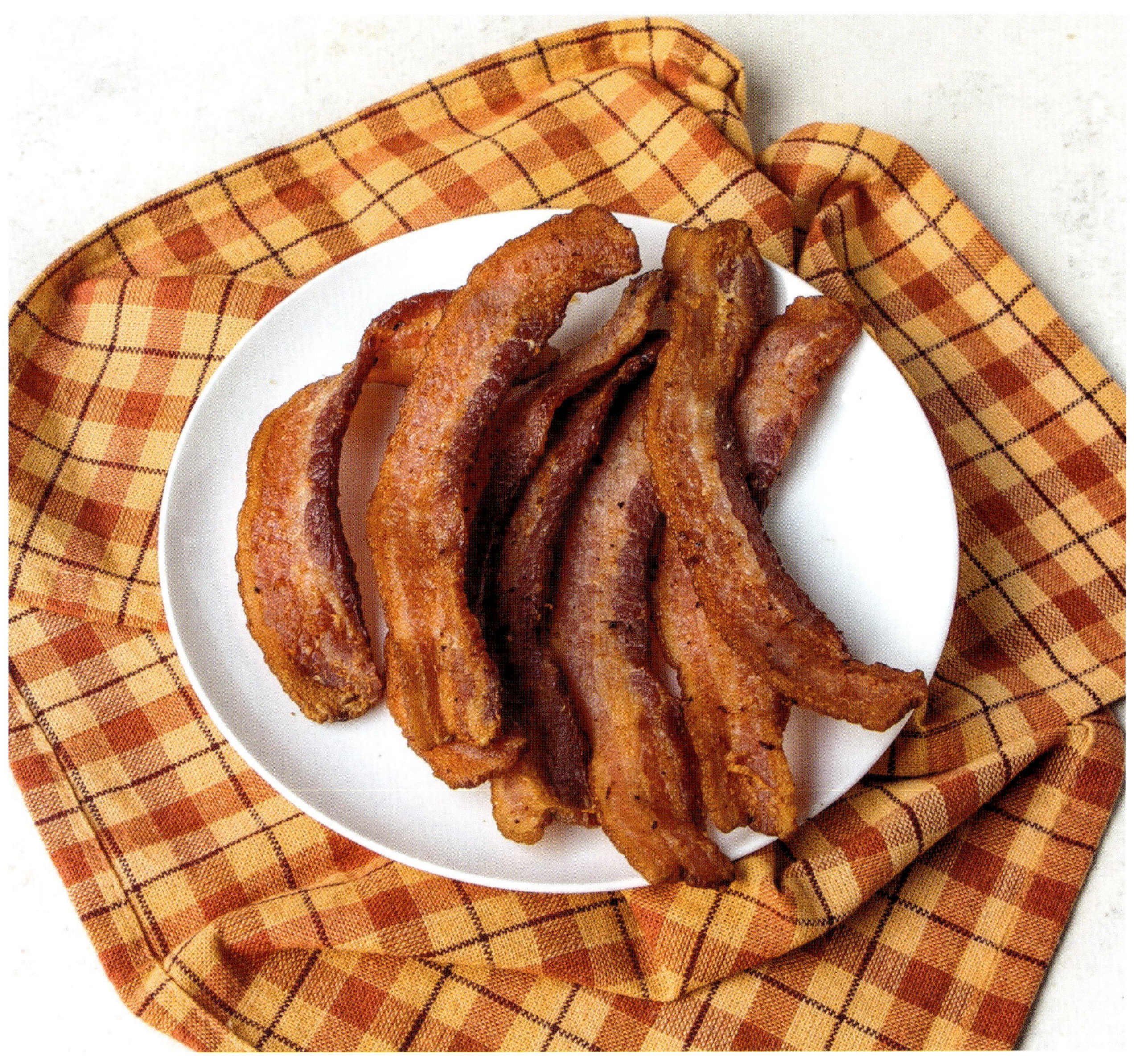

NOTES: If you want to cook a large batch of bacon, the oven method is more efficient because most air fryer baskets cannot accommodate more than 3 or 4 slices. In fact, you can bake two pans of bacon at once, placing one pan on the bottom rack and the second on the rack just above. The top pan of bacon may require a couple extra minutes of baking time to become crispy.

When selecting bacon, avoid brands cured with sugar and read the packaging to make sure the bacon has no sugar added. One of my favorites is Pederson's No Sugar Added Hickory Smoked Uncured Bacon.

Calories	Fat	Protein	Total Carbs	Dietary Fiber	Net Carbs
296	28g	9g	1g	0g	1g

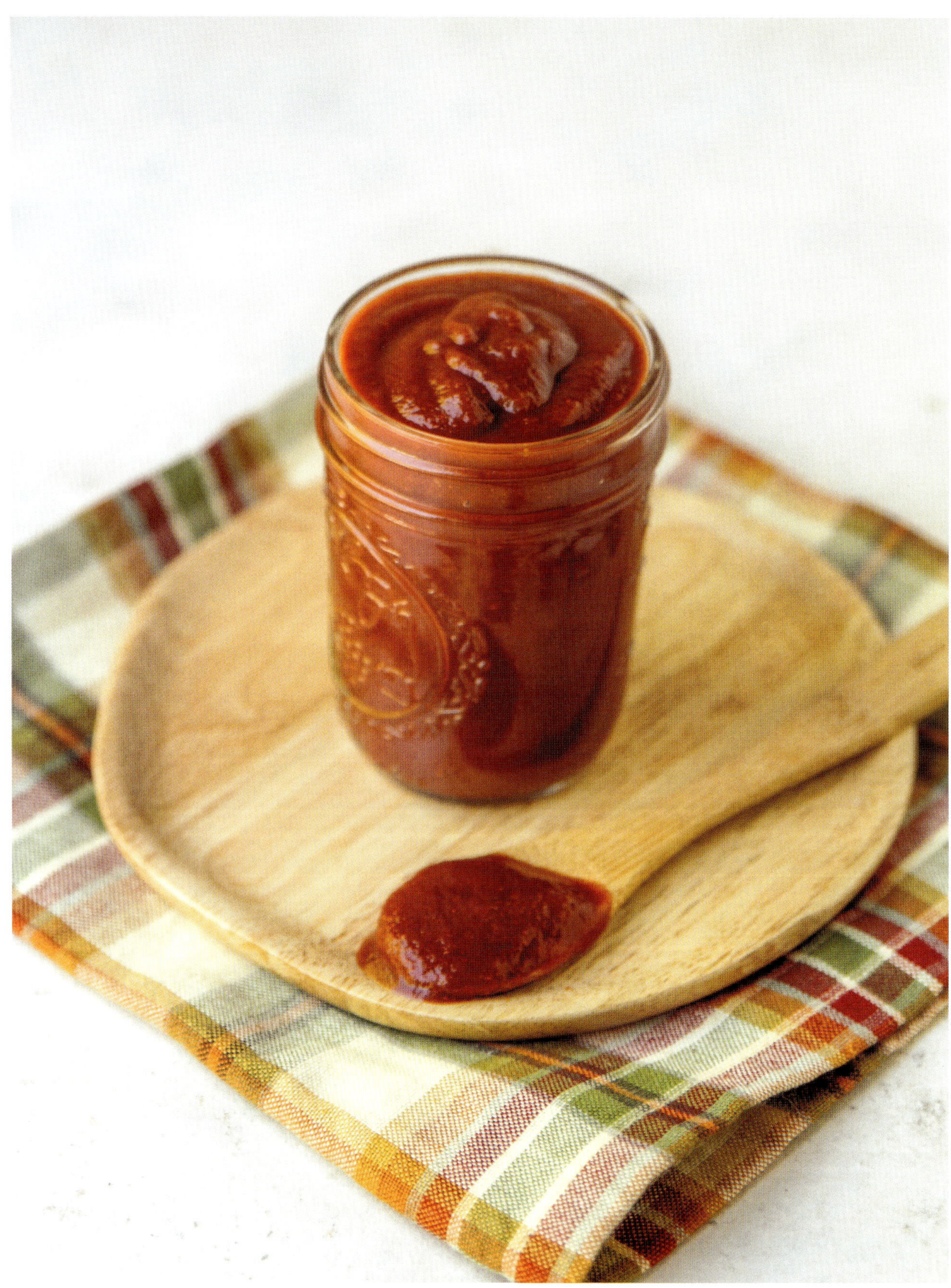

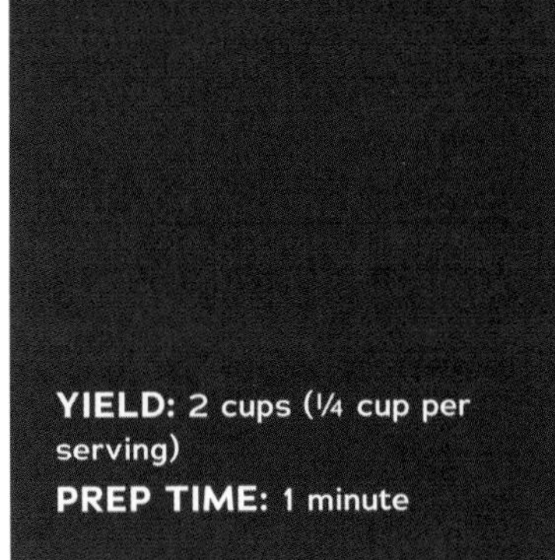

YIELD: 2 cups (1/4 cup per serving)
PREP TIME: 1 minute

KETO BBQ SAUCE

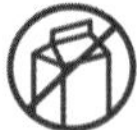   

This recipe makes a classic BBQ sauce, but you can make it spicy by adding some cayenne pepper. The smoked paprika is optional, but I recommend using it for the nice smoky flavor it adds to the sauce. If you're tight on time, simply look for a store-bought BBQ sauce that is made with avocado oil and is sweetened naturally. It's best to avoid ingredients like canola oil, soybean oil, high-fructose corn syrup, and artificial sweeteners like Splenda, aspartame, and sucralose, which can trigger cravings by spiking blood sugar.

1 1/2 cups sugar-free ketchup

1/4 cup apple cider vinegar

1/4 cup low-carb brown sugar–style sweetener or monk fruit/allulose blend

2 tablespoons smoked paprika (optional)

1 tablespoon yacón syrup or sugar-free maple syrup

1 teaspoon maple extract

Pinch of fine sea salt

NOTE: My favorite brand of store-bought BBQ sauce is Primal Kitchen.

1. Put all the ingredients in a blender and blend until smooth.
2. Taste and adjust the sweetener and salt as needed to suit your taste. Transfer to an airtight glass jar, like a mason jar, and seal with the lid. Store in the refrigerator for up to 1 month.

Calories	Fat	Protein	Total Carbs	Dietary Fiber	Net Carbs
14	0g	0g	3g	0g	3g

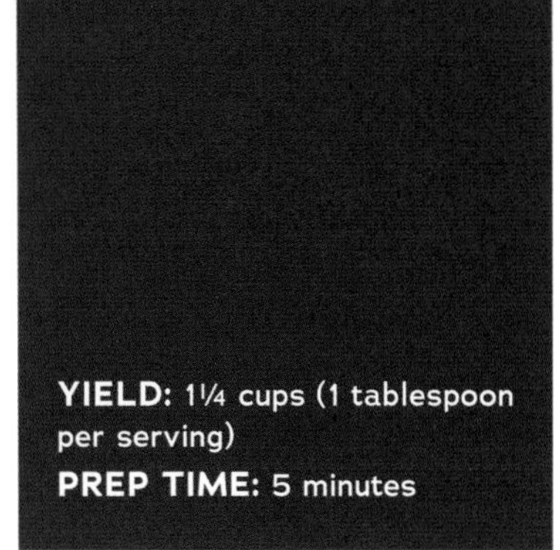

YIELD: 1¼ cups (1 tablespoon per serving)
PREP TIME: 5 minutes

TARTAR SAUCE

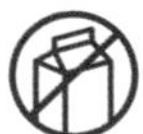  

With just a handful of ingredients, this fabulous tartar sauce takes only minutes to blend together. Enjoy this sauce whenever you're having a fish recipe.

- 1 cup avocado oil mayonnaise
- 2 tablespoons dill pickle relish
- 1 tablespoon capers, drained and chopped
- 1 tablespoon Dijon mustard
- 1 tablespoon fresh lemon juice
- ¼ teaspoon fine sea salt
- ¼ teaspoon ground black pepper
- 1 tablespoon chopped fresh parsley, or 1 teaspoon dried
- 1 tablespoon chopped scallions

Mix together all the ingredients in a small bowl. Store in an airtight container in the refrigerator for up to 5 days.

Calories	Fat	Protein	Total Carbs	Dietary Fiber	Net Carbs
82	10g	0.1g	1g	0.1g	0.9g

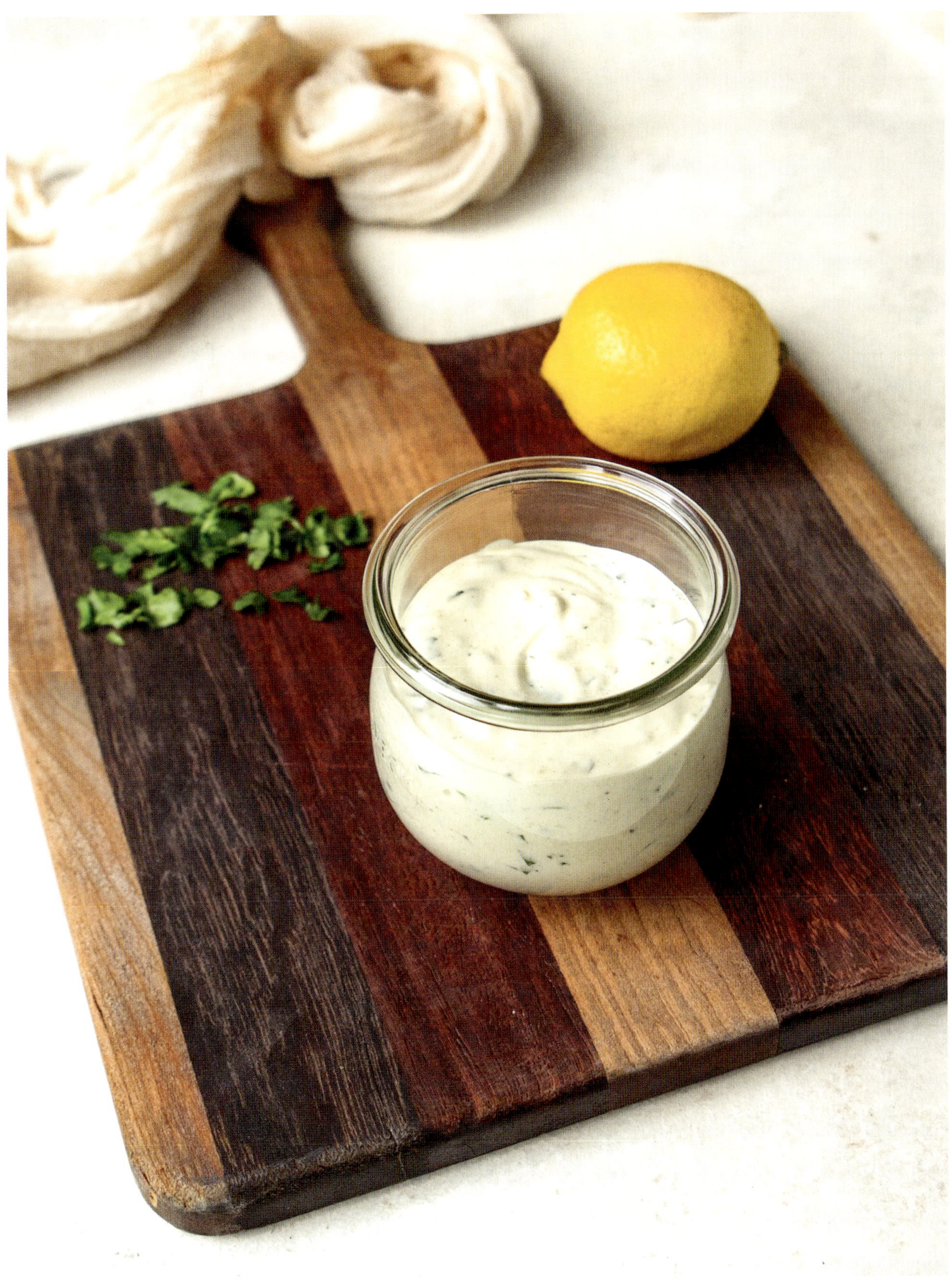

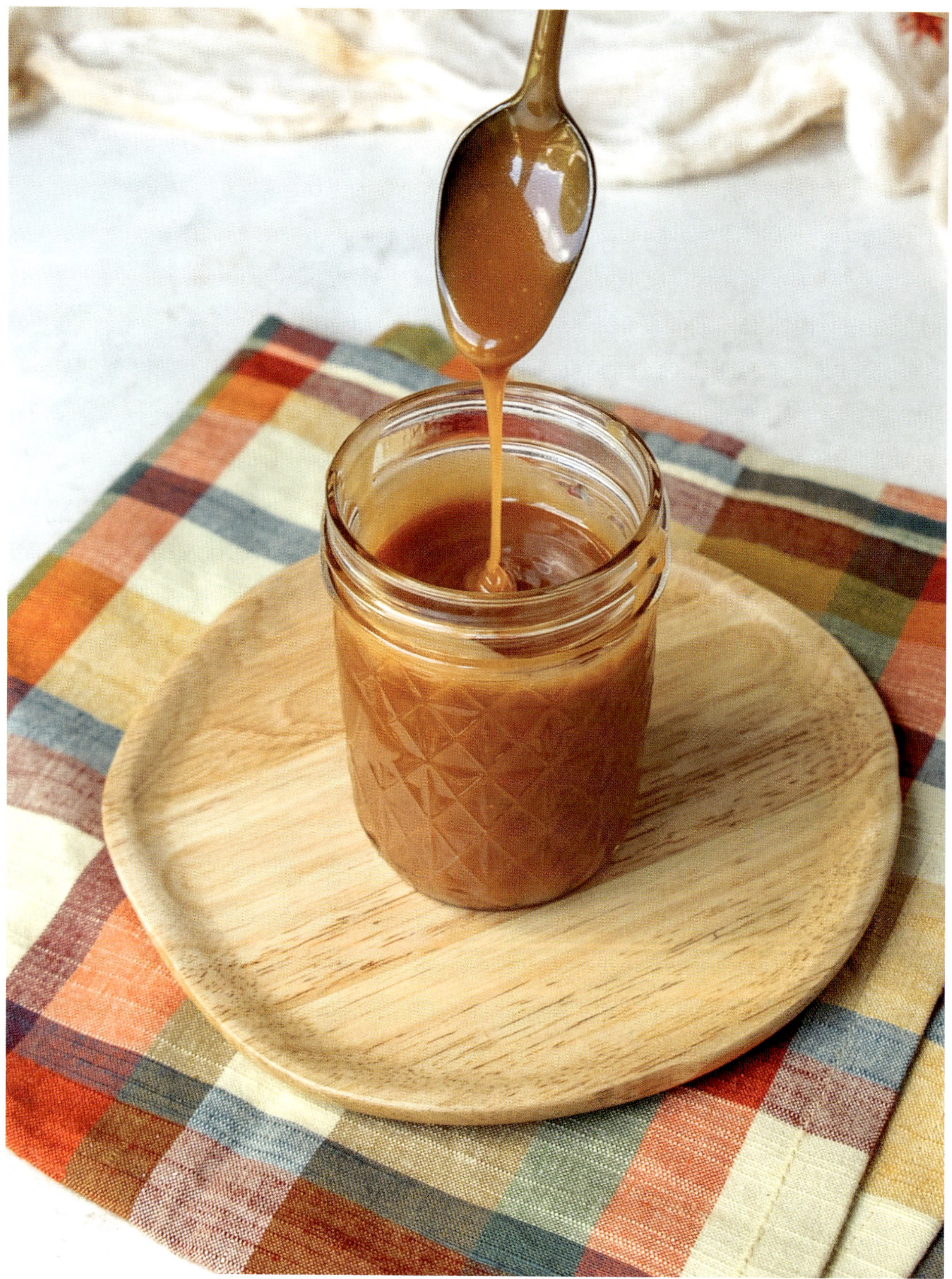

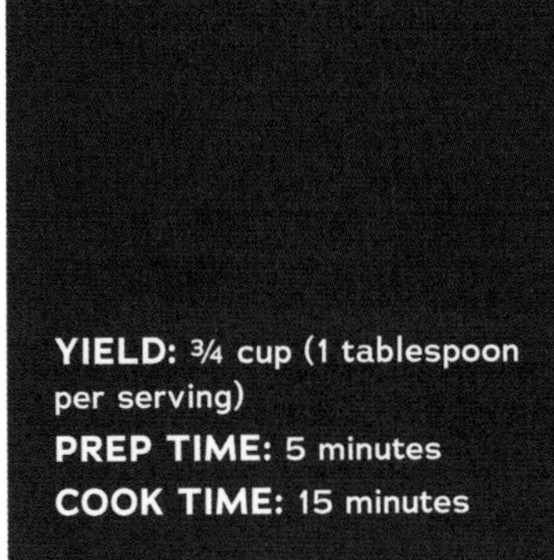

YIELD: ¾ cup (1 tablespoon per serving)
PREP TIME: 5 minutes
COOK TIME: 15 minutes

KETO CARAMEL SAUCE

This easy caramel sauce is my family's favorite recipe. It includes an extra step of browning the butter, but it's well worth the 3 or 4 minutes! We enjoy it with the Caramel Apple Scones (page 230) and on top of keto ice cream. You can use any confectioners'-style low-carb sweetener you like, but please note that a sweetener containing erythritol may cause the sauce to crystallize once refrigerated.

6 tablespoons (¾ stick) unsalted butter

½ cup confectioners'-style low-carb sweetener

½ cup heavy cream

Pinch of fine sea salt

1 teaspoon caramel extract

1. Melt the butter in a small saucepan over low heat. Once melted, whisk in the sweetener until incorporated. Cook until the butter is nicely browned, 3 to 4 minutes. When sufficiently browned, it should be the color of a chestnut.
2. Pour in the cream and salt and bring to a boil, stirring continuously. Once at a boil, reduce the heat to low and simmer until the mixture is reduced by half and thick enough to coat the back of a spoon. This should take 8 to 10 minutes.
3. Remove the pan from the heat and stir in the caramel extract.
4. Taste and adjust the sweetness if needed. Use immediately or let cool and store in a sealed glass mason jar in the fridge for up to 2 weeks. To get refrigerated sauce to a pourable consistency, heat in the microwave for 30 seconds and then whisk vigorously.

Calories	Fat	Protein	Total Carbs	Dietary Fiber	Net Carbs
84	9g	1g	1g	0g	1g

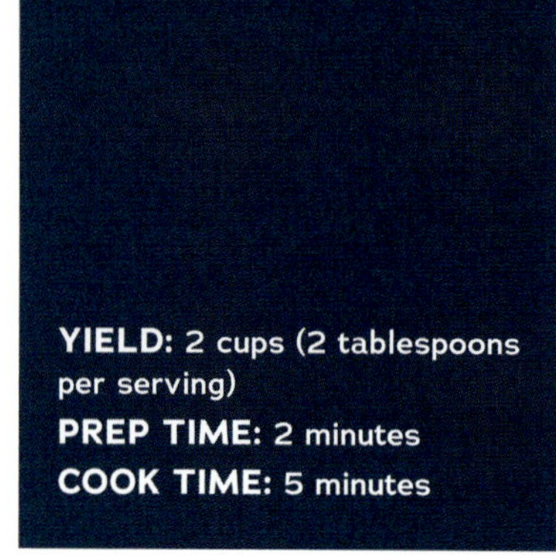

YIELD: 2 cups (2 tablespoons per serving)
PREP TIME: 2 minutes
COOK TIME: 5 minutes

GANACHE

 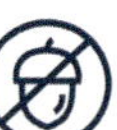 

Enjoy this easy ganache whenever you want to dazzle friends and family. Use warm to dip fruits into or drizzle over keto ice cream. Alternatively, cool it for piping onto mocha cupcakes or my no-bake cheesecake for two (pages 300 and 149).

1 cup heavy cream

1 cup sugar-free chocolate chips

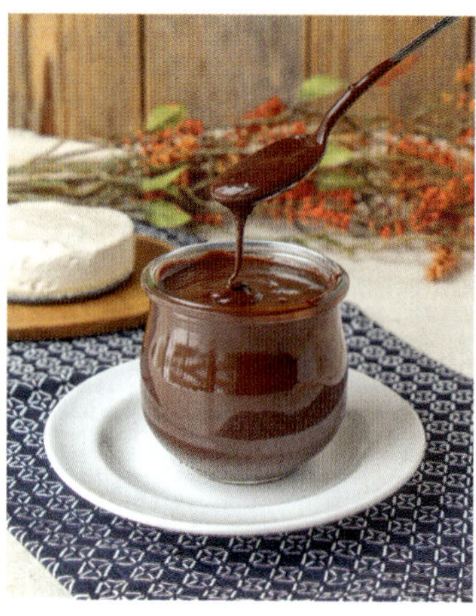

1. In a small saucepan, bring the cream to a simmer over medium-low heat. Put the chocolate chips in a small heatproof bowl.
2. Once the cream is simmering, pour it over the chocolate chips. Let stand for 5 minutes before stirring. After 5 minutes, stir until the ganache is completely smooth and there are no lumps.
3. The longer the ganache sits, the thicker it becomes. In some recipes, you may be instructed to drizzle the ganache on something like a cake while it's still warm and liquid-y; for other recipes, it's best to allow the ganache to thicken slightly so you can whisk it with an electric mixer to attain a whipped texture that you can pipe or spread with a spatula.

Calories	Fat	Protein	Total Carbs	Dietary Fiber	Net Carbs
102	10g	2g	2g	0g	2g

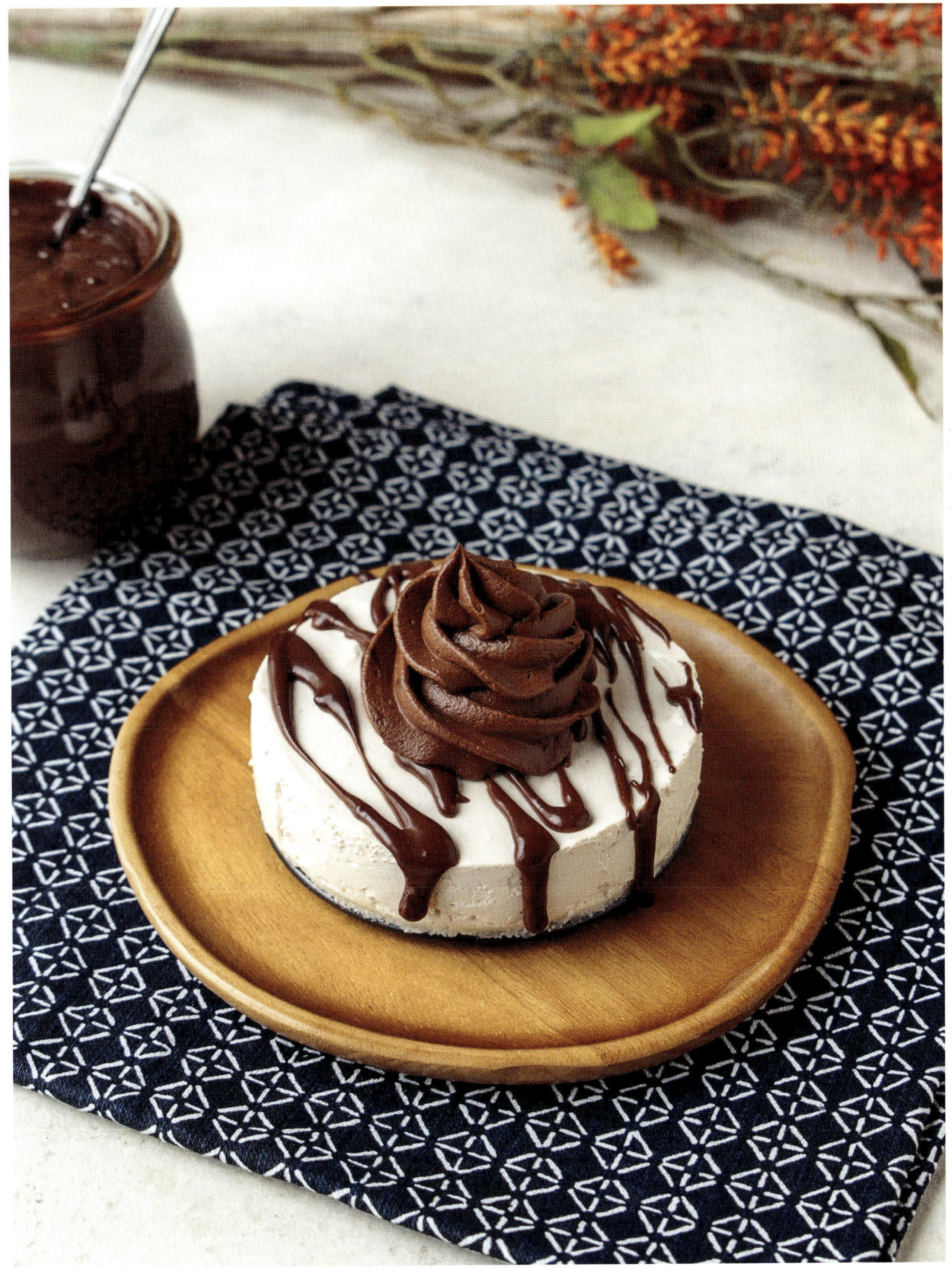

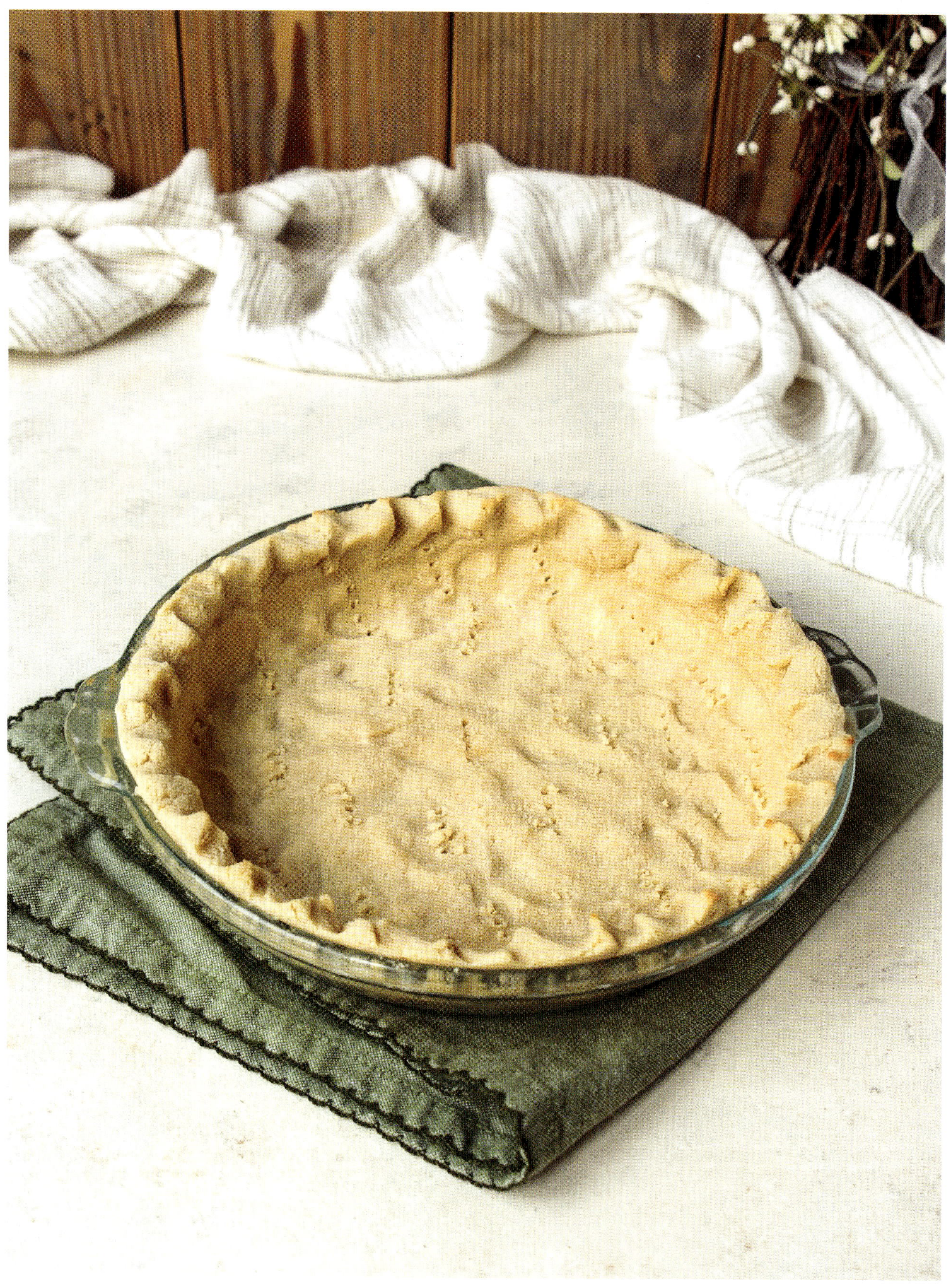

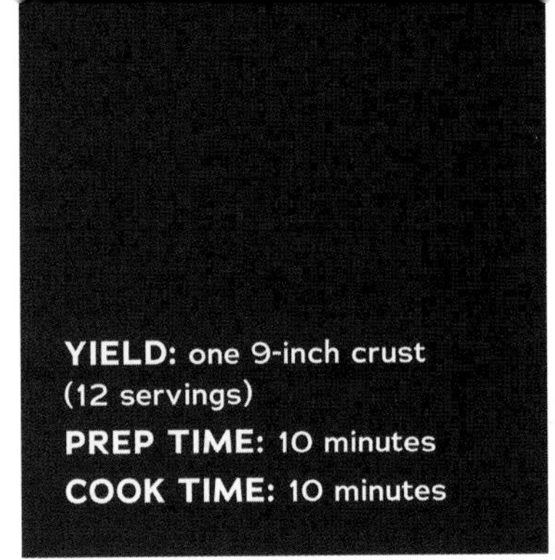

YIELD: one 9-inch crust (12 servings)
PREP TIME: 10 minutes
COOK TIME: 10 minutes

EASY KETO PIE CRUST

OPTION

Every keto cook needs a recipe for a perfectly flaky pie crust that can easily work for both sweet and savory pies. I perfected this one years ago. Even my Italian mother couldn't believe how flaky this crust is. I use it for quiche and sweet pies, and everyone, including non-keto family members and friends, loves it! The recipe below is for sweet pies. You can easily use the same base for savory recipes by omitting the vanilla extract and sweetener.

- 2 large eggs
- 1 tablespoon extra-virgin olive oil
- 1 teaspoon vanilla extract
- 1 cup (120 g) coconut flour
- 1/4 cup (56 g) low-carb granular sweetener
- 1/4 teaspoon fine sea salt
- 1/2 cup (1 stick) cold salted butter or coconut oil, cut into cubes

1. Preheat the oven to 400°F. Grease the bottom and sides of a 9-inch pie pan or line it with parchment paper.
2. Put the eggs, olive oil, and vanilla extract in a food processor and pulse until combined.
3. Add the flour, sweetener, and salt and process until combined.
4. Add the cubed butter and pulse until fine crumbles form.
5. Remove the dough from the processor and place in the prepared pie pan. Wet your hands with water. Using your fingers, press the dough out, as evenly as possible, across the bottom and up the sides of the pan. Use a fork to randomly poke holes in the bottom of the crust.
6. If you're using this crust for a pie filling that requires baking, cover the edges with aluminum foil to avoid an overly browned crust. If you will be using a no-bake filling, there is no need to cover the edges. Bake the crust for 10 minutes, or until golden. Remove from the oven and let cool.
7. Once cool, add the pie filling.

Calories	Fat	Protein	Total Carbs	Dietary Fiber	Net Carbs
129	10g	2g	5g	3g	2g

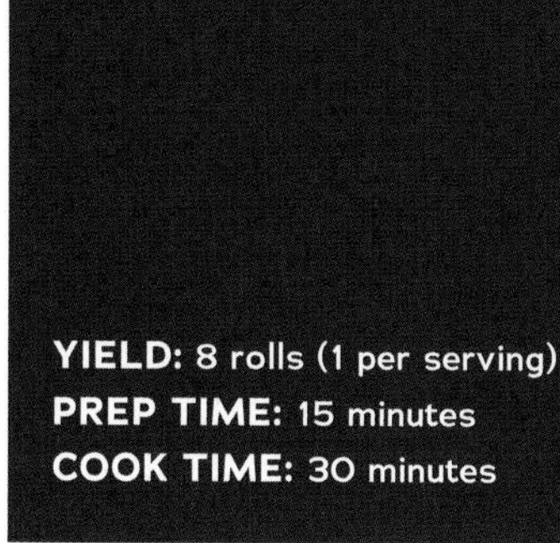

YIELD: 8 rolls (1 per serving)
PREP TIME: 15 minutes
COOK TIME: 30 minutes

COTTAGE CHEESE CLOUD BREAD ROLLS

This amazing recipe is one of my most popular on SugarFreeMom.com and for good reason. The rolls are perfect for making sandwiches or a juicy smash burger. When made ahead, these rolls can be the foundation for a plan B (see page 158) sandwich, using store-bought deli meat.

6 large eggs, separated, room temperature

1/2 teaspoon distilled white vinegar or cream of tartar

3/4 cup whey protein powder (2 1/2 scoops or 62 grams)

1/4 cup egg white protein powder (20 grams), or replace with more whey protein

1/2 cup cottage cheese (4% milkfat)

1 tablespoon low-carb sweetener (granular or confectioners' style, optional)

1/2 teaspoon baking powder

1/4 teaspoon fine sea salt

1/4 teaspoon garlic powder

1/4 teaspoon onion powder

FOR GARNISH (OPTIONAL):

Sesame seeds or everything bagel seasoning

Special equipment: **Silicone hamburger bun mold with at least 8 wells**

1. Preheat the oven to 300°F.
2. Put the egg whites and vinegar in the bowl of a stand mixer fitted with the whisk attachment or in a large metal mixing bowl for use with an electric hand mixer. Whip on high speed until stiff peaks form, 10 to 15 minutes. Set aside.
3. Put the egg yolks in a medium mixing bowl with the remaining ingredients and whisk with the hand mixer until smooth. You can also put these ingredients in a blender and blend until smooth.
4. Fold a small amount of the egg yolk mixture into the egg white mixture a little at a time until it's all incorporated, being careful not to deflate the whites.
5. Using a 1/3-cup measuring cup, scoop the batter into 8 wells of a silicone hamburger bun mold. Do not flatten the tops. To transfer the flexible mold to the oven, place it on a rimmed baking sheet.
6. Bake on the middle rack of the oven for 30 minutes, or until a toothpick or skewer inserted in the center of a roll comes out clean and the rolls are golden brown. Shut the oven off but do not open the door. Leave the pan in the oven for 10 more minutes.
7. Enjoy warm, straight from the oven, or toasted and buttered. Or allow the rolls to cool and use for sandwiches! Store leftovers in an airtight container in the fridge for up to 1 week or freeze for up to 3 months. To freeze, place the rolls between pieces of parchment paper in a zip-top bag for easier removal.

Calories	Fat	Protein	Total Carbs	Dietary Fiber	Net Carbs
101	4g	14g	2g	0.2g	1.8g

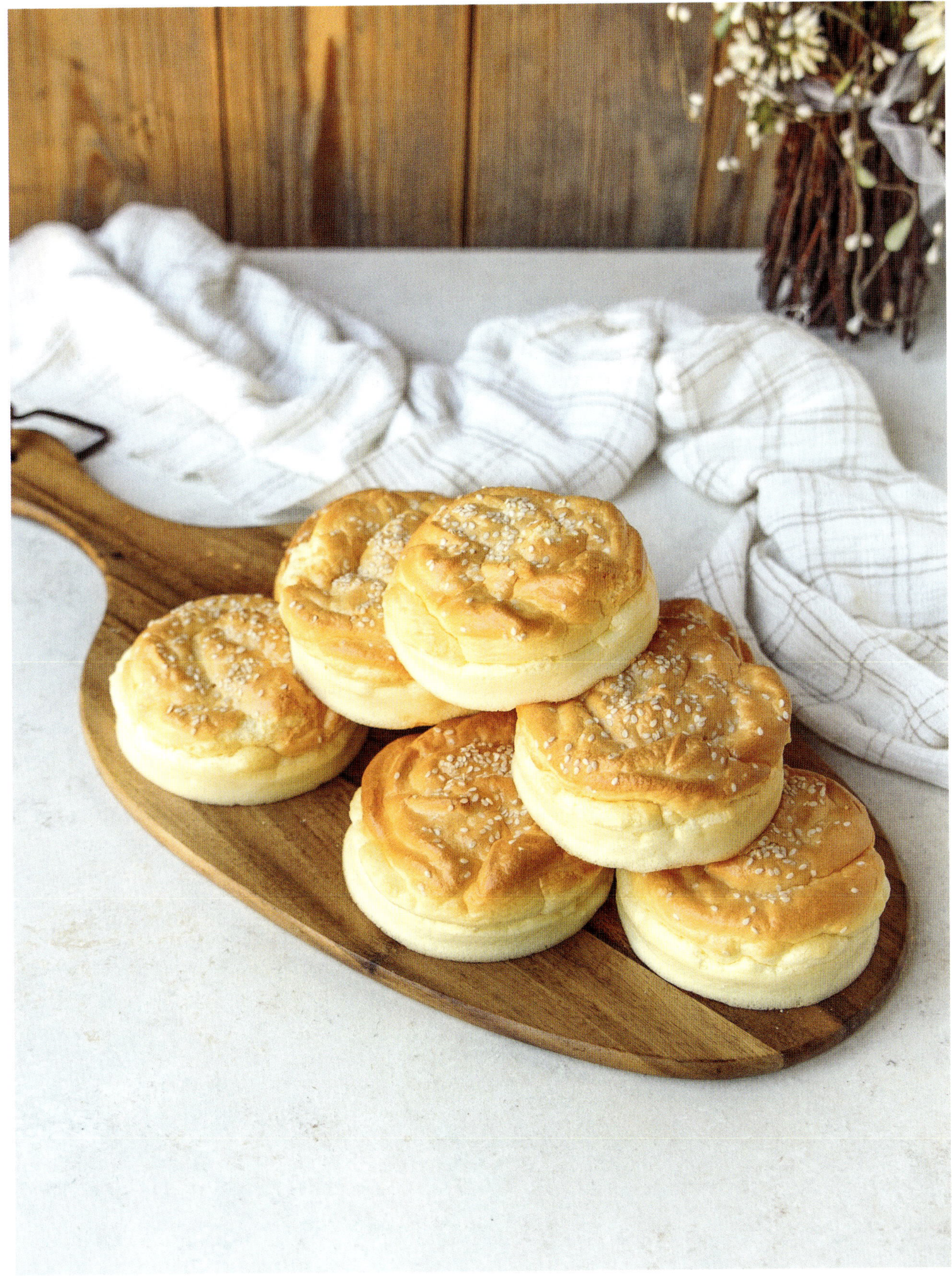

CHAPTER 6

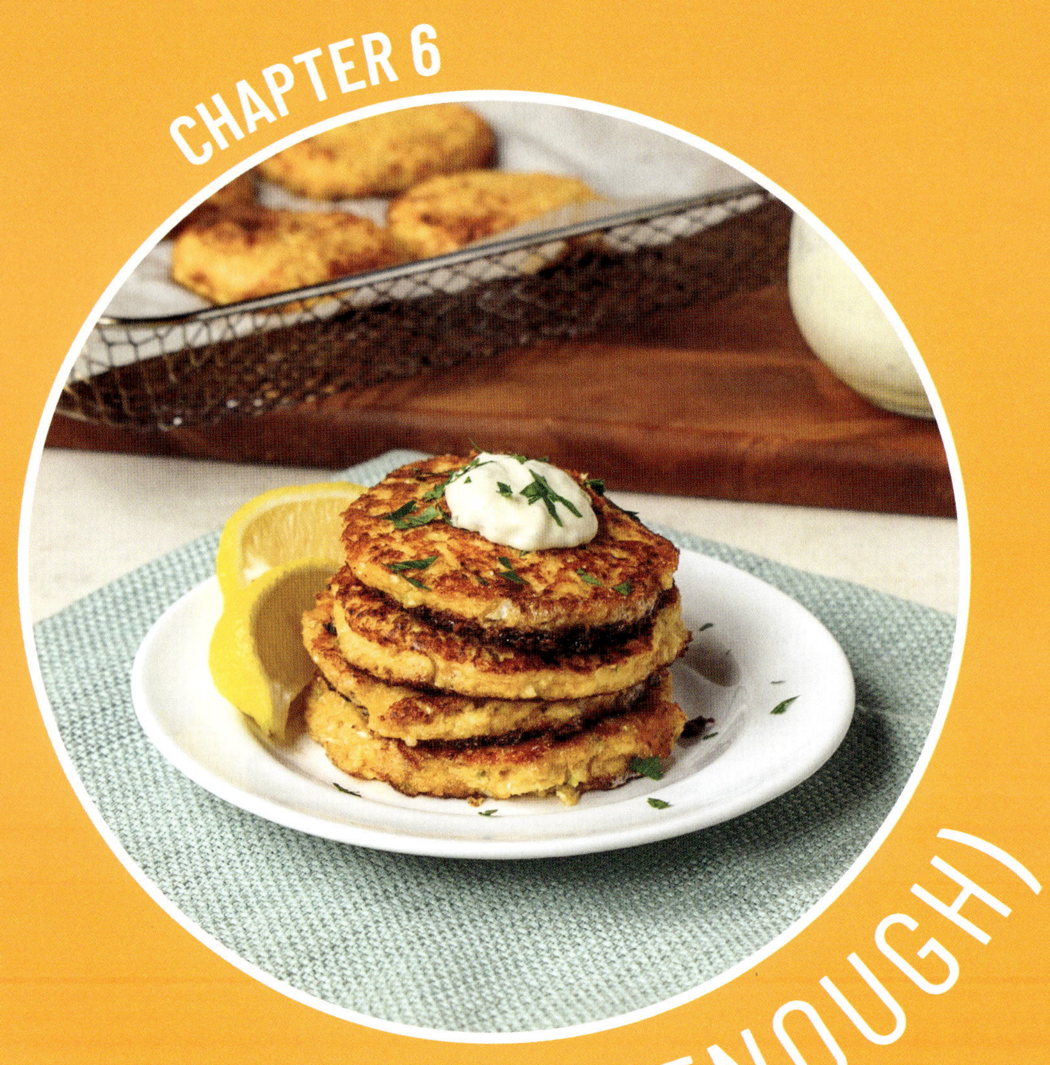

GOOD (ENOUGH)

BREAKFAST

LUNCH

DINNER & SIDES

DESSERTS

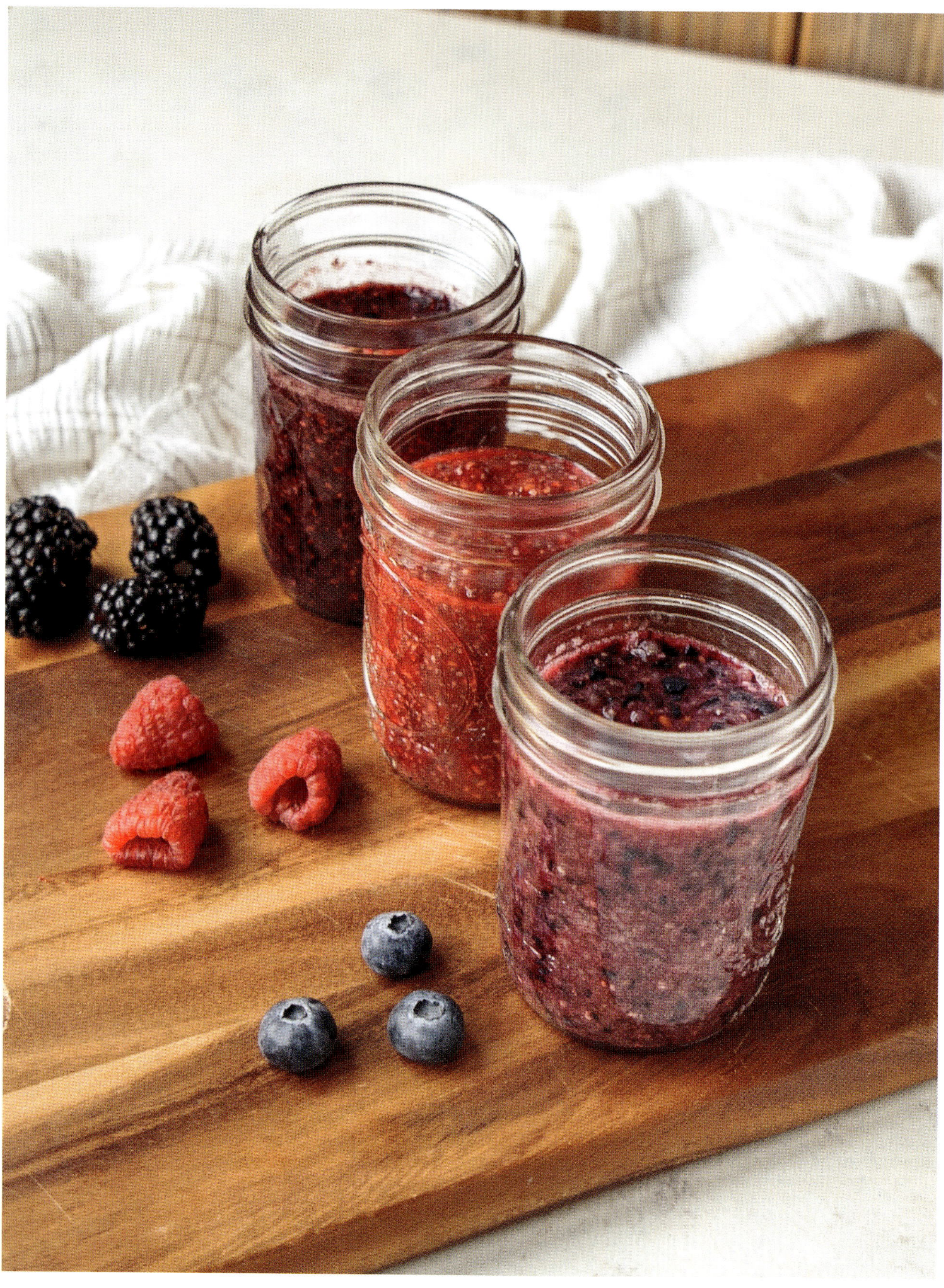

YIELD: 3/4 cup (2 tablespoons per serving)

PREP TIME: 2 minutes, plus 1 hour to chill

QUICK BERRY CHIA JAM

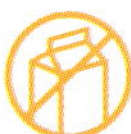  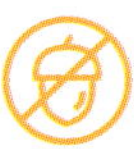 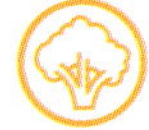

A super simple quick jam that can be made with frozen and thawed berries or fresh berries if in season.

2 cups fresh or frozen raspberries, blueberries, or blackberries, thawed if frozen

2 tablespoons fresh lemon juice

2 tablespoons confectioners'-style low-carb sweetener

1/2 teaspoon lemon liquid stevia

Pinch of fine sea salt

2 tablespoons chia seeds

1. Put all the ingredients except the chia seeds in a high-powered blender or food processor and blend on high until smooth or the desired texture. Taste and adjust the sweetness if needed.
2. Add the chia seeds and pulse 2 or 3 times to combine.
3. Pour the jam into a mason jar, cover, and refrigerate to thicken for 1 hour before using.
4. Store in the refrigerator for up to 1 week.

Calories	Fat	Protein	Total Carbs	Dietary Fiber	Net Carbs
51	2g	1g	7g	5g	2g

YIELD: 8 waffles (2 waffles per serving)

PREP TIME: 1 minute

COOK TIME: 10 minutes

COTTAGE CHEESE PROTEIN WAFFLES

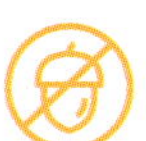 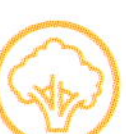 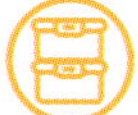

I adapted this recipe slightly from the one on my website to make the waffles a bit sturdier for using for sandwiches; I also added an extra egg so they wouldn't be dry. Perfection! These are a great meal prep option because they freeze well and can be stored in the refrigerator for up to 5 days. For variety, try flavoring them with an aromatic spice, like cinnamon or nutmeg (simply add the spice in Step 1, when combining the other ingredients). With just a little tweaking, this same recipe can be used for savory foods (see the variation below).

1 cup cottage cheese (4% milkfat)

3 large eggs

1/2 cup vanilla-flavored whey protein powder (30 grams or 1 scoop)

1 teaspoon vanilla-flavored liquid stevia

Special equipment: Waffle maker

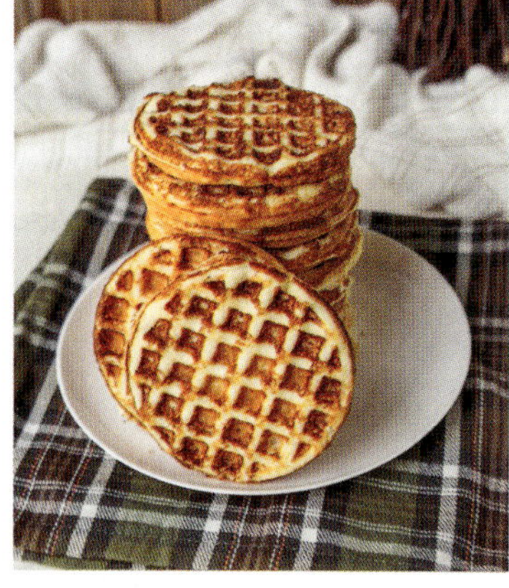

1. Put the ingredients for the waffles in a bowl and stir together until combined; the mixture will still have curds, but they won't be visible in the cooked waffles. Alternatively, you can put the ingredients in a blender and blend until smooth.
2. Preheat a waffle maker according to the manufacturer's instructions. Grease with cooking spray.
3. Place about 3 tablespoons of the batter in the center of the waffle maker. Close the lid and cook according to the manufacturer's instructions.

VARIATION: Savory Cottage Cheese Protein Waffles. Use unflavored whey protein powder instead of the vanilla-flavored and omit the stevia. If desired, add a generous pinch of onion or garlic powder.

Calories	Fat	Protein	Total Carbs	Dietary Fiber	Net Carbs
133	6g	17g	3g	0g	3g

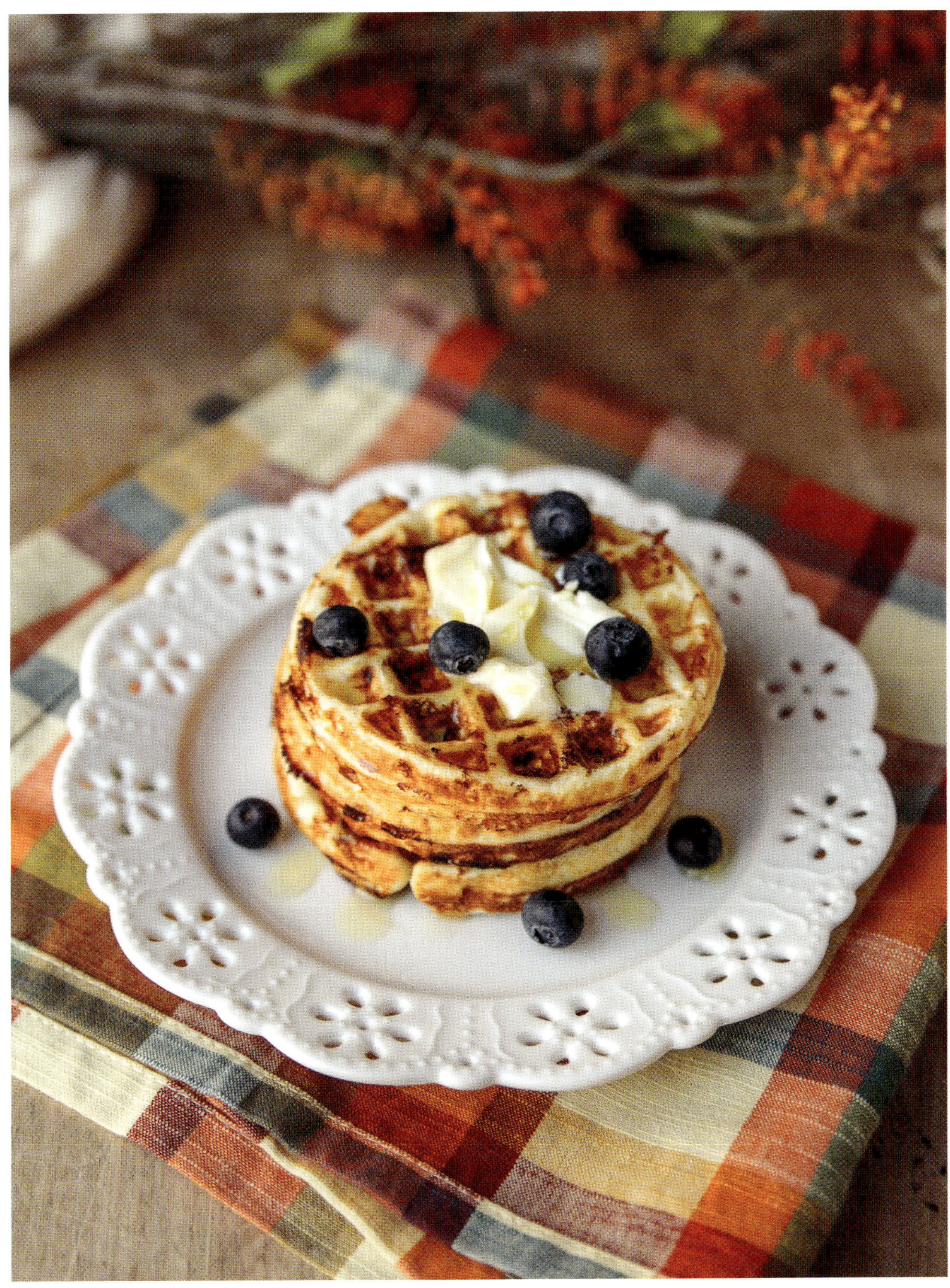

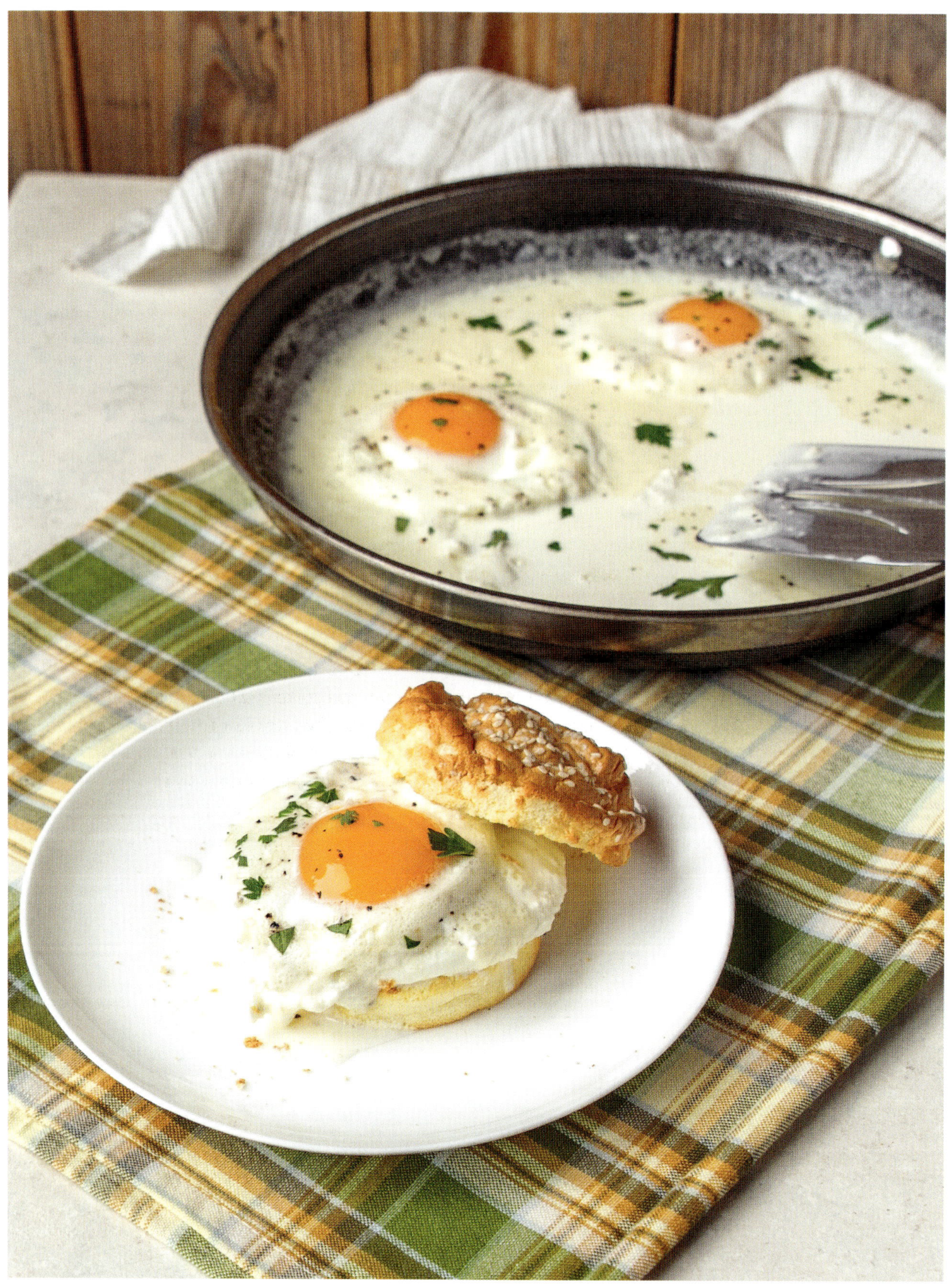

YIELD: 2 servings
PREP TIME: 2 minutes
COOK TIME: 6 minutes

QUICK CREAMED EGGS

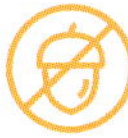
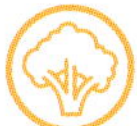

These creamy eggs don't require flipping like an omelet or the low and slow cooking used for making creamy soft-scrambled eggs. Yet they taste indulgent, like you toiled at the stove all morning. Instead of using butter or oil, you're cooking the eggs, sunny side up, in heavy cream, using a unique method best described as braising. This recipe is not recommended for making ahead; it's best enjoyed immediately. If you're making this for only one person or for the Minimal Time meal plan on page 64, simply halve the recipe.

- 1 cup heavy cream
- ¼ teaspoon salt
- ¼ teaspoon garlic powder
- ¼ teaspoon onion powder
- 4 large eggs
- 1 tablespoon chopped fresh parsley, for garnish

1. Pour the cream into an 8-inch nonstick skillet over low heat. Sprinkle in the seasonings and stir to combine.
2. Gently crack one egg at a time into the cream, trying not to crack the yolk. Turn the heat to medium-high. As the cream starts to boil, it will start to separate into buttermilk and butterfat and will thicken and caramelize around the edges of the pan. After the cream has boiled for about 3 minutes, reduce the heat to medium-low and continue cooking until the egg whites are set.
3. When the whites are set, turn off the heat, and cover the skillet to finish cooking the yolks, 2 to 3 minutes.
4. Serve garnished with chopped parsley.

Calories	Fat	Protein	Total Carbs	Dietary Fiber	Net Carbs
346	30g	13g	2g	0.1g	1.9g

YIELD: 1 serving
PREP TIME: 5 minutes
COOK TIME: 12 minutes

PARMESAN EGGS

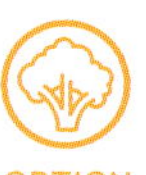
OPTION
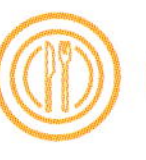
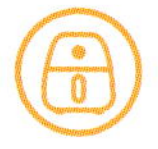

These quick, single-serving eggs take less than 5 minutes to prep, and then you let the eggs cook in your air fryer or oven while you get ready for your day. Then you can enjoy them on their own or with a low-carb English muffin (see recipe on page 100).

2 tablespoons grated Parmesan cheese

2 large eggs

Salt and pepper

1. If using an air fryer, place an 8-ounce ramekin in the air fryer basket and preheat at 350°F for 5 minutes. If using the oven, preheat the oven to 350°F and put the ramekin in the oven for 5 minutes. Spray the preheated ramekin with cooking spray.
2. Spread the Parmesan in the ramekin and then crack the eggs on top of the cheese. Sprinkle with salt and pepper.
3. Air-fry at 350°F for 8 to 10 minutes for runny yolks. Add another minute for medium-cooked yolks or add 5 extra minutes for hard yolks. If using the oven, bake at 350°F for 12 to 15 minutes for runny yolks. Add another 2 minutes for medium-cooked yolks or add 5 extra minutes for hard yolks.
4. Enjoy right from the ramekin or remove onto a plate by loosening the edges with a butter knife and using a small spatula to remove.

NOTE: If you're a strict vegetarian, make sure to use a Parmesan cheese made without animal rennet.

Calories	Fat	Protein	Total Carbs	Dietary Fiber	Net Carbs
185	12g	16g	2g	0g	2g

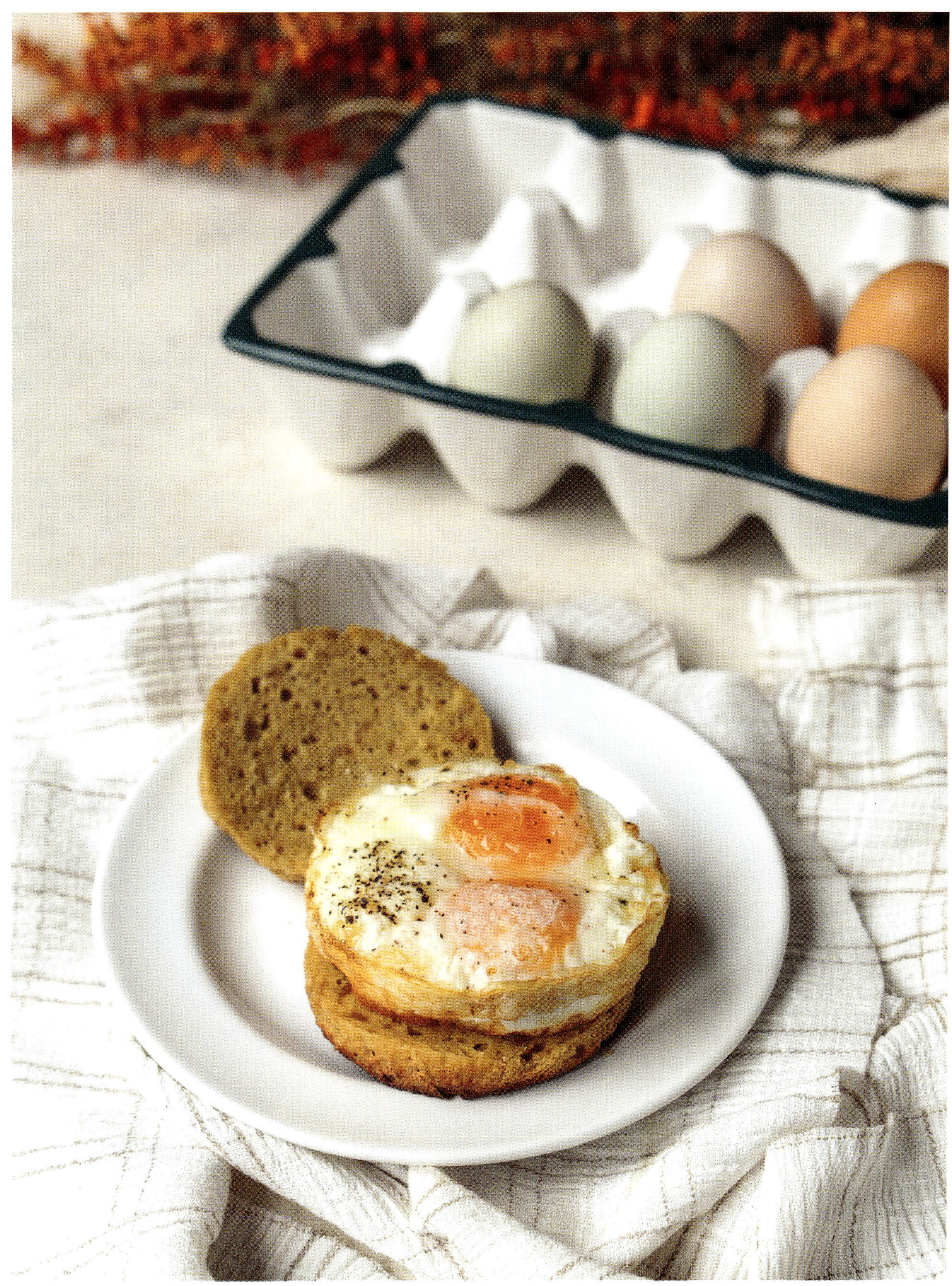

YIELD: 2 servings (2 English muffins)
PREP TIME: 1 minute
COOK TIME: 2 to 3 minutes

90-SECOND PROTEIN ENGLISH MUFFIN

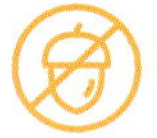

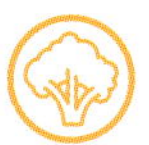

OPTION OPTION

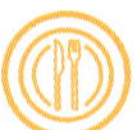

One of the most popular recipes on SugarFreeMom.com! Versatile too, with nut-free and peanut-free options included. You can make these unflavored or make a blueberry version that's lightly sweetened with stevia. If you prefer, you can bake the muffin in the oven—it will simply take longer (see below). The ideal baking dishes for this recipe are two 4- or 5-ounce quiche dishes or two 7-ounce ramekins. The larger circumference of a quiche dish works better to give you the classic shape of an English muffin, but ramekins also work. Try these toasted with butter or cream cheese and Quick Berry Chia Jam (page 93).

2 tablespoons cottage cheese (4% milkfat)

2 tablespoons blanched almond flour (or sunflower meal for nut-free)

2 tablespoons powdered peanut butter, natural peanut butter, or sunflower seed butter (see note)

1 large egg

1/2 teaspoon baking powder

FOR SWEET BLUEBERRY MUFFINS (OPTIONAL):

1 tablespoon fresh blueberries

1/2 teaspoon vanilla-flavored liquid stevia

1. Grease two 4-ounce quiche dishes or 7-ounce ramekins with cooking spray. Set aside.
2. Put the ingredients in a small bowl and stir together until combined.
3. Divide the batter evenly between the two prepared dishes. Place one dish in the microwave and cook for 1 minute. Check with a toothpick in the center. If it comes out clean, it's done; if not, cook for another 30 seconds. Repeat with the second dish.
4. Set aside until cool enough to handle. Remove and slice in half and toast to enjoy right away. Alternatively, store whole muffins in an airtight container in the fridge for up to 3 days or freeze for up to 3 months.

VARIATION: Baked English Muffin. Preheat the oven to 350°F. Follow the recipe as written, but put both filled dishes on a rimmed baking sheet and bake for 8 to 10 minutes, until a toothpick comes out clean when inserted in the center.

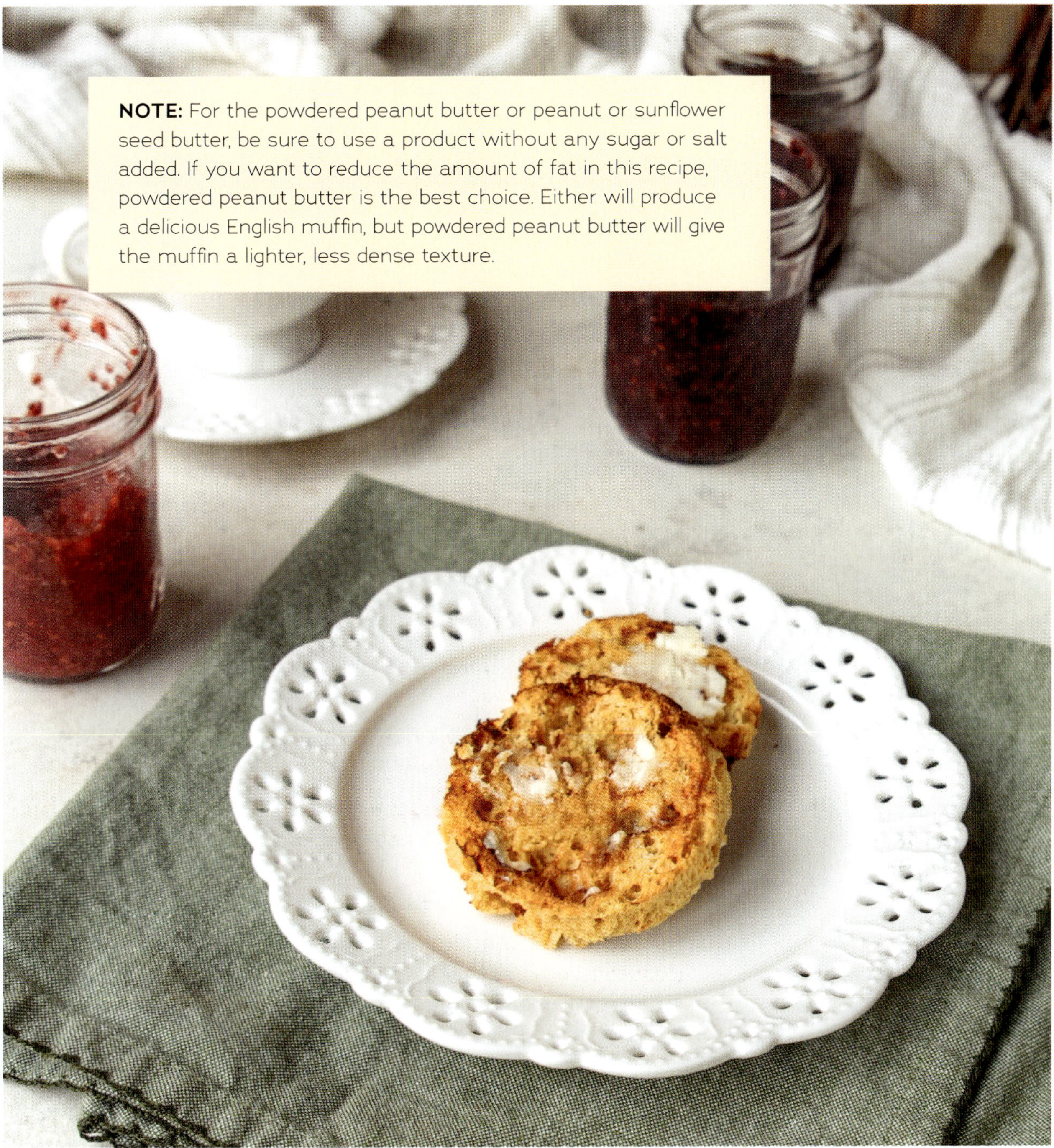

NOTE: For the powdered peanut butter or peanut or sunflower seed butter, be sure to use a product without any sugar or salt added. If you want to reduce the amount of fat in this recipe, powdered peanut butter is the best choice. Either will produce a delicious English muffin, but powdered peanut butter will give the muffin a lighter, less dense texture.

MADE WITH PEANUT BUTTER

Calories	Fat	Protein	Total Carbs	Dietary Fiber	Net Carbs
192	15g	10g	6g	2g	4g

MADE WITH POWDERED PEANUT BUTTER

Calories	Fat	Protein	Total Carbs	Dietary Fiber	Net Carbs
115	7g	9g	5g	2g	3g

YIELD: 2 muffins (1 muffin per serving)

PREP TIME: 5 minutes

COOK TIME: 3 to 20 minutes, depending on method used

STRAWBERRY PROTEIN MUG MUFFINS

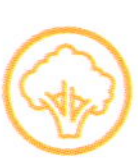
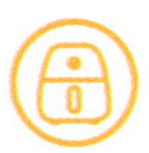
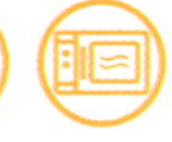

These simple protein muffins can be made ahead for easy mornings on the run! You can use a microwave, air fryer, or oven to cook them. Feel free to swap in any berries you like.

5 tablespoons blanched almond flour or sunflower seed meal

¼ cup cottage cheese (4% milkfat), unsweetened almond milk, or heavy cream

1 large egg

½ cup vanilla-flavored whey protein powder (30 grams or 1 scoop)

½ teaspoon baking powder

2 tablespoons granular allulose

2 large fresh strawberries (about 1 ounce), sliced

1. If using the oven to bake the muffins, preheat the oven to 350°F.
2. Put all the ingredients, except the strawberries, in a small bowl and mix to combine. Gently stir in the fresh strawberries.
3. Grease 2 (12-ounce) microwave-safe or ovenproof mugs. Pour the batter evenly into the mugs.
4. Cook the muffins using one of these 3 methods:

   To cook in a microwave, place 1 mug in the microwave at a time. Microwave for 1 minute to 1½ minutes. Check the center with a toothpick; if it comes out clean, it's done.

   To cook in an air fryer, place 1 mug at a time in the air fryer basket. Air-fry at 350°F for 10 minutes. Check the center with a toothpick; if it comes out clean, it's done.

   To cook in the oven, put both mugs on a small rimmed baking sheet. Bake for 15 to 20 minutes, until a toothpick inserted in the center comes out clean.
5. Once cooked and cooled, the muffins can be covered and refrigerated. Store for up to 3 days. These muffins taste great cold right out of the fridge and can easily be made ahead for busy mornings. If you prefer a warm muffin, slice in half and toast for 2 to 3 minutes.

MADE WITH COTTAGE CHEESE

Calories	Fat	Protein	Total Carbs	Dietary Fiber	Net Carbs
222	12g	22g	7g	2g	5g

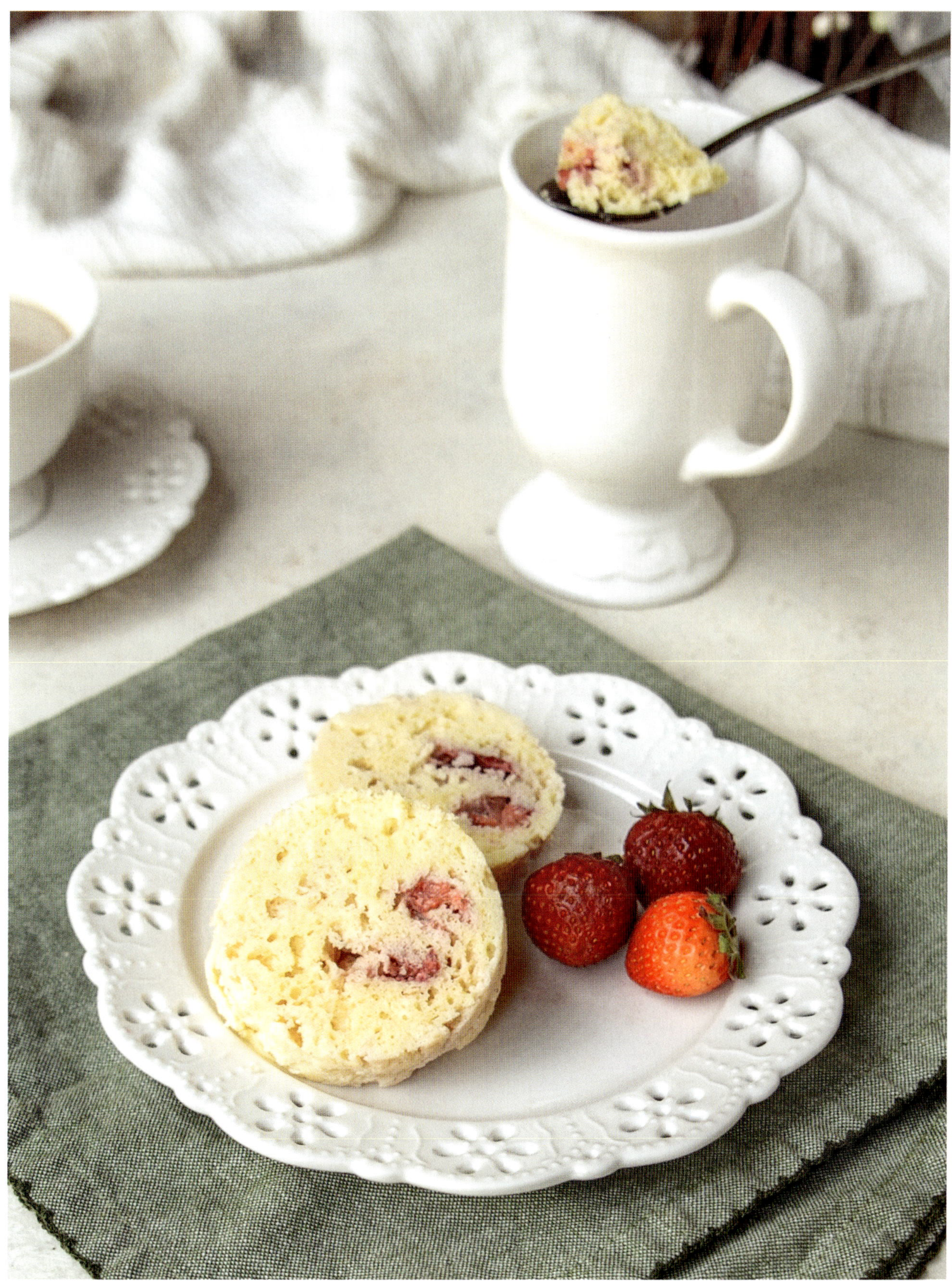

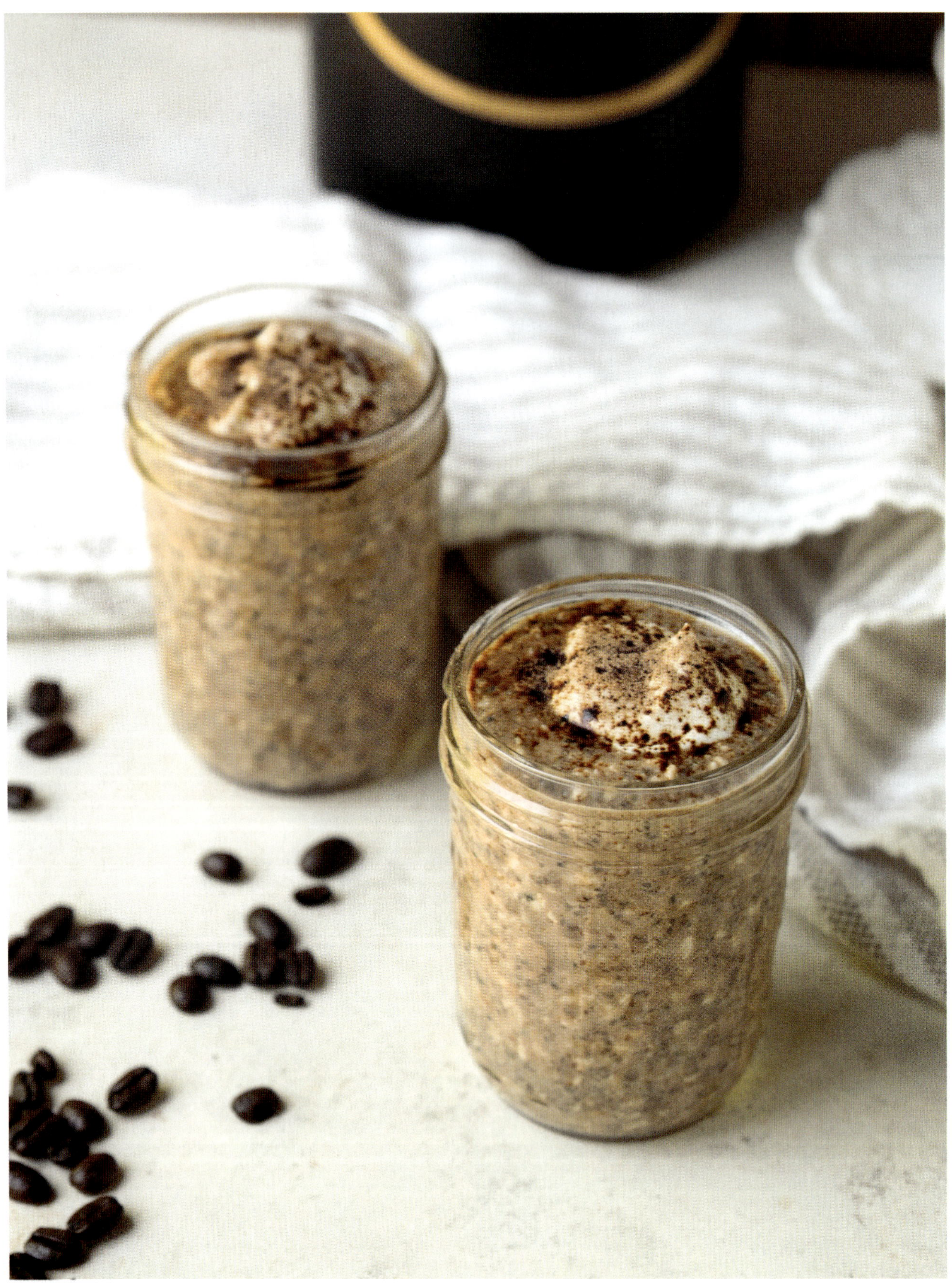

YIELD: 2 servings
PREP TIME: 5 minutes, plus 3 hours to chill and thicken

TIRAMISU OVERNIGHT "OATS"

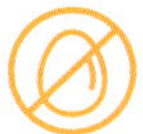 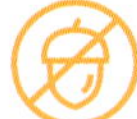

This recipe is for all those who miss the texture of overnight oats. It's fantastic to make ahead and store in the fridge to grab and take to work with you. If you don't like the flavor of coffee, you can easily make these oats straight up chocolate (see the variation below).

- 1 cup cottage cheese (4% milkfat)
- ½ cup brewed coffee, cooled
- ¼ cup hulled hemp seeds
- ¼ cup chocolate-flavored collagen peptides (27 grams)
- 2 tablespoons ground flaxseed
- 4 teaspoons chia seeds
- 1 teaspoon espresso powder
- 1 to 2 teaspoons rum extract, according to taste
- 1 to 2 teaspoons chocolate-flavored liquid monk fruit, to taste (optional)

FOR GARNISH (OPTIONAL):

- Plain Greek yogurt
- Dusting of unsweetened cocoa powder

1. Put the cottage cheese and coffee in a mixing bowl and stir to combine. Add the dry ingredients and mix well. Divide the mixture evenly between 2 (8-ounce) serving glasses or mason jars and cover.
2. Place in the fridge overnight or for at least 3 to 4 hours to thicken. If desired, garnish with Greek yogurt and cocoa powder before serving. Store in the fridge for up to 3 days.

VARIATION: Chocolate Overnight "Oats." Follow the recipe as written but swap out the coffee for unsweetened almond milk and omit the espresso powder and rum extract. If desired, garnish with Greek yogurt and cocoa powder before serving. If planning to garnish with additional low-carb toppings, such as fresh berries, chopped nuts, and/or shredded coconut, be sure to use 12-ounce mason jars to leave room at the top.

NOTE: To make this keto, you can leave out the chia seeds. The total carbs will be 10 grams, and the dietary fiber and net carbs will be 6 grams. The result will be less thick, but it will still resemble overnight oats after being chilled in the fridge.

Calories	Fat	Protein	Total Carbs	Dietary Fiber	Net Carbs
433	23g	42g	16g	8g	8g

YIELD: 1 serving
PREP TIME: 3 minutes

VANILLA PROTEIN POWER SMOOTHIE

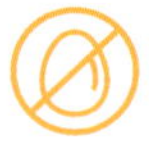
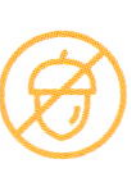
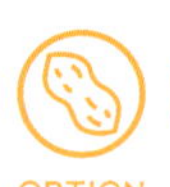
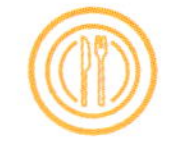

OPTION OPTION

A quick, powerful, and mighty way to get your protein on the go!

1/2 cup unsweetened almond milk or coconut milk

1/2 cup cottage cheese (4% milkfat) or plain yogurt

1/3 cup vanilla-flavored collagen peptides (30 grams)

1 tablespoon unsweetened peanut butter, almond butter, or sunflower seed butter

1 tablespoon plus 1/2 teaspoon unflavored gelatin powder (10 grams)

1/2 teaspoon vanilla-flavored liquid stevia

1/2 cup ice

SUGGESTED ADD-INS/ TOPPINGS:

2 tablespoons frozen or fresh berries of choice

1 tablespoon hulled hemp seeds (aka hemp hearts)

1 tablespoon unsweetened peanut butter, almond butter, or sunflower seed butter

1. Put the milk, cottage cheese, and collagen in a blender and blend until smooth.
2. Once well blended, add the rest of the ingredients to the blender and blend until smooth. If adding the berries and/or hulled hemp seeds, add them now.
3. Taste and adjust the sweetener if needed. If desired, garnish with a drizzle of peanut, almond, or sunflower seed butter. Pour into a 12-ounce glass and enjoy!

Calories	Fat	Protein	Total Carbs	Dietary Fiber	Net Carbs
351	16g	43g	8g	1g	7g

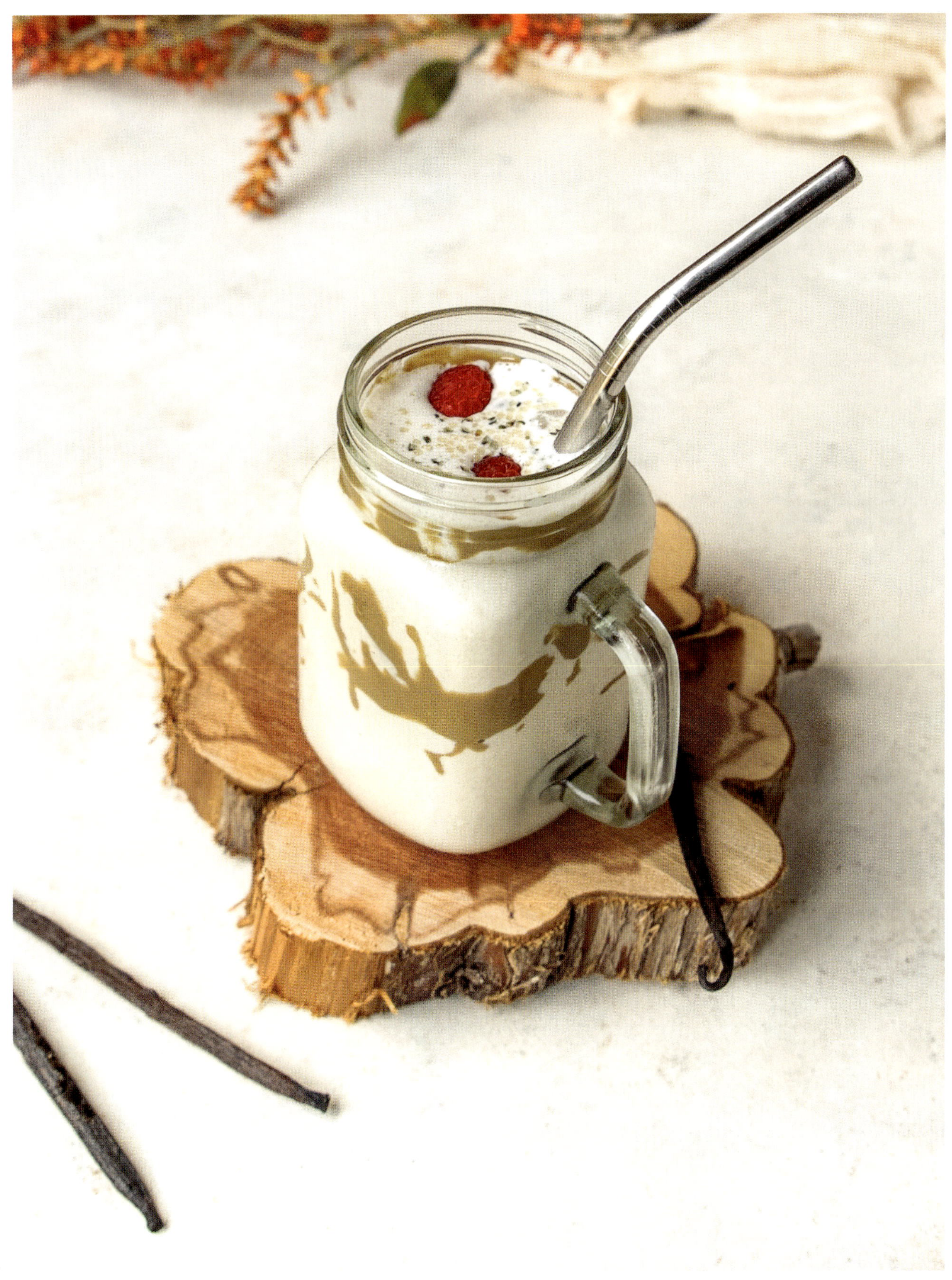

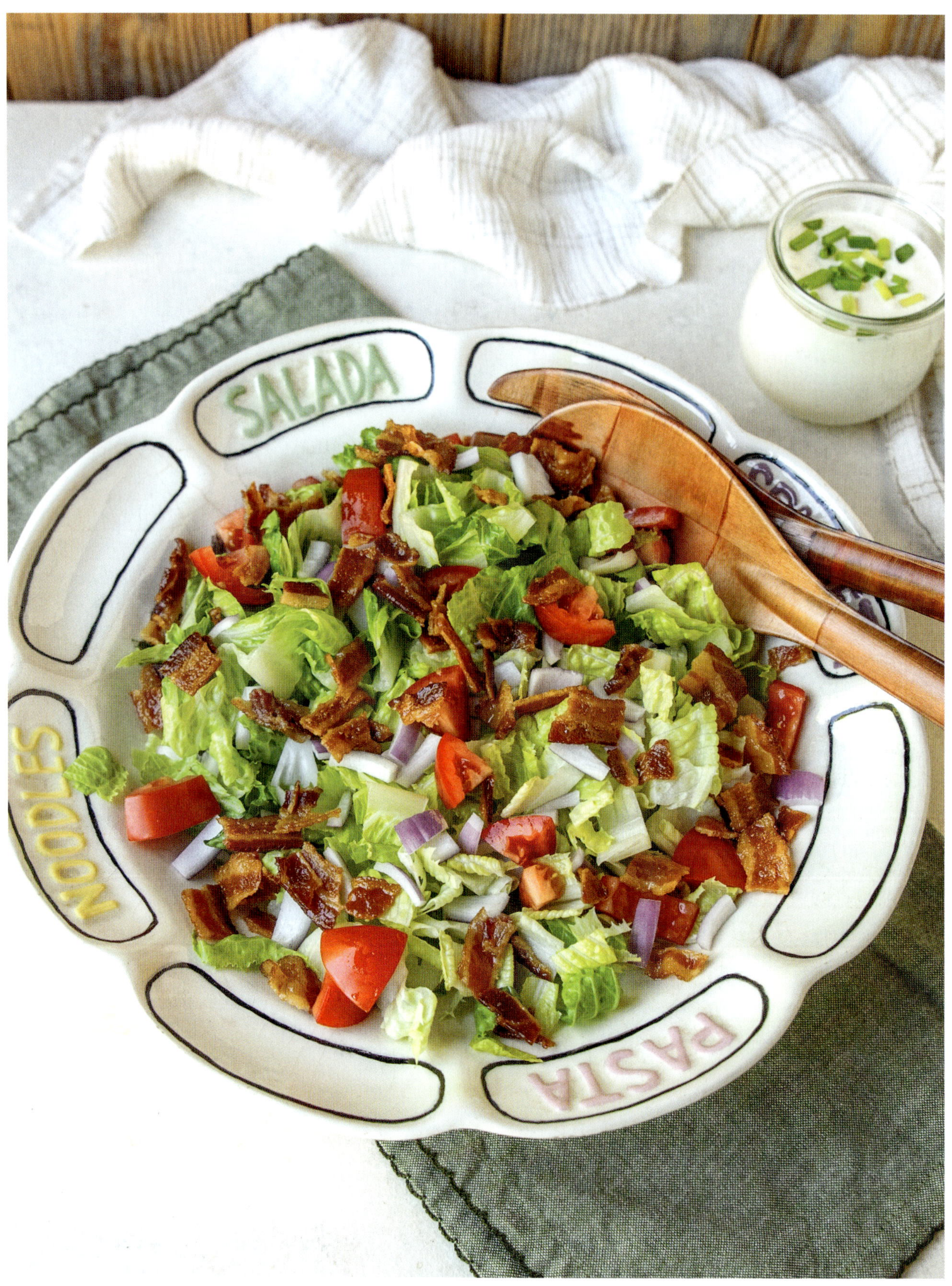
SALADA
NOODLES
PASTA

YIELD: 4 servings
PREP TIME: 10 minutes (not including time to cook bacon)

GOOD ENOUGH BLT SALAD

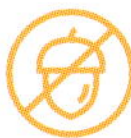
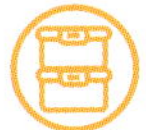

All the goodness of the sandwich tossed with a creamy mayonnaise-based dressing, but without the bread!

- 2 romaine lettuce hearts (about 11 ounces)
- 8 ounces bacon, baked (see page 76)
- 2 large Roma tomatoes (about 6 ounces)
- 1 small red onion (about 1¾ ounces)

FOR THE DRESSING:

- ¼ cup avocado oil mayonnaise
- ¼ cup sour cream
- 1 tablespoon extra-virgin olive oil
- 1 clove garlic, minced
- ¼ teaspoon sea salt
- ¼ teaspoon ground black pepper
- 2 tablespoons sliced scallions

1. Chop the lettuce and put in a large serving bowl or in 4 individual storage containers if meal prepping. Chop the bacon, tomatoes, and onion. Toss with the lettuce.
2. Whisk together all the dressing ingredients in a small bowl.
3. When ready to serve, toss the salad with the dressing. If meal prepping, store the dressing and salad fixings in separate containers and dress the salad just before serving. When stored separately, the salad and dressing will keep for up to 3 days.

Calories	Fat	Protein	Total Carbs	Dietary Fiber	Net Carbs
247	23g	6g	7g	2g	5g

YIELD: 1 serving
(1 muffin per serving)
PREP TIME: 5 minutes

COTTAGE CHEESE LUNCH BOWL

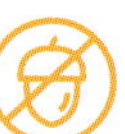
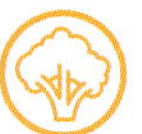
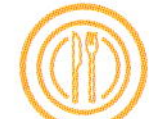

No cooking required for this fast and easy lunch! I like to serve this with pork rinds for scooping up the cottage cheese. For extra pizzazz, try seasoning the salad with everything bagel seasoning, instead of just salt and pepper.

- 1 cup chopped romaine lettuce
- ⅓ cup half-moon-sliced cucumbers
- ¼ cup halved cherry tomatoes
- 1 tablespoon chopped red onions
- 1 cup cottage cheese (4% milkfat)
- 2 tablespoons distilled white vinegar
- 1 tablespoon extra-virgin olive oil
- Salt and pepper
- ½ ounce pork rinds, for dipping (optional)

1. Put the salad fixings (lettuce, cucumbers, tomatoes, and red onion) in a shallow serving bowl. Top with the cottage cheese.
2. Drizzle with the vinegar and olive oil and season to taste with salt and pepper. Enjoy immediately with the pork rinds on the side.

NOTE: If you'd like to make this salad ahead, keep the salad fixings and cottage cheese separate until right before serving; likewise, don't dress the salad with oil and vinegar until ready to eat.

To make a keto bowl, omit the red onion and tomato, which will reduce the total carbs to 10 grams, the fiber to 1 gram, and the net carbs to 9 grams.

WITHOUT PORK RIND DIPPERS

Calories	Fat	Protein	Total Carbs	Dietary Fiber	Net Carbs
359	23g	25g	10g	2g	8g

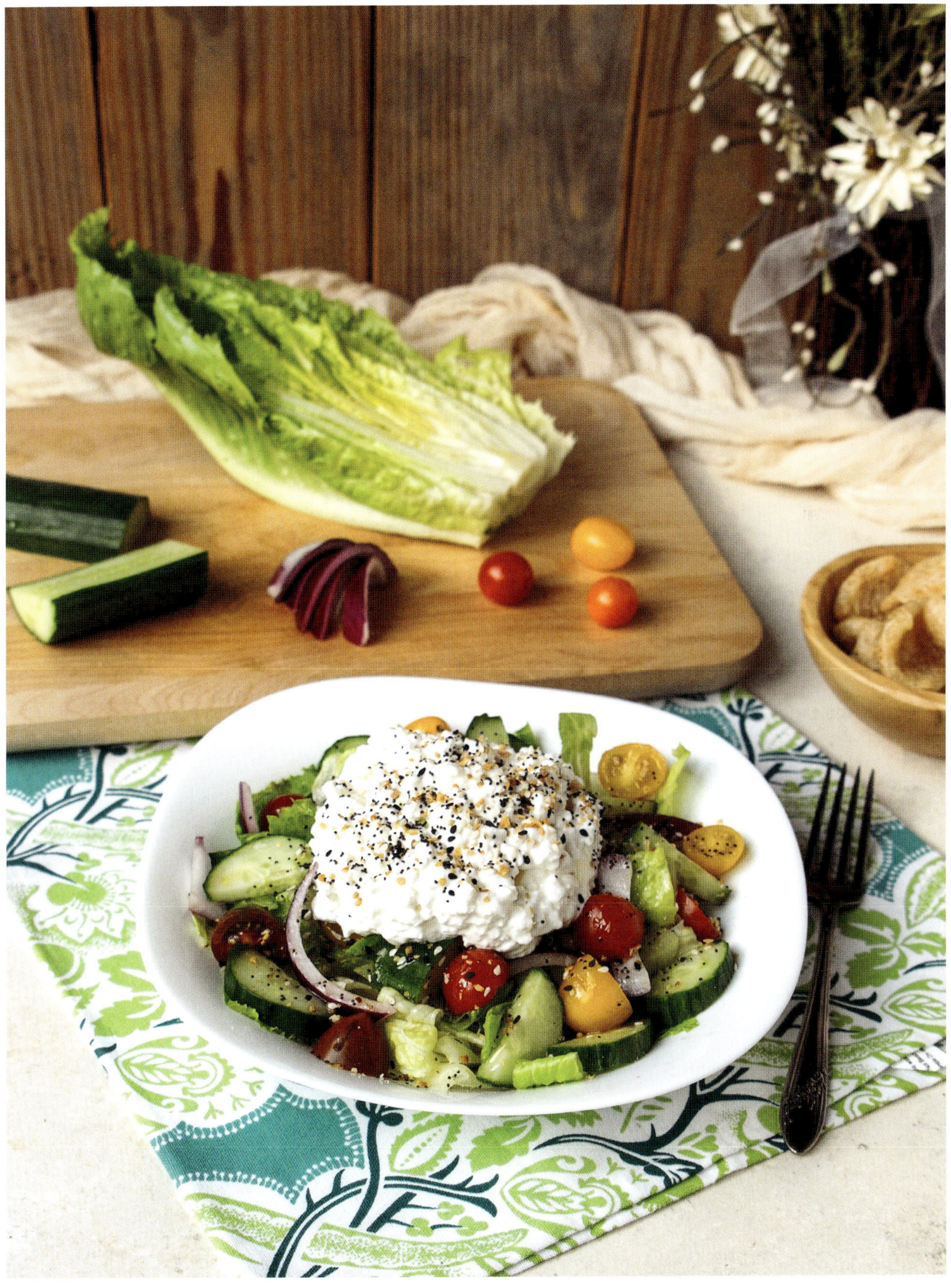

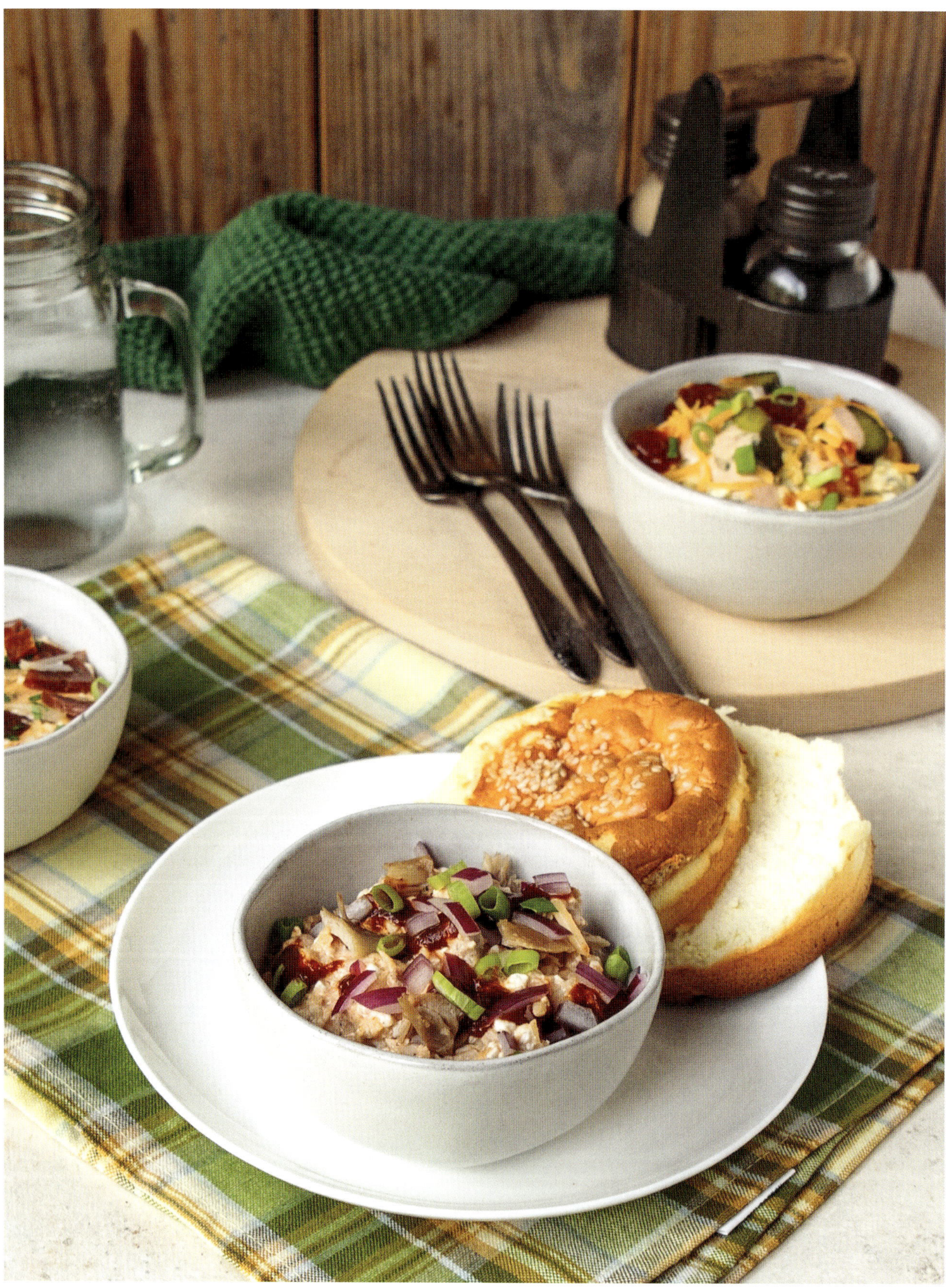

YIELD: 1 serving

PREP TIME: 5 minutes (not including time to cook chicken)

COOK TIME: 1 or 6 minutes, depending on method

HOT BBQ CHICKEN COTTAGE CHEESE BOWL

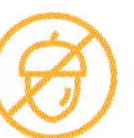
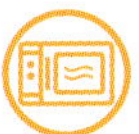
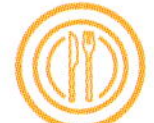

Whenever you have leftover cooked chicken, make this easy BBQ chicken lunch bowl. Another option is to purchase a rotisserie chicken or frozen grilled chicken strips. And the easiest option? If you happen to have leftover Batch-Cooked BBQ Pulled Chicken (page 260), you can use that to make this bowl. Simply omit the BBQ sauce and onion powder listed below and mix ⅓ cup of the leftover pulled chicken with the cottage cheese, mozzarella cheese, and salt. This bowl is heated until warmed. I like to garnish with red onion and scallion for some crunch and color.

- ½ cup cottage cheese (4% milkfat)
- ¼ cup shredded mozzarella cheese (part skim)
- ¼ teaspoon onion powder
- ¼ teaspoon fine sea salt
- 1 (3-ounce) boneless, skinless chicken thigh, cooked and chopped or shredded
- 1 tablespoon sugar-free BBQ sauce, store-bought or homemade (page 79)

FOR GARNISH (OPTIONAL):

- 1 tablespoon chopped red onions
- 1 tablespoon chopped scallions

1. If heating the bowl in the oven, preheat the oven to 400°F.
2. Put all the ingredients in a 12-ounce microwave-safe bowl or ovenproof ramekin or other comparably sized baking dish. Mix until well combined.
3. Microwave for 1 minute or place in the oven and bake for 6 to 8 minutes, until heated through.

Make It Better: Serve this as a filling sandwiched between a split store-bought or homemade cloud bread roll (see page 88).

NOTE: If you'd like to prep this bowl ahead, complete Step 2, cover, and refrigerate for up to 4 days. When ready to serve, heat the bowl following the instructions above. If using the oven, put the refrigerated ramekin in a cold oven and set the oven temperature to 400°F so that the ramekin and oven heat up at the same time. (Putting a chilled dish in a hot oven can cause it to break.) Note that the oven heating time will likely be doubled.

Calories	Fat	Protein	Total Carbs	Dietary Fiber	Net Carbs
369	23g	32g	7g	0.1g	6.9g

YIELD: 1 serving (1 muffin per serving)

PREP TIME: 5 minutes (not including time to cook burger)

COOK TIME: 1 or 6 minutes, depending on method

HOT CHEESEBURGER COTTAGE CHEESE BOWL

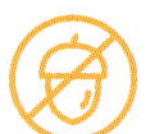  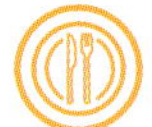

This popular bowl is now made even better with the addition of cottage cheese. To make this very easy, purchase frozen precooked hamburger patties or quickly brown some ground beef patties in a pan and freeze for later, then make a lunch bowl whenever you want.

½ cup cottage cheese (4% milkfat)

¼ cup shredded cheddar cheese, plus more for garnish if desired

1 (3-ounce) 90/10 hamburger patty, cooked and chopped

1 tablespoon sugar-free ketchup

1 tablespoon avocado oil mayonnaise

¼ teaspoon onion powder

¼ teaspoon fine sea salt

1 small dill pickle, sliced, for garnish

1 tablespoon sliced scallions, for garnish (optional)

1. If heating the bowl in the oven, preheat the oven to 400°F.
2. Put all the ingredients, except the pickle and scallions (if using), in a 12-ounce microwave-safe bowl or ovenproof ramekin or other comparably sized baking dish. Mix until well combined.
3. Microwave for 1 minute or place in the oven and bake for 6 to 8 minutes, until heated through. To serve, top with the pickle and, if desired, scallions and extra cheese.

Make It Better: Serve this as a filling sandwiched between a split store-bought or homemade cloud bread roll (see page 88 for recipe).

NOTE: If you'd like to prep this bowl ahead, complete Step 2, cover, and refrigerate for up to 4 days. When ready to serve, heat and then garnish the bowl following the instructions above. If using the oven to heat the bowl, put the refrigerated ramekin in a cold oven and set the oven temperature to 400°F so that the ramekin and oven heat up at the same time. (Putting a chilled dish in a hot oven can cause it to break.) Note that the oven heating time will likely be doubled.

Calories	Fat	Protein	Total Carbs	Dietary Fiber	Net Carbs
485	35g	35g	7g	0.5g	6.5g

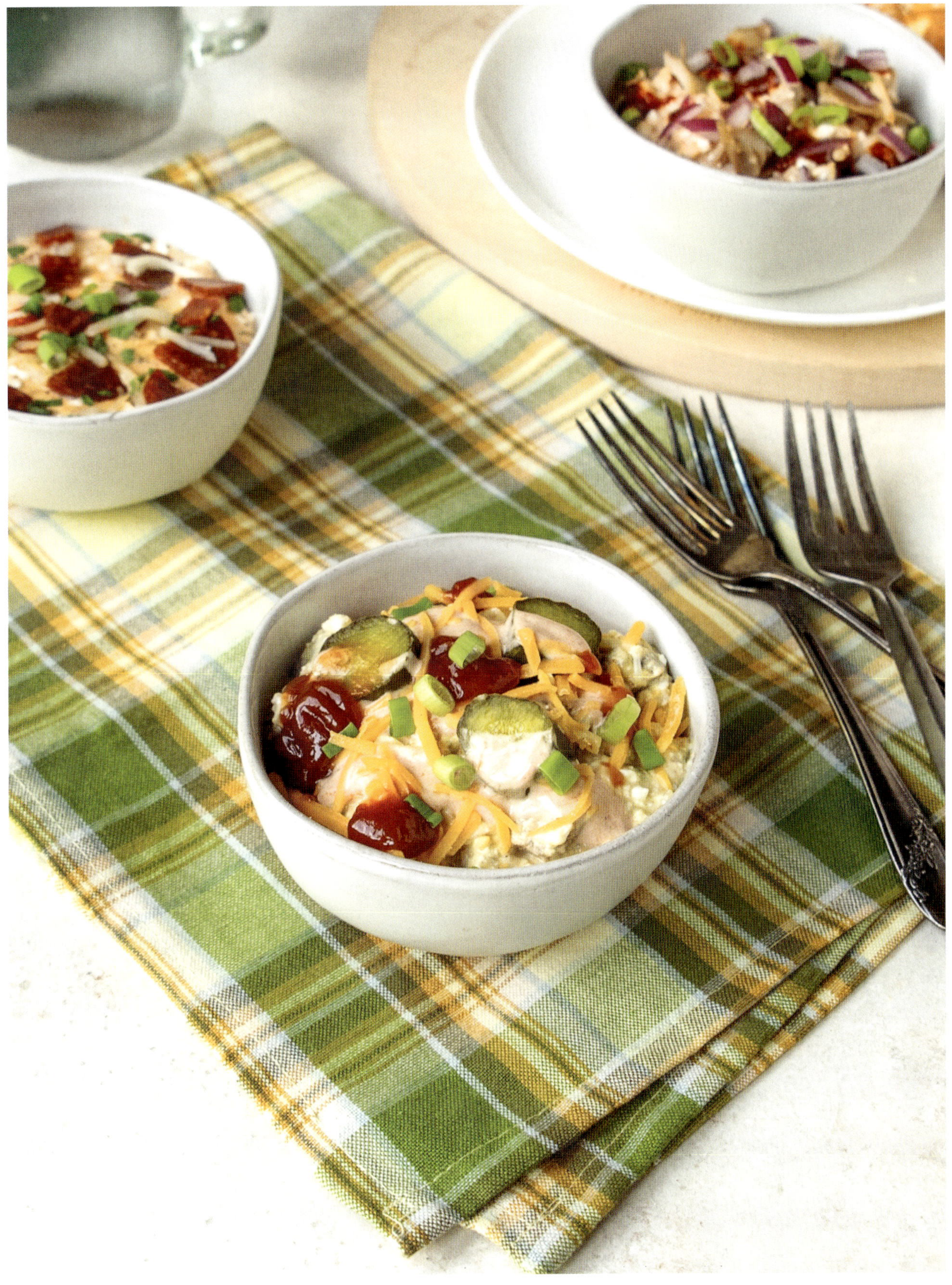

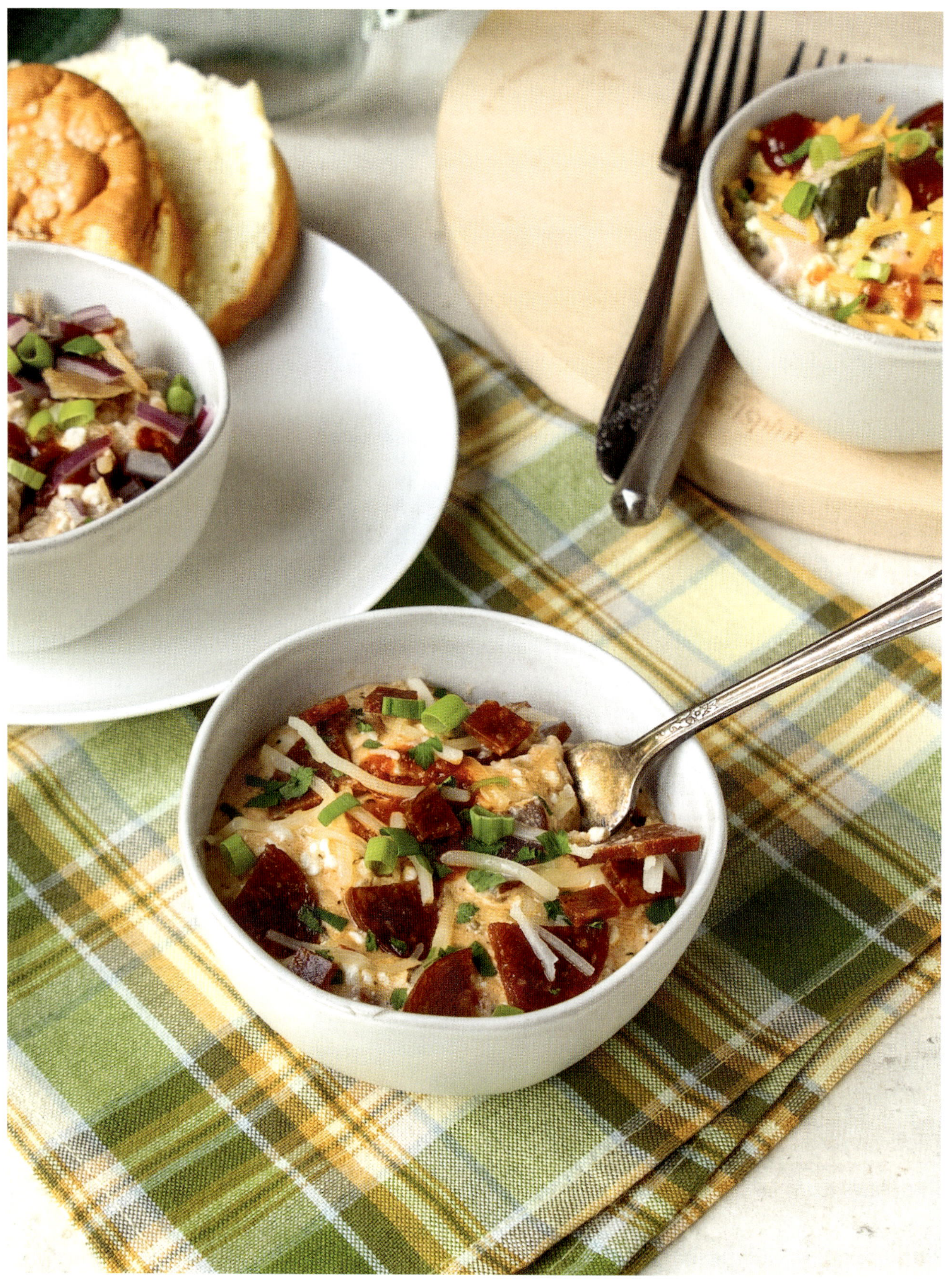

YIELD: 1 serving
PREP TIME: 5 minutes
COOK TIME: 1 or 6 minutes, depending on method

HOT COTTAGE CHEESE PIZZA BOWL

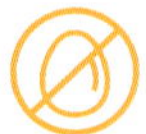  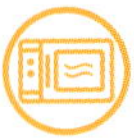 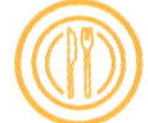

While it might not sound appealing if you've never tried it before, cottage cheese is similar to ricotta cheese and blends nicely in this recipe for a pizzalike flavor but with added protein for a hearty bowl.

- 1/2 cup cottage cheese (4% milkfat)
- 1/4 cup shredded mozzarella cheese (part skim), plus more for garnish if desired
- 1/4 teaspoon onion powder
- 1/4 teaspoon salt
- 1/4 teaspoon Italian seasoning
- 1 tablespoon low-carb marinara sauce
- 1/2 ounce pepperoni, chopped
- 1 tablespoon sliced scallions, for garnish

1. If heating the bowl in the oven, preheat the oven to 400°F.
2. Put all the ingredients in a 12-ounce microwave-safe bowl or ovenproof ramekin or other comparably sized baking dish. Mix together until well combined.
3. Microwave for 1 minute or bake for 6 to 8 minutes, until heated through. Garnish with extra mozzarella if desired.

Make It Better: Serve this as a filling sandwiched between a split store-bought or homemade cloud bread roll (see page 88 for recipe).

NOTE: If you'd like to prep this bowl ahead, complete Step 2, cover, and refrigerate for up to 4 days. When ready to serve, heat the bowl following the instructions above. If using the oven, put the refrigerated ramekin in a cold oven and set the oven temperature to 400°F so that the ramekin and oven heat up at the same time. (Putting a chilled dish in a hot oven can cause it to break.) Note that the oven heating time will likely be doubled.

Calories	Fat	Protein	Total Carbs	Dietary Fiber	Net Carbs
259	17g	21g	6g	0.4g	5.6g

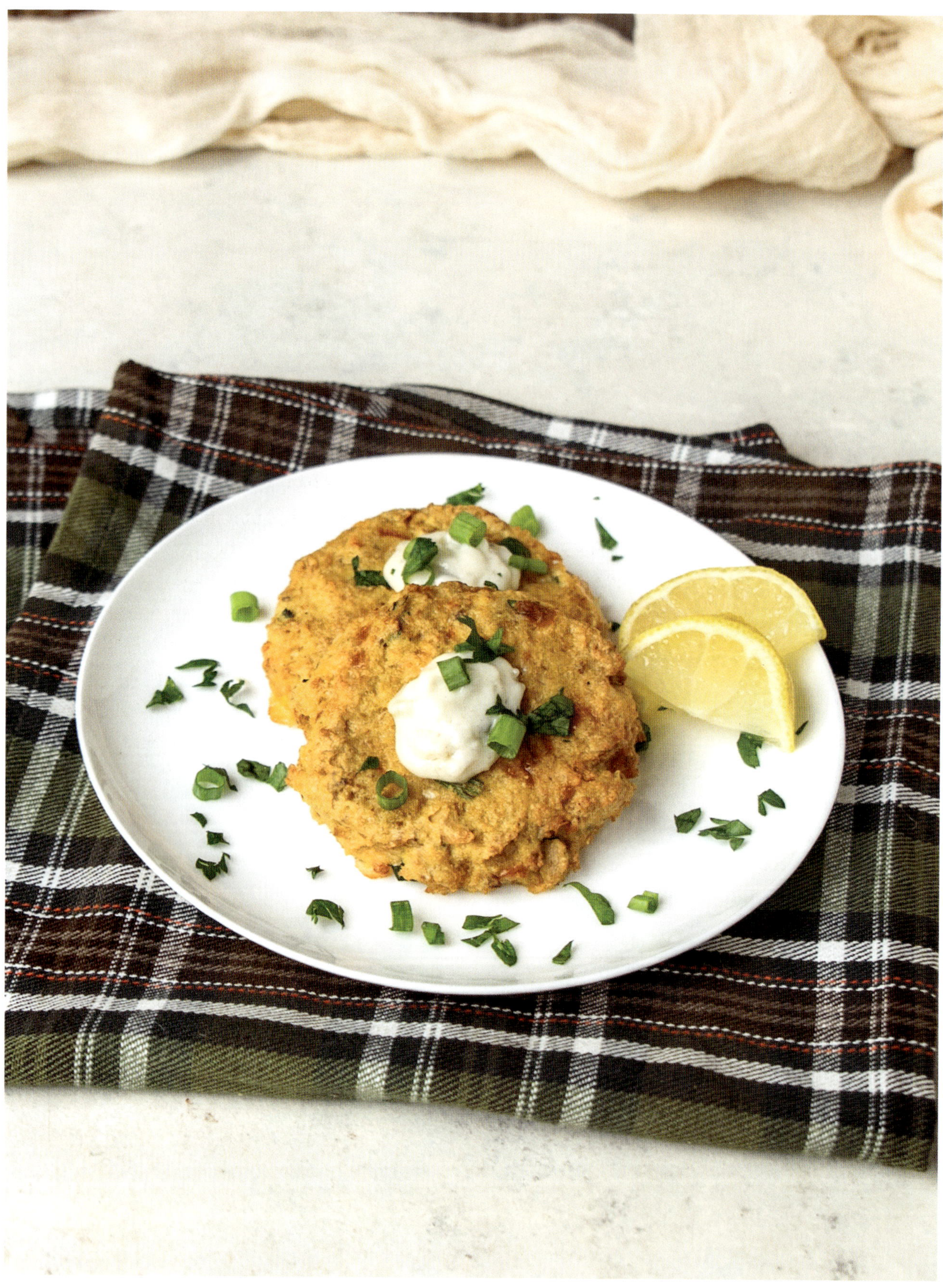

YIELD: 1 serving
PREP TIME: 5 minutes
COOK TIME: 10 to 15 minutes, depending on method

SALMON PATTIES

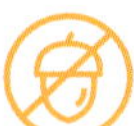 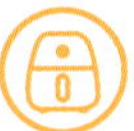 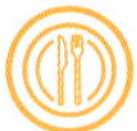

This is an easy hot lunch. Air-fry for a super quick high-protein meal. The oven is nearly as fast! This recipe is versatile too. Don't like salmon? Replace it with canned tuna (packed in water) or 5 ounces cooked chicken.

5 ounces canned salmon, drained

¼ cup pork rind panko

¼ cup shredded cheddar cheese

1 large egg

1 teaspoon fresh lemon juice

1 teaspoon chopped fresh parsley

FOR SERVING/GARNISH (OPTIONAL):

Tartar Sauce (page 80)

Chopped fresh parsley and/or sliced scallions

Lemon slices

1. If using the oven to cook the patties, preheat the oven to 425°F.
2. Put all the ingredients in a small bowl and stir to combine. Form into 2 equal patties about ½ inch thick and 4 inches in diameter.
3. *To air-fry the patties,* place them in the air fryer basket in a single layer. Air-fry at 400°F for 5 minutes, carefully flip over, and air-fry for another 5 minutes, or until the edges are nicely browned.

   To bake the patties in the oven, place them on a small rimmed baking sheet and bake for 10 to 15 minutes, until golden brown.
4. If desired, serve the patties with a dollop of tartar sauce, a sprinkle of fresh parsley and/or scallions, and lemon slices alongside.

Calories	Fat	Protein	Total Carbs	Dietary Fiber	Net Carbs
253	15g	30g	1g	0.1g	0.9g

YIELD: 4 servings
PREP TIME: 5 minutes
COOK TIME: 10 minutes

HOT SHRIMP DIP

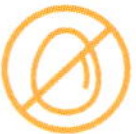
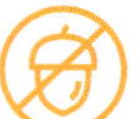

Enjoy this as a hot lunch or light dinner with slices of low-carb vegetables or pork rinds on the side for dipping. I've listed cucumber slices below for serving with the dip. Celery and bell peppers are two other good low-carb vegetable options for scoopers. Keep in mind, however, if you use another scooper, it will affect the nutrition information.

- 1 pound frozen cooked and peeled shrimp (any size), defrosted
- 1 (8-ounce) package cream cheese, softened
- 1 cup shredded cheddar cheese
- 1/3 heaping cup roughly chopped scallions
- 1/4 cup fresh lemon juice
- 1/2 teaspoon fine sea salt
- 1/2 teaspoon ground black pepper
- 8 ounces sliced cucumbers

1. Preheat the oven to 350°F.
2. Put all the ingredients in a food processor and pulse just until the mixture is combined and the shrimp are finely chopped; you want the final texture to remain a bit chunky. Taste and adjust the seasonings if needed.
3. Spread in a 6-inch cast-iron or other ovenproof skillet. Bake for 10 minutes, or until bubbly around the edges. Best served fresh.

Calories	Fat	Protein	Total Carbs	Dietary Fiber	Net Carbs
424	30g	33g	7g	1g	6g

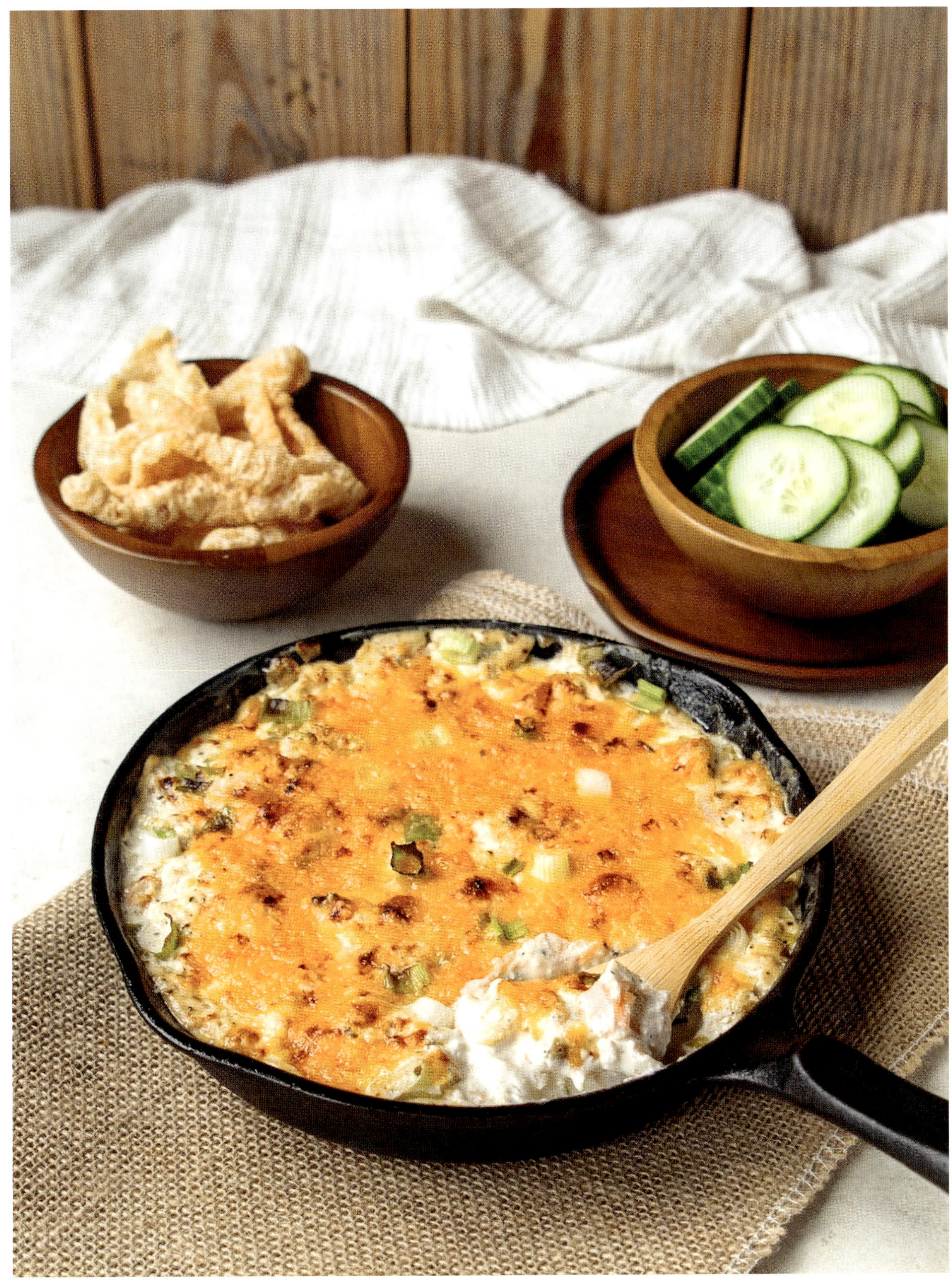

YIELD: 12 patties (3 per serving)

PREP TIME: 5 minutes

COOK TIME: 15 to 30 minutes, depending on method

TUNA CABBAGE PATTIES

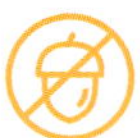
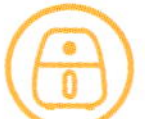

The cabbage gives these tuna patties a little extra crunch, and they are very filling. You have 3 choices for cooking them: oven, air fryer, or stovetop. Though the air fryer takes longer than an oven when cooking larger recipes like this one, I prefer it because it gives the patties a crispier exterior.

- 8 ounces green cabbage (about 1/2 small head)
- 2 (5-ounce) cans tuna (packed in water), drained
- 3 large egg yolks
- 2 cups shredded cheddar cheese
- 2 tablespoons chopped scallions
- 1/4 teaspoon sea salt
- 1/4 teaspoon ground black pepper
- 4 tablespoons avocado oil, for the stovetop method

FOR GARNISH/SERVING (OPTIONAL):

- Tartar Sauce (page 80)
- Chopped fresh parsley
- Lemon wedges

1. If cooking the patties in the oven, preheat the oven to 400°F and line a rimmed baking sheet with parchment paper.
2. Put the cabbage in a food processor and process until finely shredded, or finely shred the cabbage by hand with a sharp knife and place in a large bowl. (If you used a food processor, leave the shredded cabbage in the processor.)
3. Add the remaining ingredients to the food processor and process until combined, then remove the chopping blade from the processor. Alternatively, add the remaining ingredients to the bowl with the shredded cabbage and mix with a spoon until combined.
4. Form the tuna mixture into 12 patties about 2 1/2 inches in diameter and 1/2 inch thick, using about 1/4 cup per patty.
5. Cook the patties using one of these three methods:

   To cook in the oven, place the patties on the prepared pan, leaving space between them. Bake for 15 minutes, or until golden brown.

   To cook in an air fryer, line the air fryer basket with parchment paper. Working in batches so no patties overlap, set the patties on the prepared basket. Air-fry at 400°F for 10 minutes, or until golden brown.

   To cook on the stovetop, heat 2 tablespoons of avocado oil in a large skillet over medium-high heat. Working in two batches, to avoid crowding, cook the patties in the hot oil for 3 to 5 minutes on each side, until golden brown. Heat the remaining 2 tablespoons of avocado oil in the skillet before adding the second batch of patties.
6. Serve garnished with a dollop of tartar sauce and a sprinkle of parsley, with lemon wedges on the side, if desired.

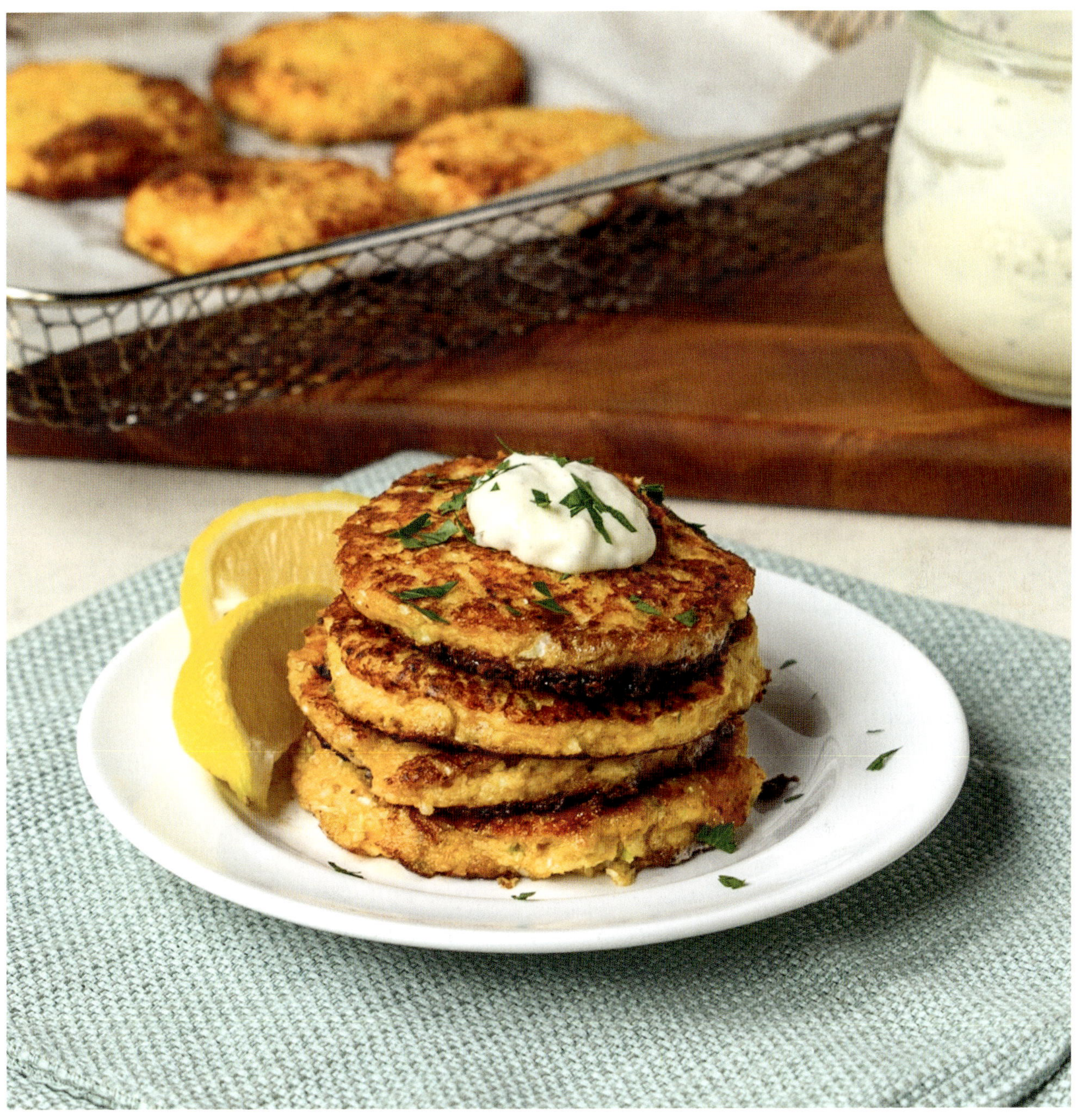

7. The patties can be stored in the refrigerator for up to 5 days or frozen for up to 3 months. Using moderate heat, reheat in a skillet, air fryer, or oven until heated through and crispy, flipping over halfway through. This should take 10 to 15 minutes, depending on the method. If freezing the patties, defrost them in the refrigerator before reheating.

Calories	Fat	Protein	Total Carbs	Dietary Fiber	Net Carbs
442	31g	35g	7g	2g	5g

YIELD: 8 burgers (1 per serving)
PREP TIME: 10 minutes
COOK TIME: 10 to 20 minutes, depending on method

SHEET PAN RANCH BURGERS

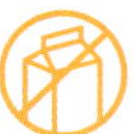 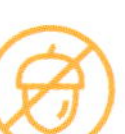  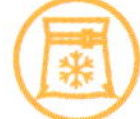

Cook this entire batch of preformed ranch burgers on a sheet pan for a no-fuss meal, or grill or pan-fry them in a skillet if you prefer. Seasoning the ground beef with the ranch seasoning and forming the mixture into patties ahead of time makes it easy to have a good (enough) meal on the table quickly. All you need to remember to do is thaw the patties before cooking.

FOR THE BURGERS:

2 pounds 80/20 ground beef

1/3 cup mayonnaise

2 tablespoons dried parsley

2 teaspoons garlic powder

2 teaspoons onion powder

2 teaspoons dried minced onion

1 teaspoon dried dill weed

1 teaspoon fine sea salt

1 teaspoon ground black pepper

ADD-ONS (OPTIONAL):

Bacon slices (for sheet pan cooking method)

Cheese slices

NOTE: The internal temperature for medium (slightly pink) burgers is 145°F. Well-done is 160°F.

1. Put all the ingredients for the burgers in a large bowl and, using clean hands, mix to combine.
2. Form into 8 patties about 3½ inches in diameter and ½ inch thick.
3. If freezer prepping, wrap each patty in parchment paper and place in a large freezer bag for up to 3 months. Thaw in the refrigerator for several hours or overnight before cooking. Remove the parchment wrapping before cooking.
4. To cook the burgers in the oven, preheat the oven to 425°F. Place the burgers on a rimmed baking sheet. If you would like to serve bacon burgers, put the bacon slices on the pan to cook alongside the burgers. Bake the burgers for 18 to 20 minutes for medium done burgers. The bacon will take 15 to 20 minutes to cook, depending on thickness and how crisp you like your bacon. Remove the bacon when done. Top the burgers with cheese if desired and broil for 1 minute to melt the cheese.
5. Alternatively, you can grill the burgers over high heat or pan-fry them in a couple of batches in a large skillet over medium-high heat. Grill or pan-fry for 5 minutes, then flip over and continue cooking for another 5 minutes for medium-done burgers. Top with cheese, if desired, about a minute before the burgers are done cooking.

Calories	Fat	Protein	Total Carbs	Dietary Fiber	Net Carbs
293	23g	20g	1g	0.2g	0.8g

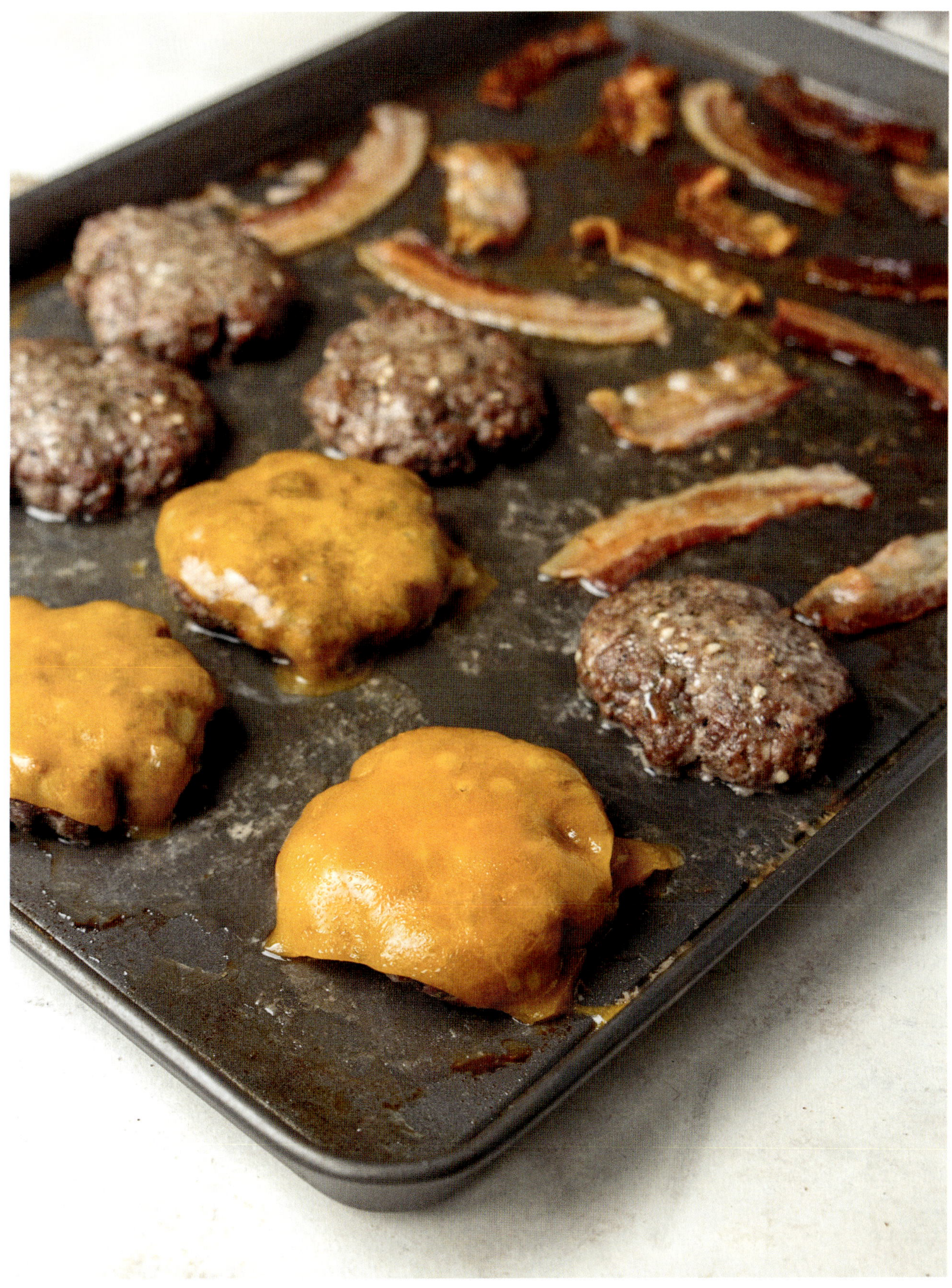

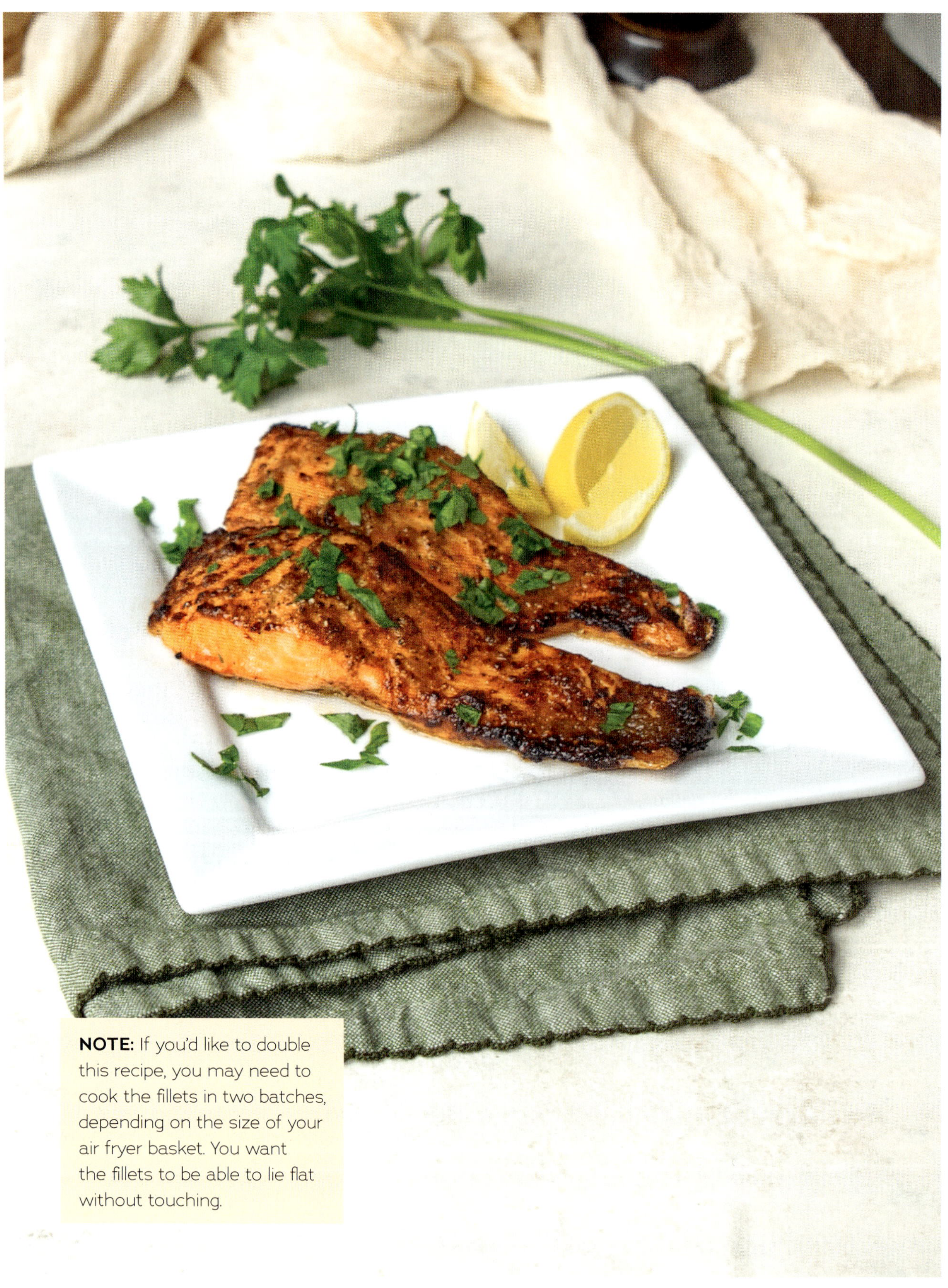

NOTE: If you'd like to double this recipe, you may need to cook the fillets in two batches, depending on the size of your air fryer basket. You want the fillets to be able to lie flat without touching.

YIELD: 2 servings
PREP TIME: 5 minutes
COOK TIME: 10 minutes

AIR FRYER SALMON

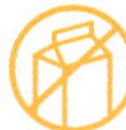
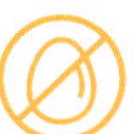
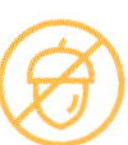
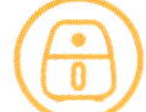

Simply the best thing to cook in your air fryer! Ready in under 15 minutes, this super simple salmon dish is a healthy, super low-carb, high-protein dinner or lunch recipe.

2 (6-ounce) skin-on salmon fillets (about 1 inch thick)

FOR THE DRESSING:

1 tablespoon extra-virgin olive oil

1 tablespoon coconut aminos or soy sauce

1 teaspoon distilled white vinegar, red wine vinegar, or lime juice

1 teaspoon Dijon mustard

½ teaspoon garlic powder, or 1 clove garlic, minced

¼ teaspoon fine sea salt

¼ teaspoon ground black pepper

FOR GARNISH/SERVING (OPTIONAL):

Finely chopped fresh parsley

Lemon wedges

Tartar Sauce (page 80)

1. Pat the salmon dry with paper towels.
2. Line the air fryer basket with parchment paper. Preheat the air fryer to 400°F.
3. Lay the salmon fillets in the prepared air fryer basket, skin side down.
4. Mix together all the dressing ingredients in a small bowl. Spoon the dressing over the tops of the salmon fillets.
5. Air-fry the salmon for 8 to 10 minutes, until the fish has become flaky, and the center is no longer translucent. Time will vary depending on the exact thickness of your salmon fillets and whether you used wild or farmed salmon. (The 1-inch-thick wild salmon fillets I used took 8 minutes for medium doneness.) Try not to overcook the salmon or it will become dry. Salmon also continues to cook and firms up as it rests. To be sure of doneness, check with a thermometer: The rested internal temperature should read 125°F for medium or 140°F for well-done; however, I don't recommend cooking salmon beyond medium.
6. Remove from the air fryer and let rest for 5 minutes before serving.
7. Sprinkle with fresh parsley and serve with lemon wedges and tartar sauce, if desired.
8. Best served fresh, although you can store it in an airtight container for up to 2 days in the fridge, but the skin won't be crispy when reheated. You can reheat in the air fryer at 300°F for 5 minutes.

Calories	Fat	Protein	Total Carbs	Dietary Fiber	Net Carbs
316	18g	34g	2g	0.3g	1.7g

YIELD: 4 servings
PREP TIME: 5 minutes
COOK TIME: 15 to 25 minutes, depending on method

BACON-WRAPPED CHICKEN TENDERS

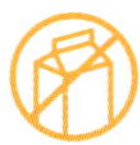
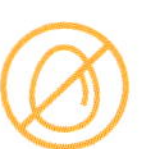

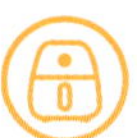
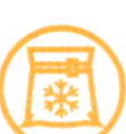

These are a family favorite and quick to prep ahead and freeze for later. And because the chicken is cut into tenders, they defrost fairly quickly. Air-fry them or bake them in the oven. My family's favorite way to eat these is dipped in barbecue sauce (see my recipe on page 79).

1 tablespoon smoked paprika

1 tablespoon ground cumin

1 teaspoon onion powder

1 teaspoon fine sea salt

2 pounds boneless, skinless chicken breasts, cut lengthwise into 12 even strips

12 slices thin-cut bacon (about 3/4 pound)

1. Put the seasonings in a large zip-top bag, close, and shake. Add the chicken tenders to the bag and shake to coat them with the seasonings. Remove one tender at a time and wrap with a slice of bacon.
2. If freezer prepping, secure the bacon to the tenders with toothpick and return the bacon-wrapped tenders to the freezer bag. Seal and freeze for up to 3 months. Thaw in the refrigerator for several hours or overnight before cooking.
3. Cook the chicken tenders using one of these two methods:

   To cook in the oven, preheat the oven to 450°F and line a rimmed baking sheet with parchment paper. Place the bacon-wrapped chicken tenders on the prepared pan, seam side down, and bake for 20 to 25 minutes, until the internal temperature of the chicken is 165°F. Broil for 1 minute to crisp the bacon.

   To cook in an air fryer, preheat the air fryer to 450°F. Arrange the bacon-wrapped chicken tenders in the air fryer basket in a single layer, seam side down. Work in batches if needed. Air-fry for 15 minutes, or until the internal temperature of the chicken is 165°F.

Calories	Fat	Protein	Total Carbs	Dietary Fiber	Net Carbs
315	11g	50g	2g	1g	1g

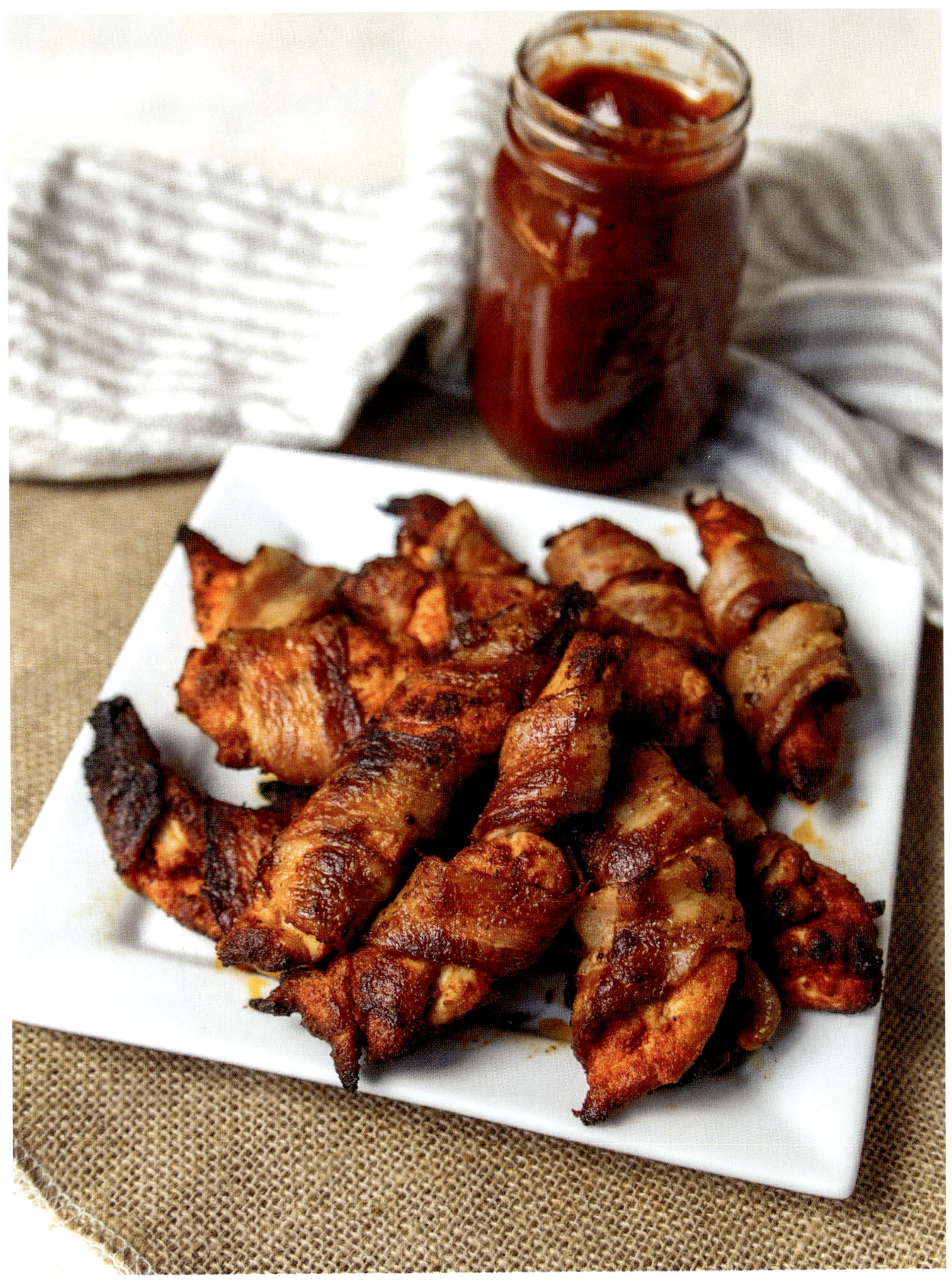

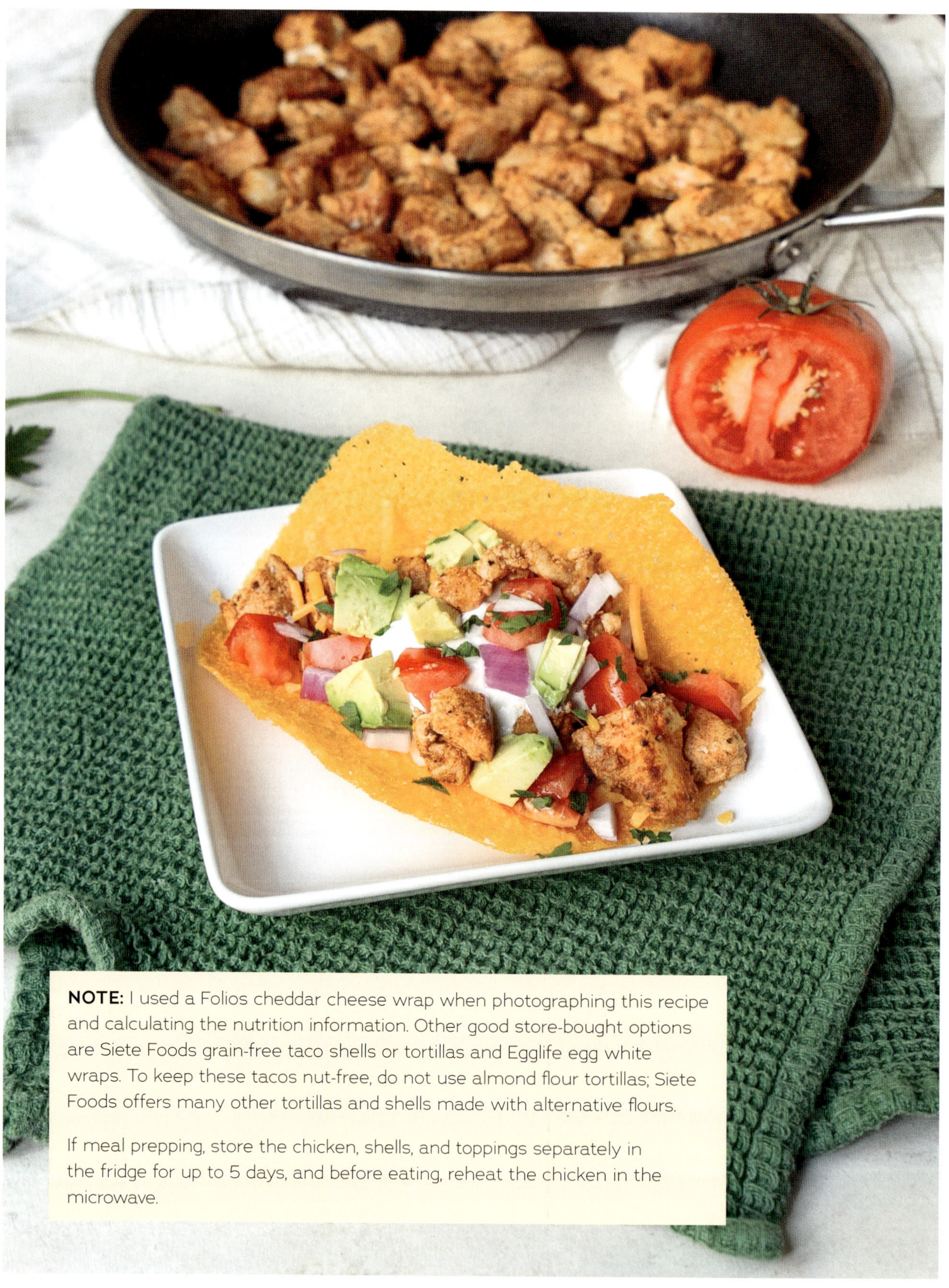

NOTE: I used a Folios cheddar cheese wrap when photographing this recipe and calculating the nutrition information. Other good store-bought options are Siete Foods grain-free taco shells or tortillas and Egglife egg white wraps. To keep these tacos nut-free, do not use almond flour tortillas; Siete Foods offers many other tortillas and shells made with alternative flours.

If meal prepping, store the chicken, shells, and toppings separately in the fridge for up to 5 days, and before eating, reheat the chicken in the microwave.

YIELD: 4 servings
PREP TIME: 5 minutes
COOK TIME: 4 minutes

CHICKEN TACOS

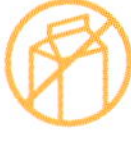

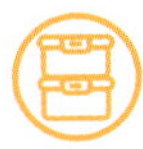

OPTION

Because of the convenience of fully cooked grilled chicken strips, you'll never make a quicker chicken taco than this recipe. These tacos are versatile and easily customizable, allowing each family member to enjoy them with toppings of their choice, and they're also seriously tasty. For a Better version of this recipe, using the same chicken taco theme, see my recipe for Chicken Taco Bowls (page 201). In that version, you cook up some raw chicken breast instead of using precooked and replace the taco shells/tortillas with freshly made red cabbage slaw.

1 teaspoon paprika

1/2 teaspoon chili powder

1/2 teaspoon garlic powder

1/2 teaspoon onion powder

1/2 teaspoon fine sea salt

1/4 teaspoon ground black pepper

1/4 teaspoon cayenne pepper

2 pounds frozen ready-to-eat grilled chicken strips (not breaded), thawed

2 tablespoons extra-virgin olive oil, for the pan

8 store-bought low-carb taco shells, tortillas, wraps, or lettuce leaves, for serving (see note)

SUGGESTED TOPPINGS:

Sour cream

Chopped red onion

Diced tomato

Diced avocado

Shredded cheese of choice

Chopped fresh cilantro

Squeeze of lime juice

1. Put the seasonings in a large bowl and mix to combine.
2. Cut the thawed chicken strips into 1-inch pieces. Add the chicken to the bowl with the seasonings and stir to coat.
3. Pour the olive oil into a large skillet and set over medium-high heat.
4. When the oil is hot, add the seasoned chicken to the skillet and sauté until heated through, about 4 minutes.
5. Serve with taco shells, tortillas, or wraps and the toppings of your choice.

Calories	Fat	Protein	Total Carbs	Dietary Fiber	Net Carbs
260	12g	36g	1g	0.4g	0.6g

YIELD: 4 servings
PREP TIME: 10 minutes
COOK TIME: 18 minutes,

TURKEY SAUSAGE PEPPER ZUCCHINI SKILLET

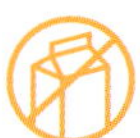 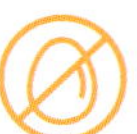 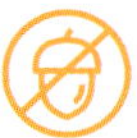 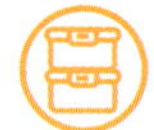

My family loves this simple skillet recipe that's quick for dinner on a busy night. Feel free to swap out turkey sausage with chicken, Italian sausage, or another protein you have on hand. This recipe is a good meal prep candidate because it freezes well.

- 2 tablespoons extra-virgin olive oil
- 1 pound turkey sausage links
- 2 cups sliced red bell peppers
- 2 cups half-moon-sliced zucchini
- 1/2 cup chopped yellow onions
- 1/2 teaspoon fine sea salt
- 1/2 teaspoon garlic powder
- 1/4 teaspoon ground black pepper

1. Pour the olive oil into a large skillet over medium-high heat. Add the sausage and cook until browned and cooked through, 5 to 8 minutes. Remove from the pan, slice into rounds, and keep warm. Leave the cooking fat in the pan.
2. Using the same pan, cook the bell peppers, zucchini, and onions over medium heat until tender, about 10 minutes. Sprinkle in the salt, garlic powder, and black pepper and stir to combine.
3. Return the sausage to the pan and toss with the vegetables, then serve.

Calories	Fat	Protein	Total Carbs	Dietary Fiber	Net Carbs
276	17g	23g	9g	3g	6g

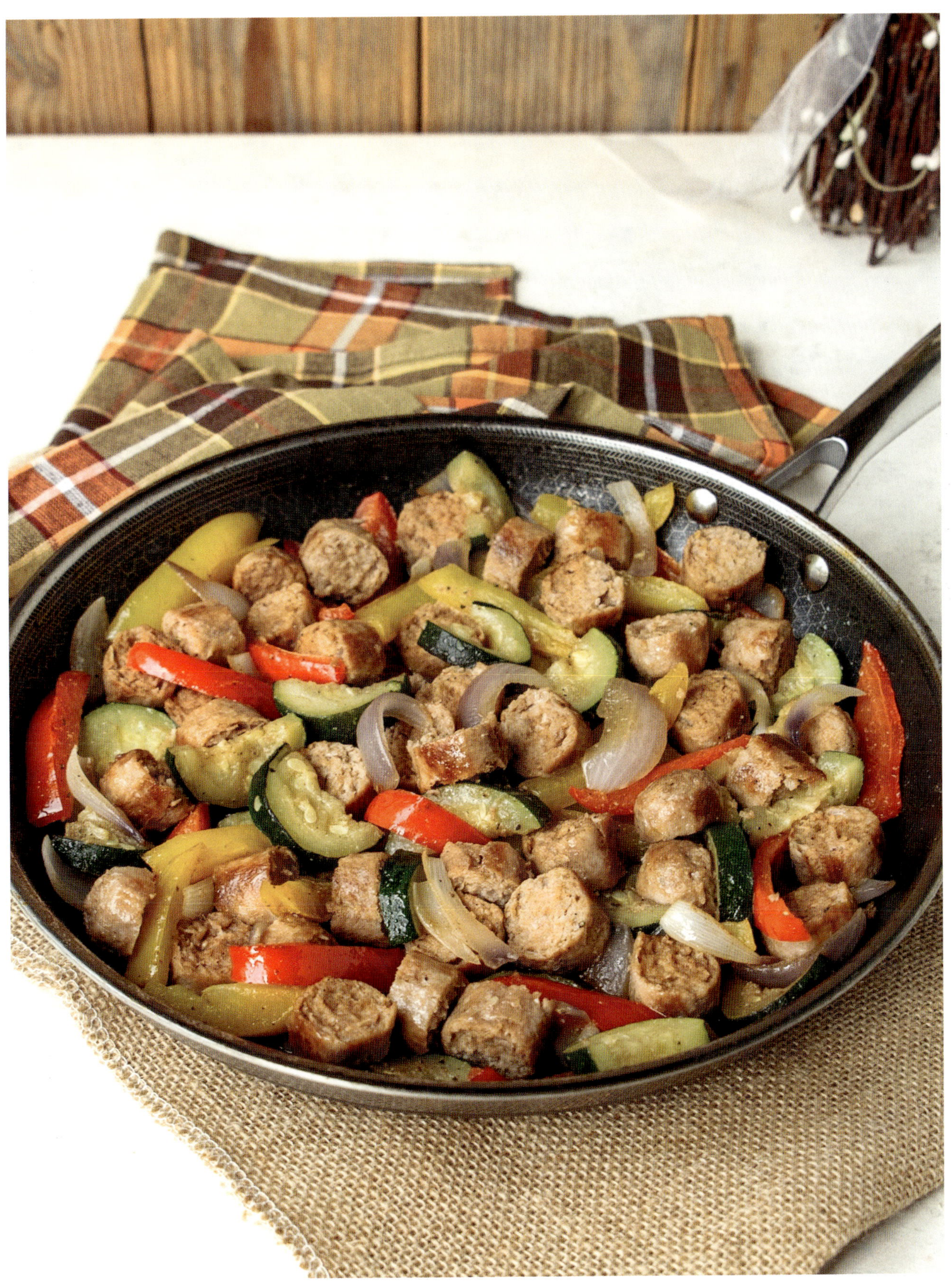

YIELD: 4 double smash burgers (1 per serving)
PREP TIME: 10 minutes
COOK TIME: 8 minutes

SHEET PAN DOUBLE SMASH CHEESEBURGERS WITH SECRET SAUCE

These are our new favorite burgers, I think because we love how thin they are, and stacking two makes them very satisfying. We like to put cheese and onion between the thin patties for a surprise filling. Between that and the sauce that really makes them extra good, we're addicted!

2 pounds 80/20 ground beef

1 teaspoon fine sea salt

1/2 teaspoon ground black pepper

4 slices cheddar cheese

4 thin, large-diameter slices red onion

FOR THE SECRET SAUCE:

1 cup avocado oil mayonnaise

1/4 cup distilled white vinegar

2 tablespoons prepared yellow mustard

1 tablespoon sugar-free ketchup

1 teaspoon garlic powder

1/2 teaspoon onion powder

1/4 teaspoon fine sea salt

1/4 teaspoon ground black pepper

FIXINGS (OPTIONAL):

Lettuce leaves

Tomato slices

Dill pickle chips

1. Weigh out 4 ounces of ground beef. Roll into a ball. Repeat, making a total of 8 balls (you will use 2 patties per burger).
2. Use a meat mallet or spatula to smash each burger into a thin patty. Don't worry about it being round; jagged edges are good! I place a piece of parchment paper over the balls to smash them so the meat doesn't stick to the tool I'm using. Place the patties on a plate in the fridge until ready to cook.
3. Place the sauce ingredients in a small bowl and whisk to combine. Taste and add more salt if needed. Refrigerate until ready to serve.
4. Place 2 rimmed baking sheets in the oven, one on the top rack and the other on the next rack down. Set the broiler to high and let the pans heat up for about 5 minutes to get them really hot.
5. Pull the top pan out of the oven and quickly place 4 burger patties on it. You should hear a sizzle. Immediately put the pan back under the broiler. Broil for 2 to 3 minutes, until the burgers are nicely browned.
6. Pull the burgers out of the oven and place 1 slice of cheese each on two of the burgers, then top with half of the onion slices, dividing them evenly between the two cheese-topped burgers. Stack the other 2 burgers on top. Place the pan back under the broiler just long enough to melt the cheese, about 1 minute, then remove. Repeat these steps with the second pan, using the remaining patties and placing the pan in the top position in the oven. Finish with the remaining cheese and onion slices to make another 2 double smash burgers.
7. Serve with the secret sauce and, if desired, fixings of your choice.

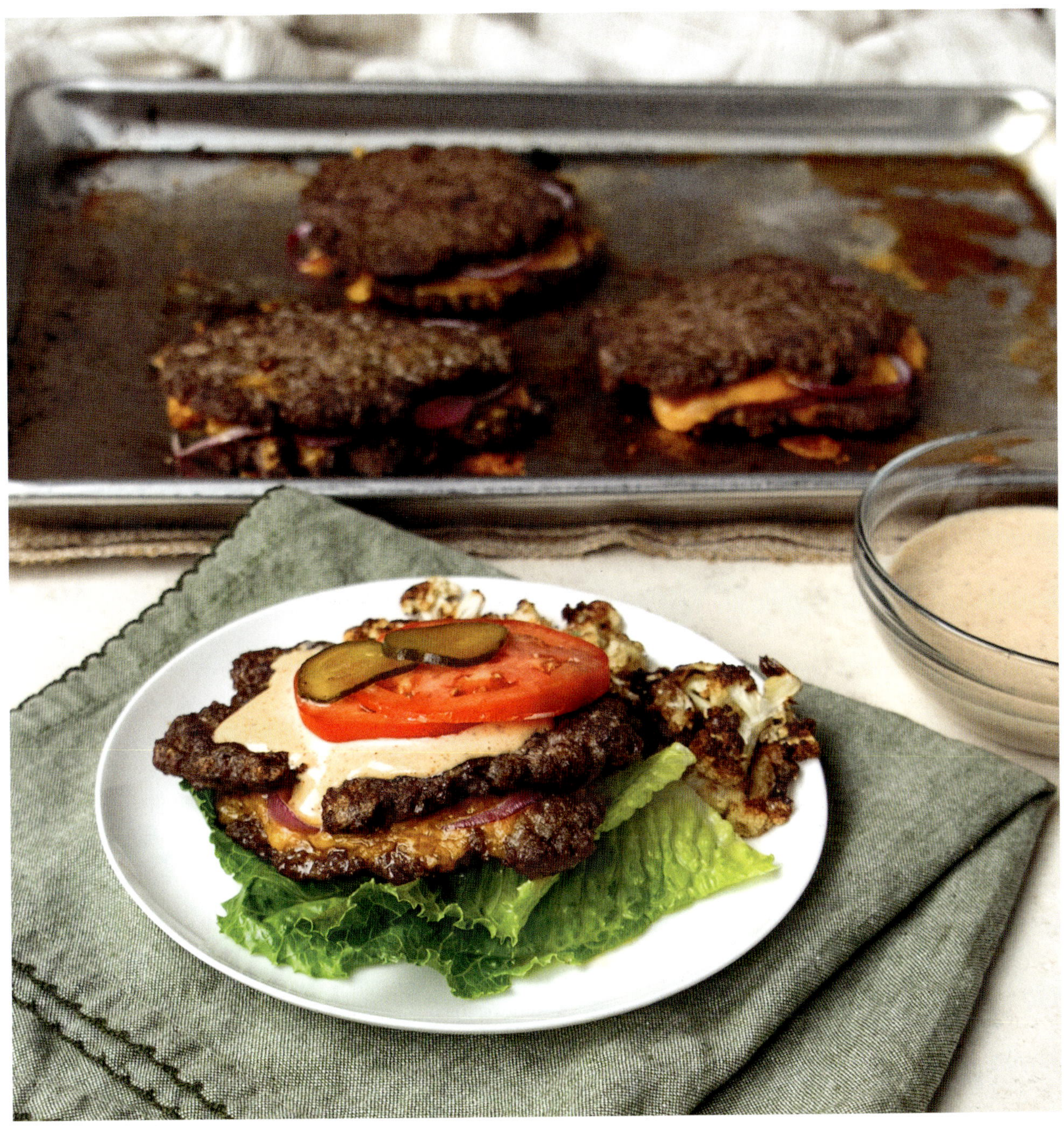

Make It Better: Though these smash burgers make a hearty meal and don't require a side, when I have time, I like to make my Crispy Smashed Cauliflower (page 271) for serving alongside.

Calories	Fat	Protein	Total Carbs	Dietary Fiber	Net Carbs
1,066	99g	44g	4g	1g	3g

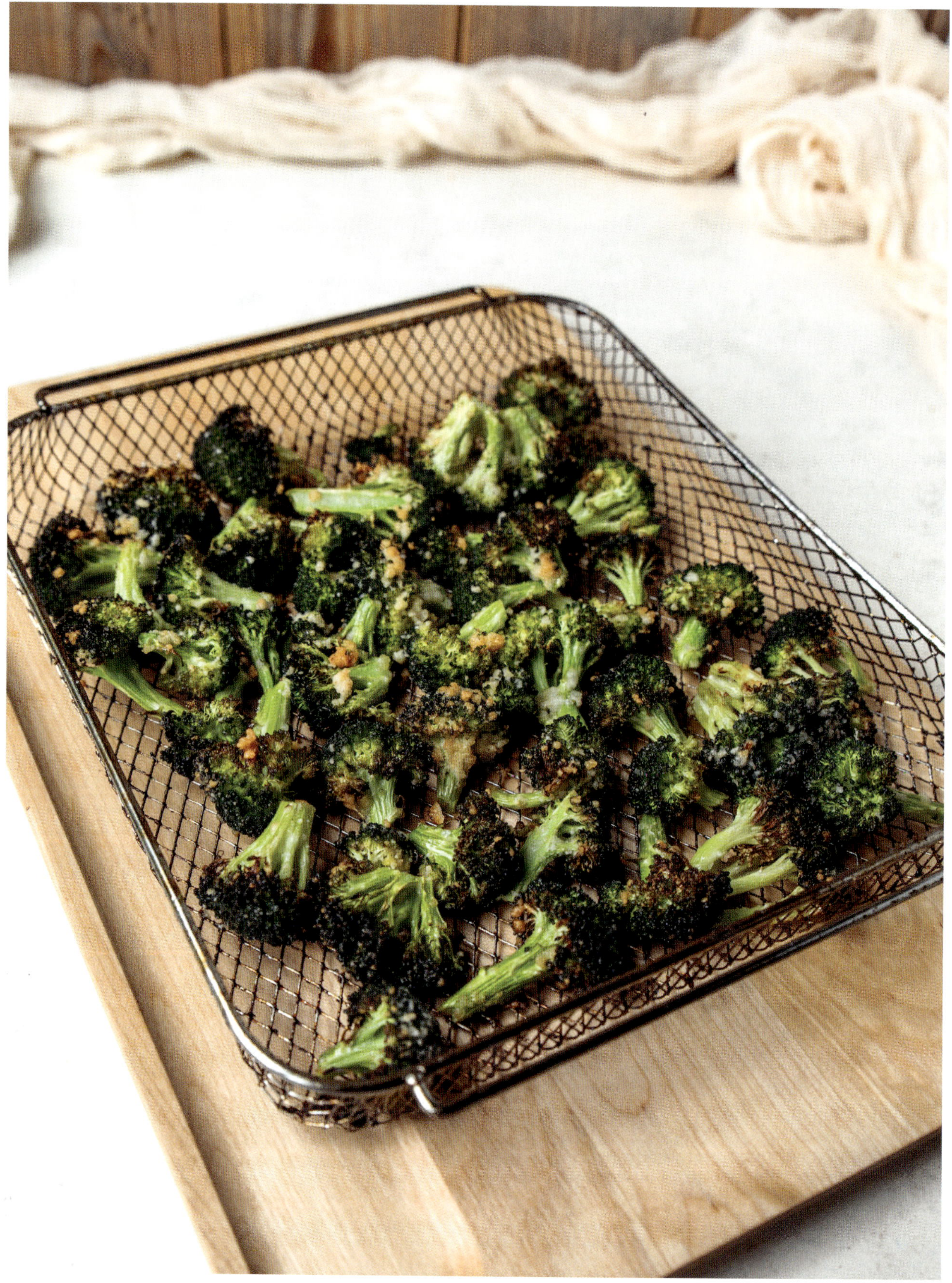

YIELD: 6 servings
PREP TIME: 5 minutes
COOK TIME: 15 minutes

GARLIC PARMESAN BROCCOLI

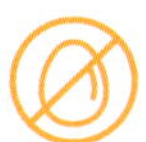 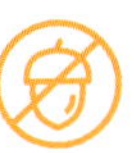 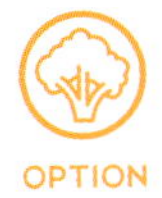

OPTION

My kids and I love a crispy broccoli with garlic and Parmesan! Broccoli is high in calcium.

- 1 pound broccoli florets
- 2 tablespoons extra-virgin olive oil
- ¼ cup grated Parmesan cheese
- 1 teaspoon garlic powder
- ½ teaspoon fine sea salt
- ¼ teaspoon ground black pepper

1. Preheat the oven to 425°F.
2. Place the florets on a rimmed baking sheet. Drizzle the olive oil over the florets and toss to coat. Sprinkle with the cheese and seasonings and toss again.
3. Roast for 12 to 15 minutes, until golden brown and tender.
4. Store in an airtight container in the refrigerator for up to 5 days.

NOTE: If you're a strict vegetarian, make sure to use a Parmesan cheese made without animal rennet.

Calories	Fat	Protein	Total Carbs	Dietary Fiber	Net Carbs
85	6g	4g	6g	2g	4g

YIELD: 4 servings
PREP TIME: 10 minutes
COOK TIME: 9 to 10 minutes, depending on method

GARLIC GREEN BEANS

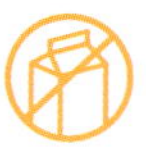 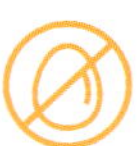 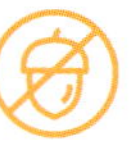 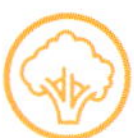
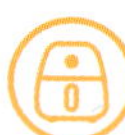

These delicious garlicky blistered green beans go with any main dish and can be prepared in two ways, both of which take very little time.

- **12 ounces green beans, trimmed**
- **2 tablespoons extra-virgin olive oil**
- **2 teaspoons minced garlic**
- **½ teaspoon fine sea salt**
- **¼ teaspoon ground black pepper**
- **Lemon wedges, for serving (optional)**

1. *To cook the beans in an air fryer,* put the green beans in a bowl and toss with the oil, garlic, salt, and pepper. Spread the beans in the air fryer basket in a single layer. Air-fry at 375°F for 8 to 10 minutes, until blistered and tender.

   To cook the beans on the stovetop, heat the oil in a large skillet over medium-high heat. Add the green beans to the hot skillet in a single layer and do not stir. Allow to cook undisturbed for 4 to 5 minutes, then stir and add the garlic, salt, and pepper. Cover and reduce the heat to medium-low. Cook for 3 to 4 minutes, until blistered and tender.
2. Serve with lemon wedges, if desired.

Calories	Fat	Protein	Total Carbs	Dietary Fiber	Net Carbs
91	7g	2g	7g	2g	5g

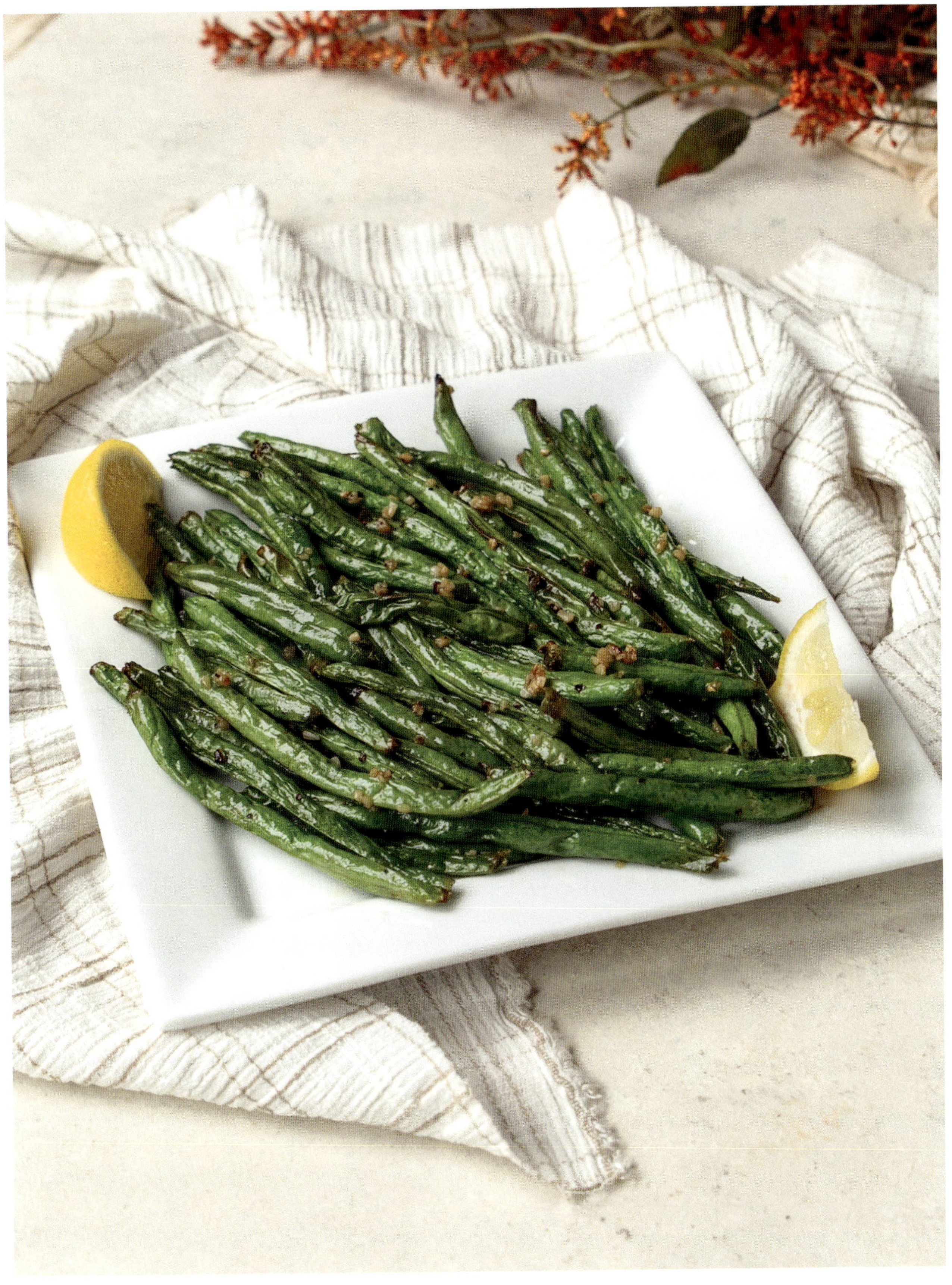

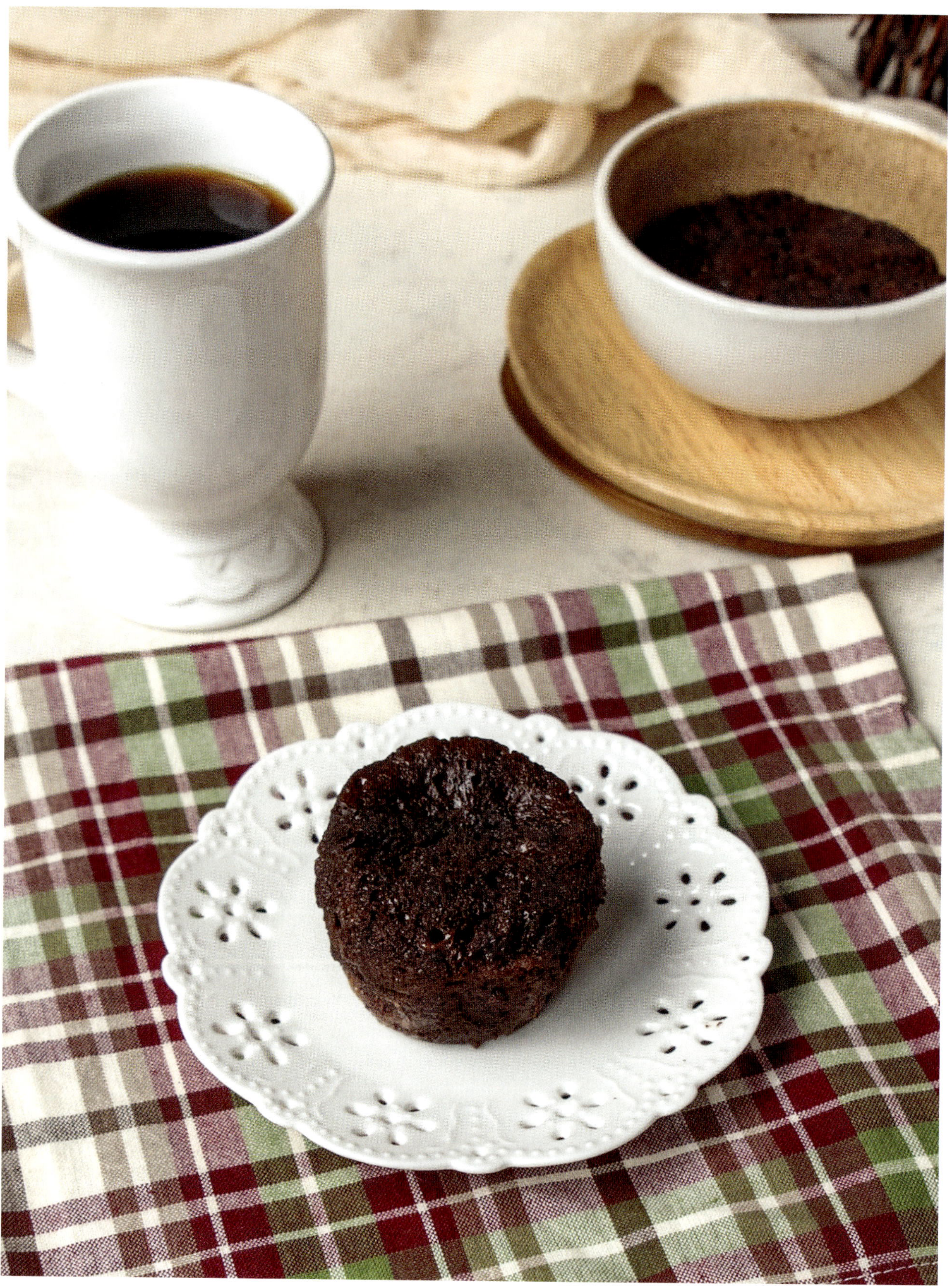

YIELD: 1 serving
PREP TIME: 5 minutes
COOK TIME: 1 minute or 10 to 15 minutes, depending on method

CHOCOLATE PROTEIN CAKE

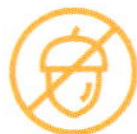  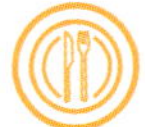

With just 5 minutes prep and 1 minute in the microwave, you can have an easy chocolate protein cake with 14 grams of protein! You can make a thinner cake or a taller one; it just depends on whether you use a bowl or a tall mug. If you prefer, you can bake this cake in the oven.

1 large egg

2 tablespoons cottage cheese (4% milkfat)

1 tablespoon unsweetened cocoa powder

1 tablespoon chocolate-flavored collagen peptides

1 tablespoon low-carb brown sugar–style sweetener

½ teaspoon instant espresso powder (optional)

¼ teaspoon baking powder

1. *If using the oven,* preheat it to 350°F and grease a 12-ounce ramekin.

   If using the microwave, spray a 12-ounce microwave-safe bowl, ramekin, or mug with cooking spray. If you'd like a taller cake, use a tall 16-ounce mug. A bowl or ramekin will produce a thinner cake.
2. In a small bowl, whisk together the egg and cottage cheese until well blended. Add the remaining ingredients and whisk to combine.
3. Pour the batter into the prepared ramekin or bowl.
4. *If using the microwave,* microwave on high power for 1 minute, or until a toothpick comes out clean when inserted in the center.

   If using the oven, place in the oven and bake for 10 to 15 minutes, or until a toothpick comes out clean when inserted in the center.
5. Enjoy immediately right from the ramekin or bowl or remove to a small plate if you prefer. If not eating right away, store in the fridge for up to 3 days and enjoy chilled.

Calories	Fat	Protein	Total Carbs	Dietary Fiber	Net Carbs
141	7g	14g	7g	3g	4g

YIELD: 1 servings
PREP TIME: 2 minutes

NO-COOK CHOCOLATE PROTEIN PUDDING

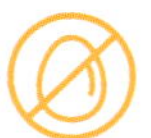 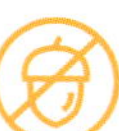 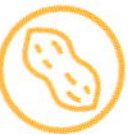 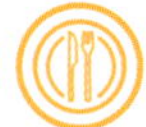

It tastes like a traditional pudding, but no cooking is required. You can also use part-skim ricotta cheese or full-fat plain Greek yogurt in place of the cottage cheese. Using cottage cheese in this no bake pudding gives it a texture similar to tapioca pudding. If you prefer, you can use an immersion blender to give the pudding a smooth texture.

¼ cup cottage cheese (4% milkfat), preferably small curd

1 tablespoon unsweetened cocoa powder

1 tablespoon powdered peanut butter (see note)

1 teaspoon chocolate-flavored liquid monk fruit or other low-carb sweetener of choice, plus more if needed

1 tablespoon chocolate-flavored collagen peptides

Sugar-free chocolate chips, for garnish (optional)

Put all the ingredients in a 6-ounce ramekin or bowl. Mix, taste, and add more sweetener if needed. Garnish with chocolate chips, if desired. Enjoy immediately or store in the fridge for up to 5 days.

NOTE: Powdered peanut butter, aka peanut butter powder, is available in a sugar-free version that's sweetened with monk fruit, which is what I used in this recipe, and in a pure form that is 100% peanuts, with no added salt or sweetener of any kind. You can use the latter type for this recipe if you like, but if you do, you'll want to add a little more low-carb sweetener.

Calories	Fat	Protein	Total Carbs	Dietary Fiber	Net Carbs
176	7g	21g	10g	3g	7g

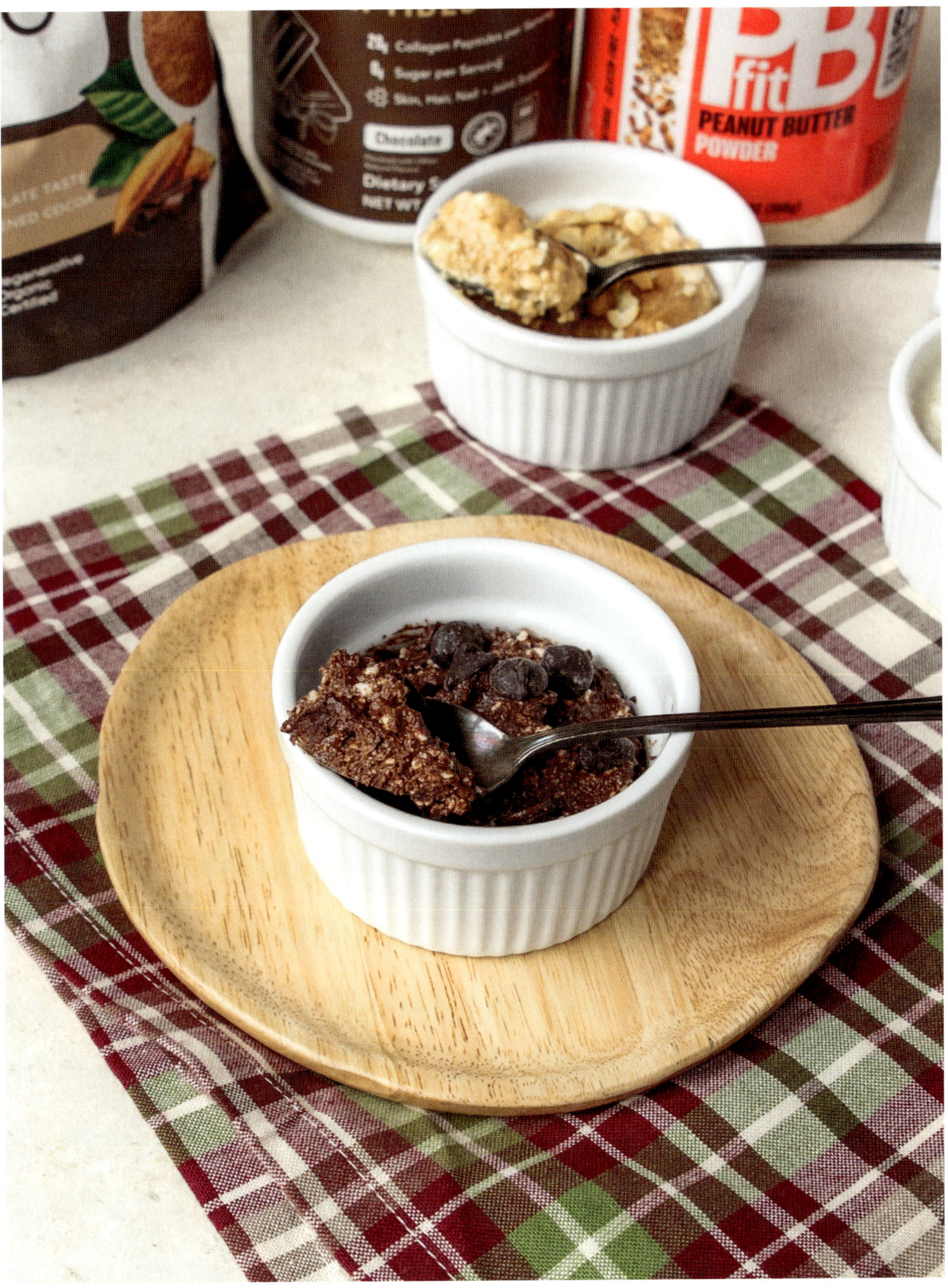
PB fit
PEANUT BUTTER
POWDER
Chocolate

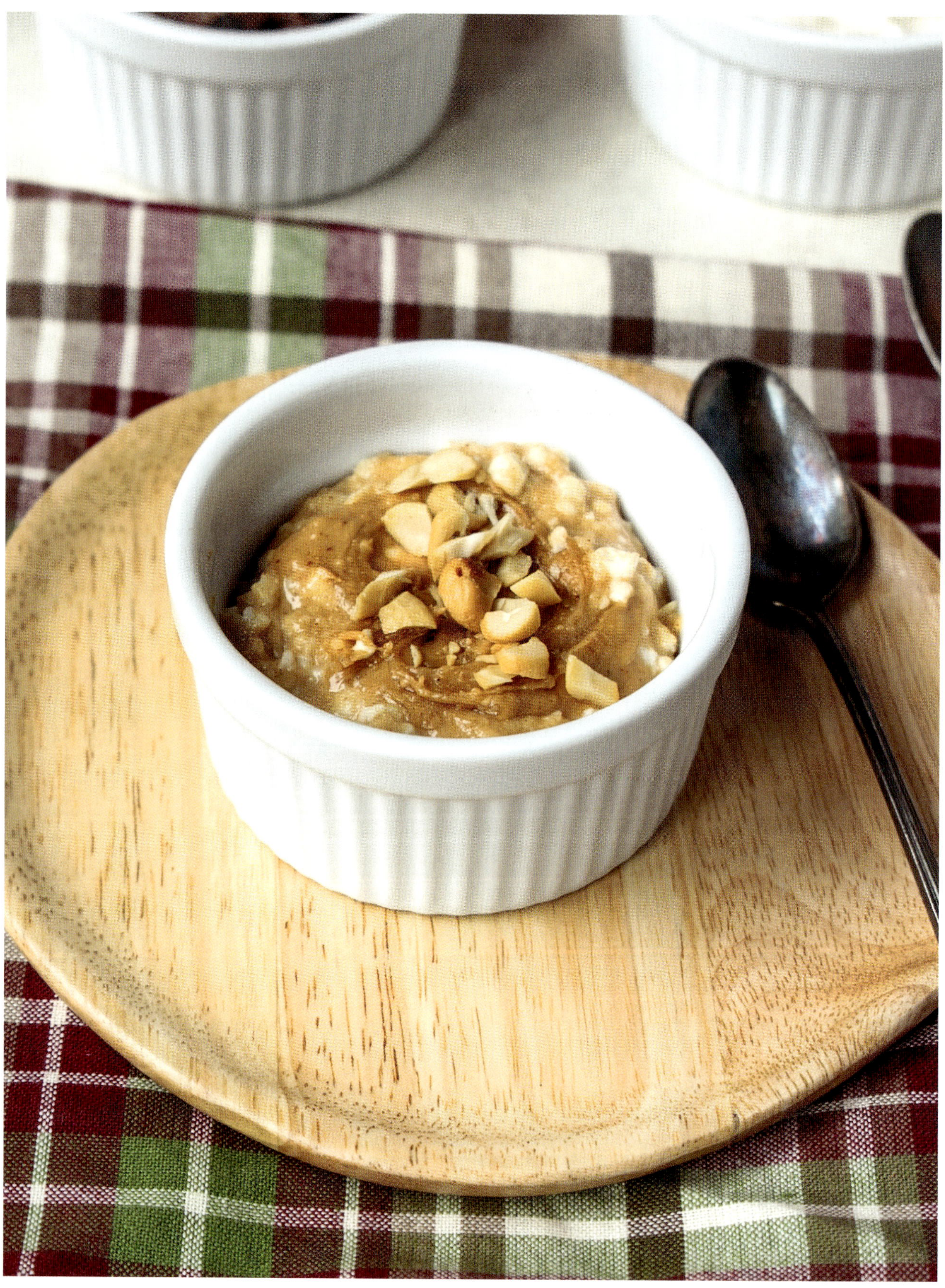

YIELD: 1 servings
PREP TIME: 2 minutes

NO-COOK PEANUT BUTTER PROTEIN PUDDING

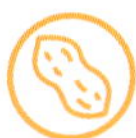
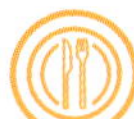

This quick protein pudding can be whipped up in a minute and enjoyed immediately or chilled in the refrigerator for a quick snack anytime. Using cottage cheese in this no-cook pudding gives it a texture similar to tapioca pudding. If you prefer, you can use an immersion blender to give the pudding a smooth texture.

- ¼ cup cottage cheese (4% milkfat), preferably small curd
- 2 tablespoons powdered peanut butter (see note, page 142)
- 2 tablespoons vanilla-flavored collagen peptides
- 1 teaspoon vanilla-flavored liquid stevia or other low-carb sweetener of choice, plus more if needed
- Chopped roasted peanuts, for garnish (optional)

Put all the ingredients in a 6-ounce ramekin or bowl. Mix, taste, and add more sweetener if needed. Garnish with chopped peanuts, if desired. Enjoy immediately or store in the fridge for up to 5 days.

Calories	Fat	Protein	Total Carbs	Dietary Fiber	Net Carbs
191	7g	25g	5g	0g	5g

YIELD: 1 serving
PREP TIME: 2 minutes

NO-COOK CHEESECAKE PROTEIN PUDDING

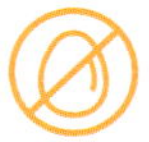 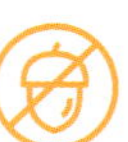 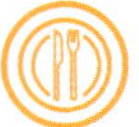

This pudding has a classic cheesecake flavor with the tanginess of the cream cheese shining through. Using cottage cheese in this no-bake pudding gives it a texture similar to tapioca pudding. If you prefer, you can use an immersion blender to give the pudding a smooth texture. If you prefer a flavored cheesecake, simply swap the vanilla-flavored collagen peptides with your favorite flavor.

¼ cup cottage cheese (4% milkfat), preferably small curd

2 tablespoons vanilla-flavored collagen peptides

1 tablespoon cream cheese, softened

1 teaspoon vanilla-flavored liquid stevia or low-carb sweetener of choice, plus more if needed

Put all the ingredients in a 6-ounce ramekin or bowl. Mix, taste, and add more sweetener if needed. Enjoy immediately or store in the fridge for up to 5 days.

Calories	Fat	Protein	Total Carbs	Dietary Fiber	Net Carbs
152	8g	16g	3g	0g	3g

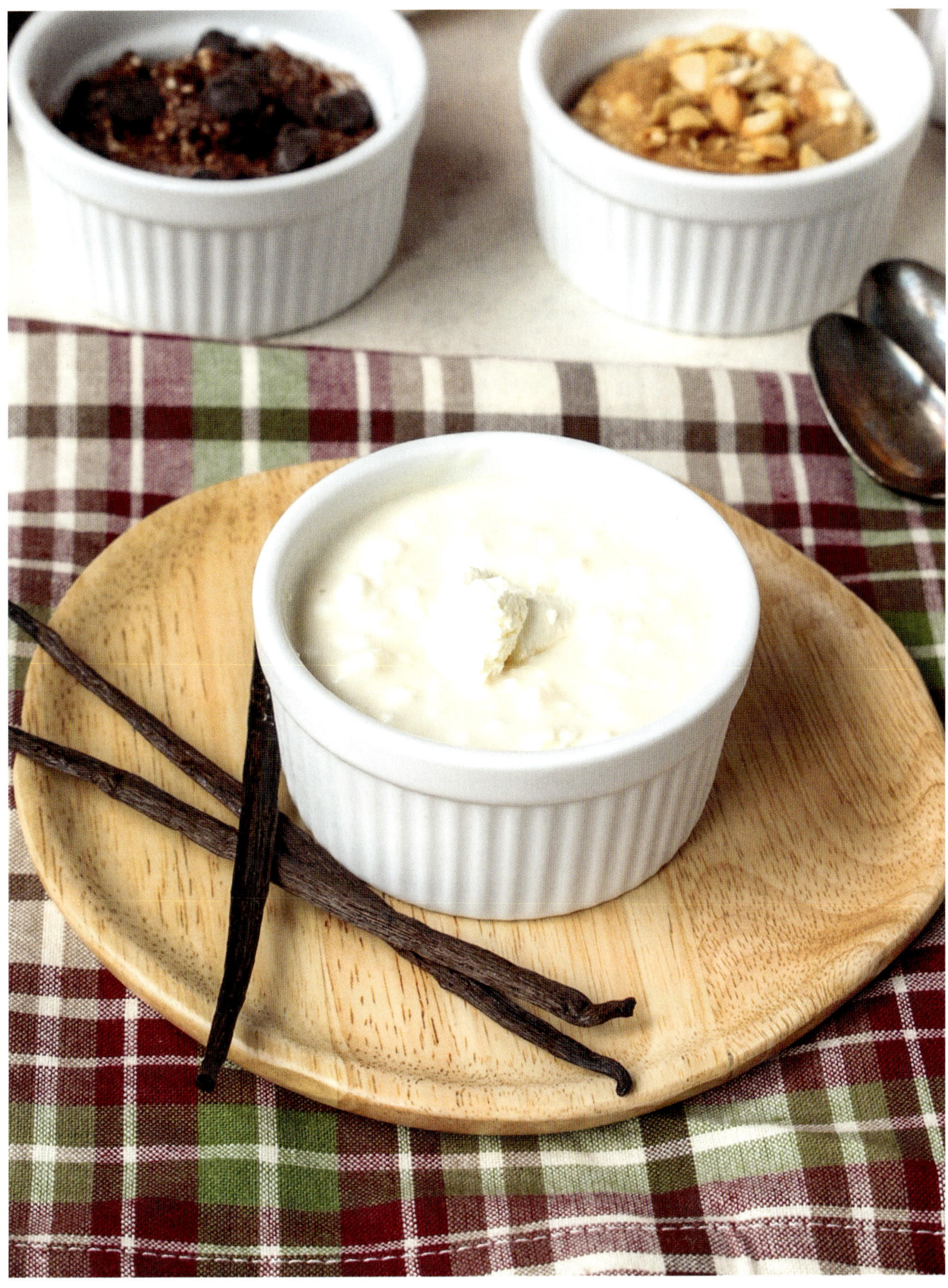

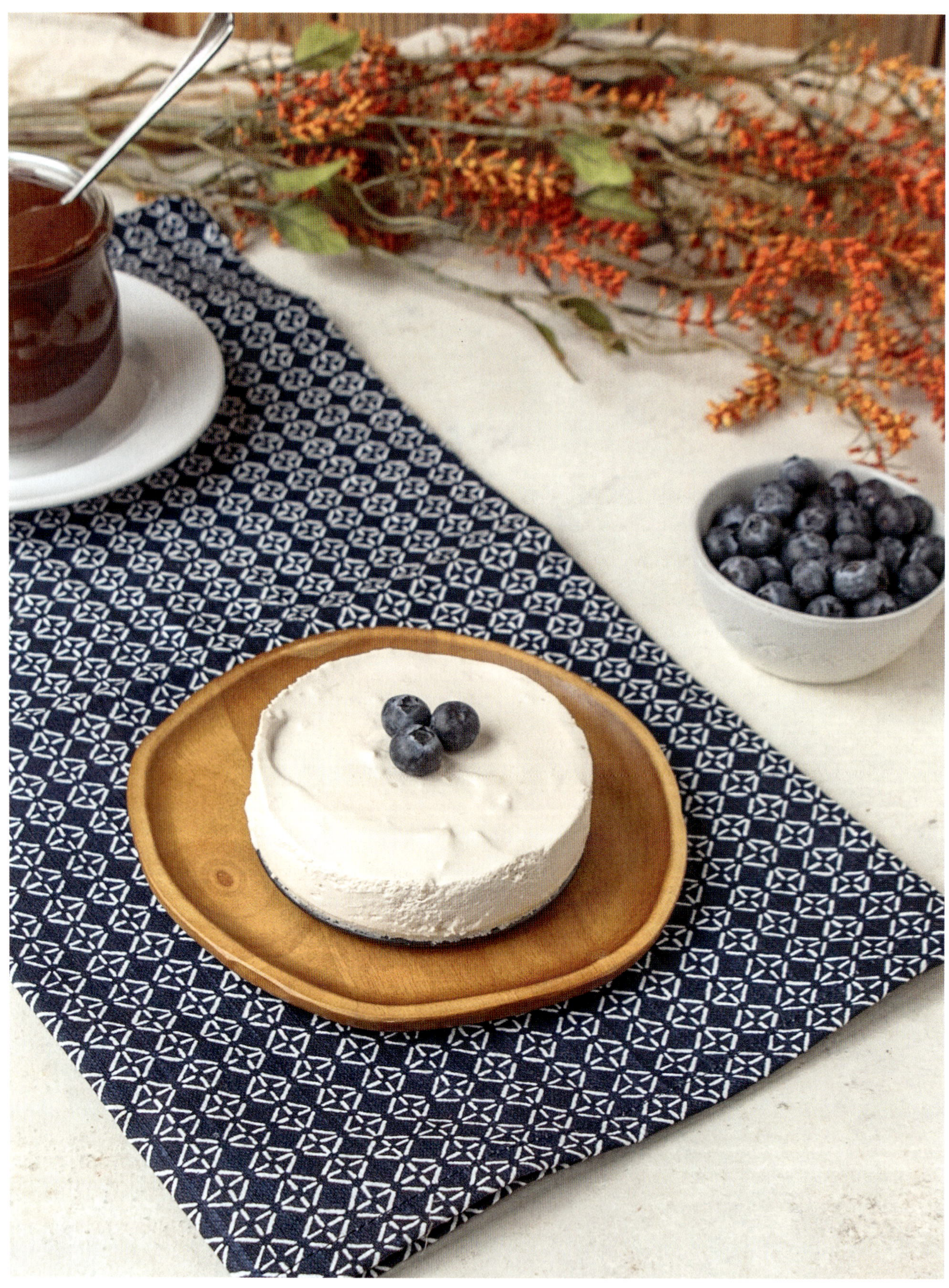

YIELD: 2 servings

PREP TIME: 10 minutes, plus 4 hours to chill

COOK TIME: 1 minute

NO-BAKE CHEESECAKE FOR TWO

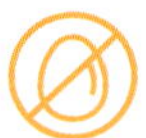 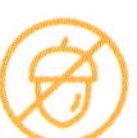 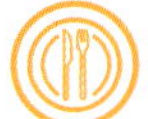

When you want some cheesecake but don't want a week's worth of leftovers to tempt you, this is just the right size. Make it ahead and store it in the fridge for an easy treat that helps you stay on track! Although cottage cheese isn't a traditional ingredient in cheesecake, it boosts the protein content of the dessert, giving it a healthier profile.

1/2 teaspoon unflavored gelatin powder

2 tablespoons water

2 ounces (1/4 cup) cream cheese, softened

3 tablespoons cottage cheese (4% milkfat)

1/2 teaspoon vanilla extract

1/4 cup heavy cream

1 teaspoon vanilla-flavored liquid stevia or liquid monk fruit

Pinch of fine sea salt

Special equipment: 4-inch springform pan

1. Sprinkle the gelatin over the water in a small microwave-safe bowl. Let sit for a minute to bloom then heat in the microwave for 1 minute. Stir until gelatin is dissolved and there are no clumps. Set aside to cool.
2. Using either a food processor, high-powered blender, or medium mixing bowl and an electric mixer, blend the cream cheese, cottage cheese, and vanilla until smooth.
3. Pour the heavy cream and sweetener into the cream cheese mixture and blend again until well combined. Taste and adjust the sweetener if needed.
4. Drizzle in the cooled gelatin mixture and blend until incorporated.
5. Spread the cheesecake batter into a 4-inch springform pan and refrigerate for 4 hours or overnight. Remove the sides of the springform pan and cut in half to make 2 servings. Store covered in the fridge for up to 5 days.

Make It Better: Serve topped with ganache (page 84).

Calories	Fat	Protein	Total Carbs	Dietary Fiber	Net Carbs
230	21g	5g	3g	0g	3g

YIELD: 16 bites
(1 per serving)

PREP TIME: 10 minutes, plus 30 minutes to chill dough

NO-BAKE COOKIE DOUGH BITES

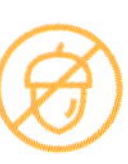
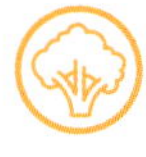
OPTION

Enjoy these quick-to-make edible cookie dough bites any time you get a craving for cookie dough. Or bake them for a warm low-carb cakelike cookie (see variation below). Try them with chocolate chips or pretty rainbow sprinkles.

½ cup (1 stick) unsalted butter, softened

1½ cups blanched almond flour or sunflower seed meal

½ cup vanilla-flavored whey protein powder (30 grams)

2 tablespoons confectioners'-style low-carb sweetener

1 teaspoon vanilla extract

¼ teaspoon fine sea salt

½ cup sugar-free chocolate chips, or ¼ cup naturally colored low-carb rainbow sprinkles (see note)

NOTE: I use Good Dee's Rainbow Sprinkles. Other brands are fine; just make sure the carb content is no higher than 3 grams per serving.

1. Put all the ingredients, except the chocolate chips or sprinkles, in a food processor and blend until you have a smooth dough. Alternatively, you can mix the ingredients in a large bowl with an electric hand mixer or a wooden spoon. Stir in the chocolate chips or sprinkles. Refrigerate for 30 minutes.
2. Scoop up a tablespoon of the dough, form into a ball, and place on a parchment paper–lined tray. Repeat to make a total of 16 balls. Dough bites will keep in the refrigerator in a sealed container for up to 1 week. They can also be frozen in a single layer in an airtight container for up to 3 months.

VARIATION: Baked Cookies. Preheat the oven to 350°F. Complete the recipe as written. Place the cookie dough balls on a parchment paper–lined baking sheet, leaving 1 inch between them. Flatten slightly with wet fingers. Bake for 12 to 14 minutes, until golden brown. Cookies will keep for 2 days on the counter.

MADE WITH CHOCOLATE CHIPS

Calories	Fat	Protein	Total Carbs	Dietary Fiber	Net Carbs
136	13g	4g	3g	1g	2g

MADE WITH RAINBOW SPRINKLES

Calories	Fat	Protein	Total Carbs	Dietary Fiber	Net Carbs
122	11g	4g	5g	1g	4g

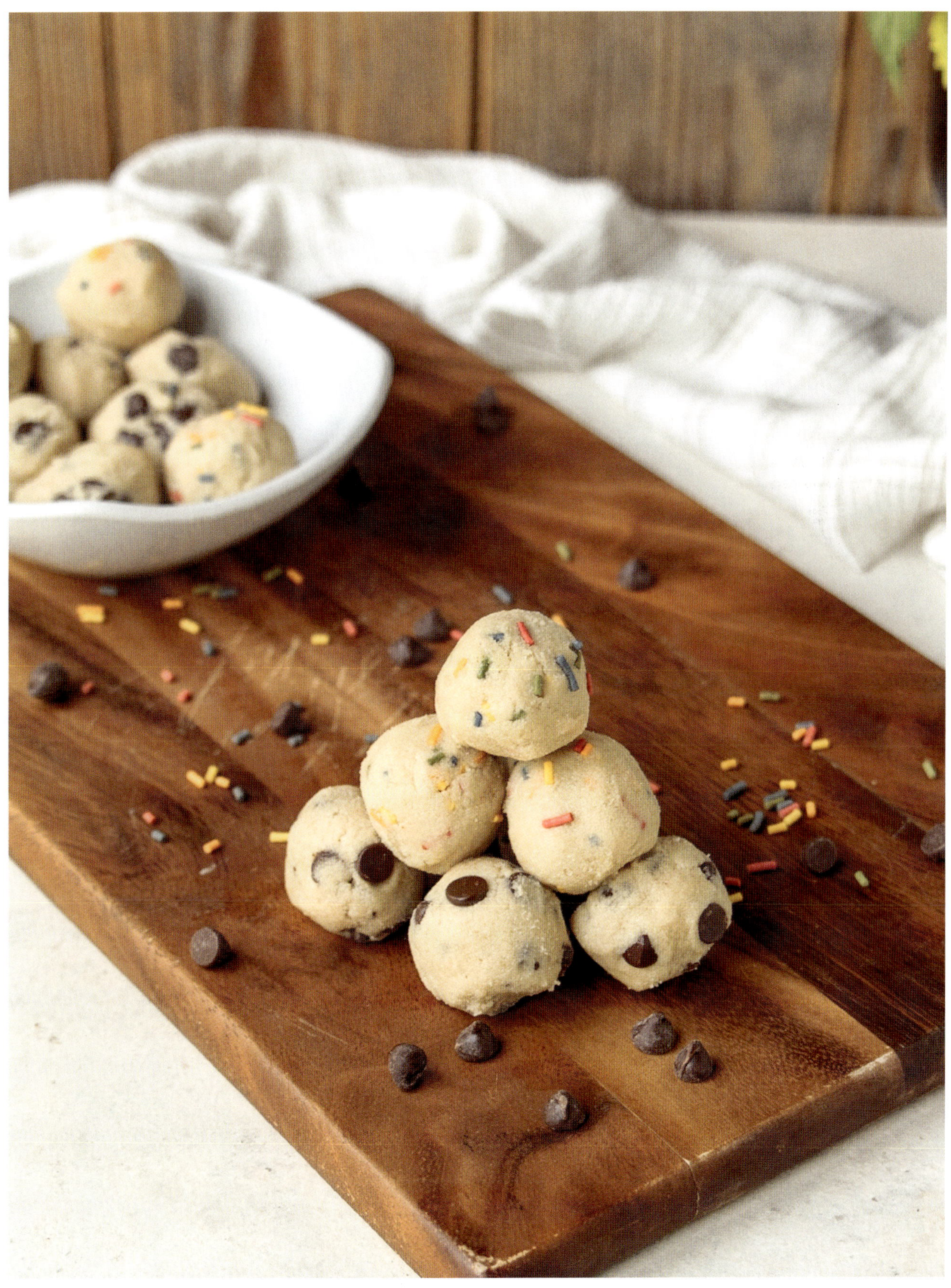

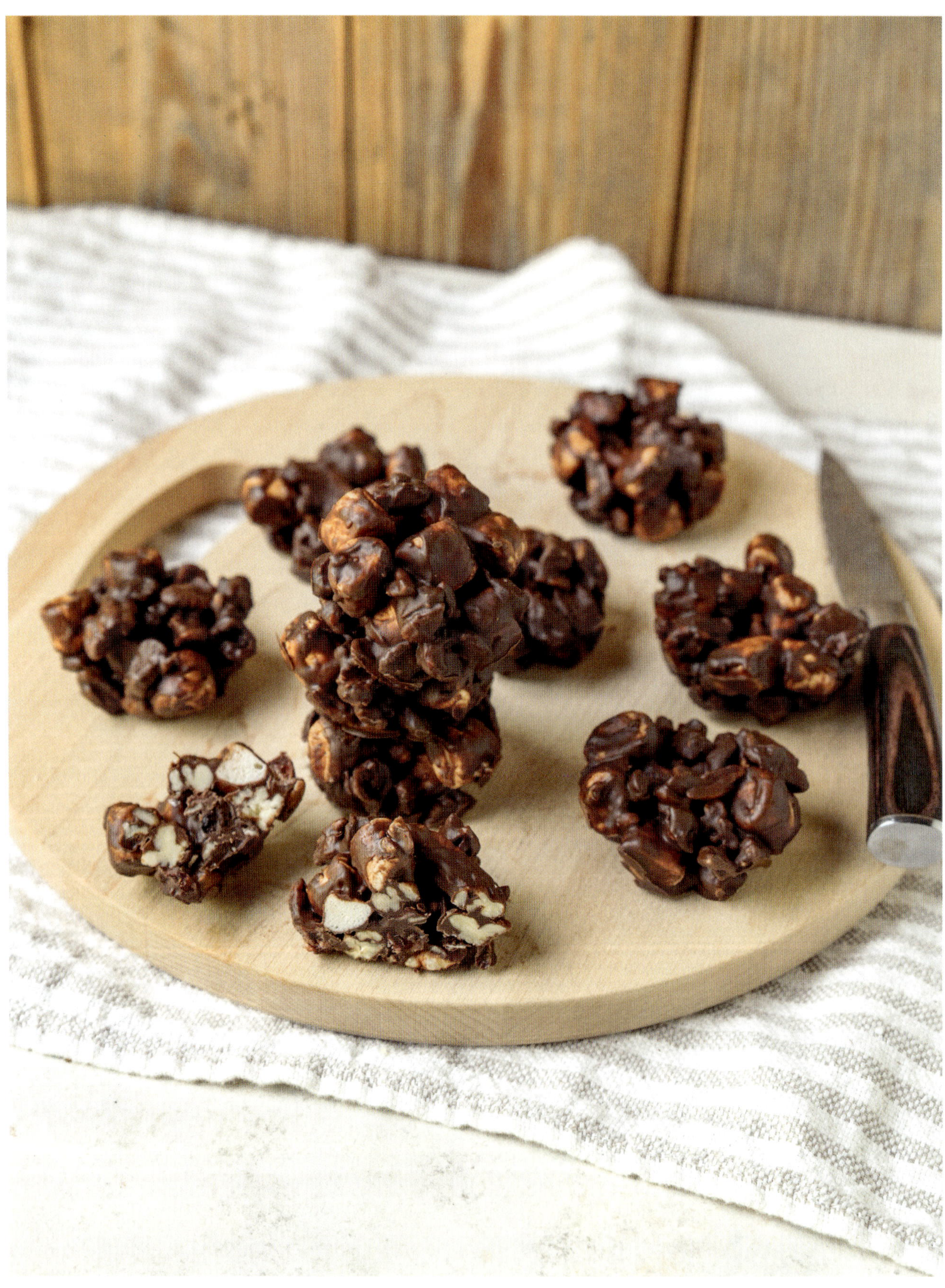

YIELD: 12 bites (1 per serving)

PREP TIME: 5 minutes, plus 30 minutes to chill

COOK TIME: 1 minute

ROCKY ROAD BITES

 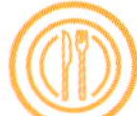

These bites are ideal for when you want a quick little treat for family and friends and don't have time to bake. I always keep the pantry items needed for these sweet morsels on hand, so that when the need (or urge) arises, I can whip up a batch.

- ¾ cup sugar-free chocolate chips
- 2 tablespoons unsalted butter
- 1 cup raw pecans, chopped
- 3⅓ cups sugar-free mini marshmallows
- ⅓ packed cup unsweetened dried cranberries, chopped

1. Have on hand a 12-well silicone muffin pan or place 12 cupcake liners in a standard muffin pan.
2. Put the chocolate chips and butter in a large microwave-safe bowl and heat in 30-second increments, stirring until melted. Once completely melted, stir until smooth, with no lumps remaining.
3. Add the pecans, marshmallows, and cranberries to the chocolate mixture and stir to coat. Pour the mixture into the wells of the muffin pan, filling each about halfway. Refrigerate for 30 minutes before serving.
4. Store in the refrigerator for up to 1 week or freeze in an airtight container for up to 3 months.

NOTE: If you don't have a 12-well muffin pan, you can make this recipe in an 8-inch square baking pan lined with parchment paper. Simply pour the mixture into the prepared pan, spread it with a rubber spatula, and refrigerate for 30 minutes. To serve, cut into 12 pieces.

Calories	Fat	Protein	Total Carbs	Dietary Fiber	Net Carbs
151	12g	2g	6g	1g	5g

YIELD: 15 or 18 truffles (1 per serving)

PREP TIME: 20 minutes, plus 30 minutes to chill filling

COOK TIME: 4 minutes

WHITE CHOCOLATE STRAWBERRY TRUFFLES—2 WAYS

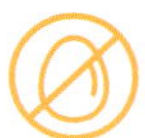 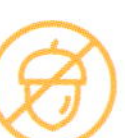 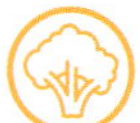

These are super quick to prepare. Once the filling is chilled, you simply form it into truffle balls and then roll them into either unsweetened shredded coconut or crushed freeze-dried strawberries! The filling of the coconut-coated truffles (version 1) uses stevia, strawberry extract, and natural food coloring to get that strawberry color and flavor; for version 2, freeze-dried strawberries provide natural strawberry flavor and sweetness as well as a natural pink color. Though the coconut-coated truffles have fewer calories and carbs than the other, it's nice to know there's an all-natural option.

FOR THE BASE:

1 cup sugar-free white chocolate chips

¼ cup (½ stick) unsalted butter

3 tablespoons heavy cream

FOR VERSION 1:

½ teaspoon berry- or vanilla-flavored stevia

½ teaspoon strawberry extract

3 drops natural red food coloring (optional)

Pinch of fine sea salt

½ cup unsweetened shredded coconut, for coating truffles

1. Line a rimmed baking sheet with parchment paper. If making version 2, finely chop the freeze-dried strawberries using a sharp knife or a food processor until you have a fine crumb texture. Set aside.
2. Make the base: In a small saucepan, heat the chocolate chips, butter, and cream over low heat, stirring constantly, until melted, about 3 or 4 minutes. Remove the pan from the heat.
3. *If making version 1,* stir in the stevia, strawberry extract, food coloring (if using), and salt. Once thoroughly combined, check the color and, if it is not as pink as you'd like, stir in another drop or two of food coloring.

   If making version 2, stir in ½ cup of the crushed freeze-dried strawberries and salt. Taste and decide if it needs more sweetness. If it does, simply crush more freeze-dried strawberries and stir in.
4. Place the filling in the fridge for 30 minutes to firm up. To prepare for the coating step, put the shredded coconut or remaining crushed freeze-dried strawberries in a shallow bowl.
5. Using a 1-tablespoon measuring spoon, scoop the chilled filling onto the prepared pan. If making version 1, you should be able to make 18 mounds; if making version 2, you will only get 15 mounds. Roll the mounds into balls, then roll them in the coconut or crushed strawberries.

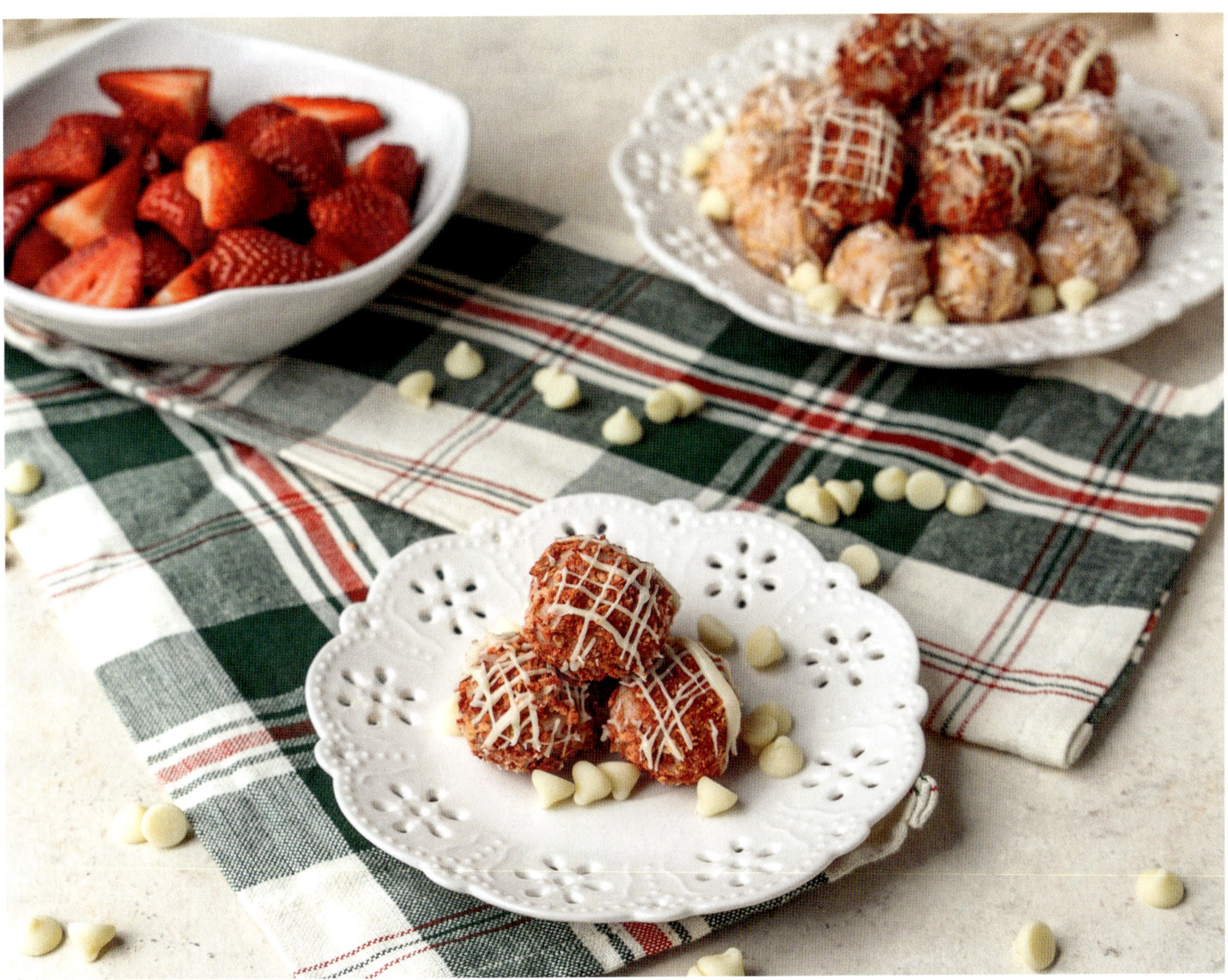

FOR VERSION 2:

1 ounce freeze-dried strawberries (about 1 cup), plus more if needed

Pinch of fine sea salt

FOR DRIZZLE (OPTIONAL):

¼ cup sugar-free white chocolate chips

6. If you want to drizzle the truffles with chocolate, melt the ¼ cup of white chocolate chips in the microwave for 30 seconds or in a small saucepan over low heat on the stovetop. Stir until smooth. Using a small spoon, drizzle the melted chocolate over the truffles, moving your hand back and forth to create a zigzag pattern.
7. Store in an airtight container in the refrigerator for up to 1 week or freeze for up to 3 months.

VERSION 1

Calories	Fat	Protein	Total Carbs	Dietary Fiber	Net Carbs
96	9g	1g	8g	3g	5g

VERSION 2

Calories	Fat	Protein	Total Carbs	Dietary Fiber	Net Carbs
108	9g	0.2g	11g	4g	7g

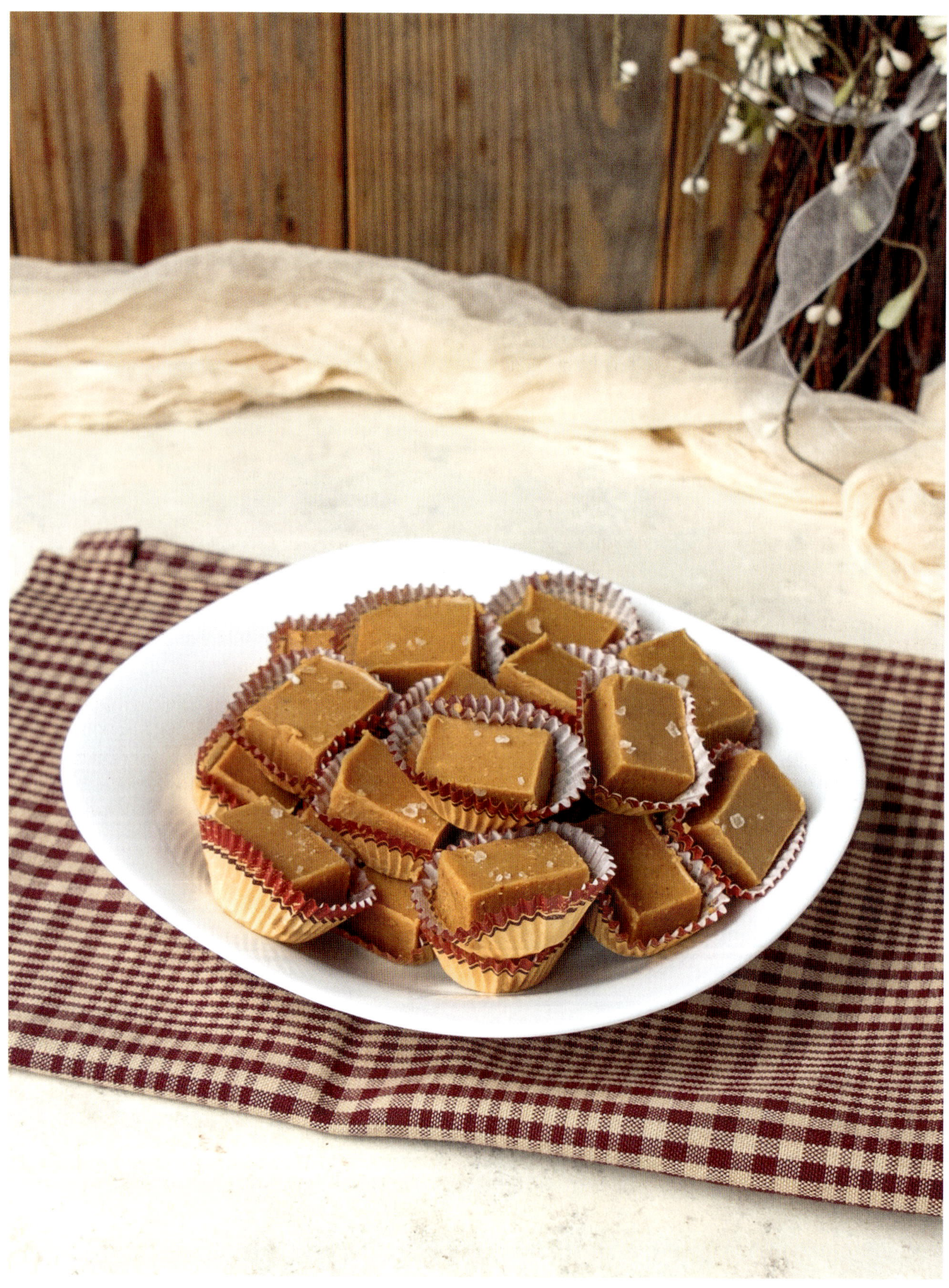

YIELD: 12 bites (1 per serving)
PREP TIME: 5 minutes, plus 2 hours to set
COOK TIME: 3 minutes

SALTED CARAMEL PEANUT BUTTER FUDGE

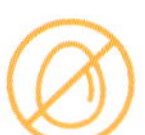 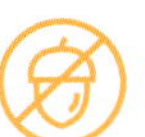 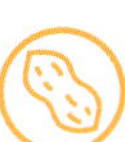 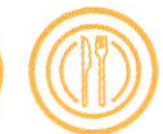

Most everyone loves peanut butter, and most everyone loves caramel. You might be surprised by how delicious the two are together! If you have the time to make my recipe for sugar-free caramel sauce, it really takes the flavor of this fudge up a notch!

1 cup unsweetened peanut butter (salted or unsalted)

½ cup (1 stick) unsalted butter

½ cup sugar-free caramel sauce, homemade (page 83) or store-bought, or maple-flavored allulose syrup

2 teaspoons caramel extract

1 teaspoon caramel-flavored liquid stevia, or low-carb sweetener of choice to taste

Pinch of salt (if using unsalted peanut butter)

Flaky sea salt, for garnish

1. Line an 8 by 5-inch loaf pan with parchment paper, allowing the paper to hang over the sides for easy removal.
2. Slightly melt or soften the peanut butter and butter together in the microwave for 1 minute or in small saucepan on the stovetop over low heat for about 3 minutes.
3. Transfer the peanut butter mixture to a blender and add the rest of the ingredients. Blend until combined.
4. Pour into the prepared loaf pan. Refrigerate until set, about 2 hours. To serve, cut into 12 pieces. Store in an airtight container in the fridge for up to 1 week. You can also freeze it for up to 3 months: After slicing the fudge into 12 pieces, store it in an airtight container between pieces of parchment paper for easy removal later.

MADE WITH KETO CARAMEL SAUCE, PAGE 83

Calories	Fat	Protein	Total Carbs	Dietary Fiber	Net Carbs
190	19g	3g	3g	1g	2g

BACKUP PLAN B

GOOD (ENOUGH) MEALS

This handy list of backup meals is the way to conquer those days when things don't go as planned for that recipe you'd hoped to make. I know what it's like to fail at dinner. When I was a teacher and young mother of my first child, I was super proud of myself for making a meal in the slow cooker to have ready for hubby and me when we got home from work. It was a beautiful pork tenderloin with veggies, and I was excited for it! After I picked up my son at day care, we arrived home. Instead of being greeted by the lovely aromas of the slow-cooked meal I was anticipating, there was no smell at all! I was positive I had turned the slow cooker on. I discovered that yes, I had turned it ON, but I sadly never plugged it in! These situations are why you need a plan B.

Having some prepared items in your pantry, fridge, and freezer will be a lifesaver when you need to make quick meals for you and the family. Most of the ingredients for the plan B meals included here can be purchased fully cooked and ready to use. No prep work needed. These quick meals practically cook themselves! Note that basic pantry items like cooking oil and seasonings are not included in these lists, so please review the instructions to make sure you have everything you need before you start cooking.

MEAL 1

SHRIMP STIR-FRY

Frozen cooked shrimp

Frozen broccoli

Frozen cauliflower rice

Remove the frozen shrimp from the bag and put in a bowl, then cover with cold water and set aside to defrost while you prepare the vegetables. In a medium skillet, heat about 2 tablespoons of avocado oil, olive oil, or coconut oil over medium-high heat. Add the broccoli and cauliflower rice and toss to coat in the oil. Cover the pan, then lower the heat to medium and steam until tender. Sprinkle with some seasonings of your choice, like garlic powder, onion powder, salt, and/or pepper. Remove the shrimp from the cold water and toss into the skillet with the vegetables. Let cook long enough just to heat through. I like topping this quick shrimp stir-fry with a sprinkle of sesame seeds and coconut aminos.

MEAL 2

QUICK QUESADILLA

Frozen ready-to-eat grilled chicken strips (about 3 per wrap)

Bagged shredded cheddar cheese

Egg white wraps*

*My favorite brand of egg white wraps is Egglife. You can find them in the refrigerator section of your grocery store.

Defrost the grilled chicken strips in the microwave for 1 to 2 minutes or in a skillet on the stove for about 5 minutes. Set aside. Grease a large skillet with cooking spray and set over medium heat. Working with two egg wraps at a time, place them in the skillet. Heat the wraps for about 30 seconds, then add an even layer of shredded cheese onto half of each wrap. Place an even layer of chicken strips on top of the cheese, using about 3 strips per wrap. Fold the other side of the wrap over the chicken and cheese to form a semi-circle and continue to cook for 1 to 2 minutes, until browned on the underside. Then flip the wrap over to cook for another 1 to 2 minutes to brown the other side.

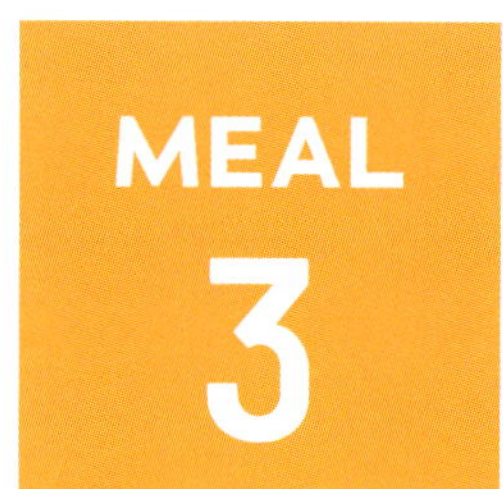

BACON BURGERS

Frozen precooked hamburgers*

Precooked bacon (or homemade equivalent, see page 76)**

Sliced cheese of choice (optional)

Frozen "Cloudies" Cloudbread,* defrosted (or homemade equivalent, see page 88)**

Condiments and burger fixings of choice

Place frozen precooked hamburgers in a skillet over medium-high heat. Add precooked bacon to the pan, placing it around the hamburgers. Cover and allow to heat through for about 5 minutes. Flip the hamburgers over and cook for 3 to 4 more minutes. If using cheese, top with cheese and cover to melt. Place the burgers between split and toasted cloud rolls and top with the bacon. Serve with condiments and burger fixings of your choice.

*I suggest the Ball Park brand packages of frozen fully cooked flame grilled beef patties, available at Walmart and other stores. Or use your own homemade stash of frozen precooked burgers. To speed prep time, you can use ready-to-cook preformed patties.

**Precooked bacon is sold in the refrigerated sections of grocery stores. Or you can batch-cook bacon at home and freeze it for later!

***Cloudies is a trademarked name for cloud bread rolls made by The Cloud Bread Company. You can order them online, directly from the company's website, or look for them at in the freezer sections of most supermarkets. I've found them at Walmart, Super Stop & Shop, and Market Basket.

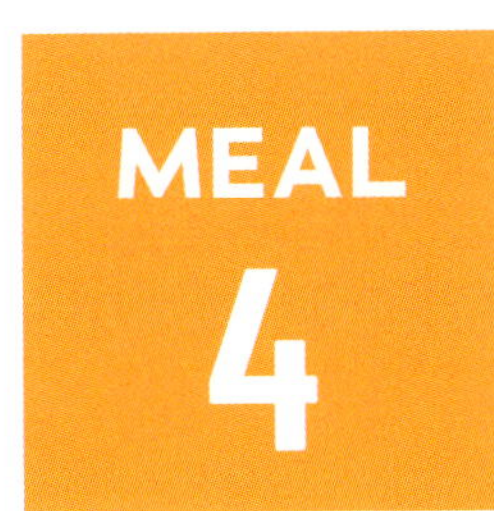

LOW-CARB PIZZA—2 WAYS

PEPPERONI PIZZA

Cauliflower pizza crust*

Rao's marinara sauce

Bagged shredded part-skim mozzarella cheese

Pepperoni slices

Follow the instructions on the package of cauliflower pizza crust for heating. Once the crust is heated through, spread some marinara over the crust. Top with mozzarella cheese and pepperoni slices.

BACON RANCH CHICKEN PIZZA

Cauliflower pizza crust

Frozen ready-to-eat grilled chicken strips

Ranch dressing**

Bagged shredded part-skim mozzarella cheese

Precooked bacon* (or homemade equivalent, see page 76), chopped**

Follow the instructions on the package of cauliflower pizza for heating. While the crust is heating in the oven, remove the frozen chicken from the bag and defrost in the microwave for 1 or 2 minutes or in a skillet on the stove for about 5 minutes. Cut the strips into smaller diced pieces. Once the crust is heated through, spread some ranch dressing over the crust. Top with grilled chicken pieces, mozzarella cheese, and bacon.

*Cauliflower pizza crust can be found in the freezer section of most grocery stores.

**Primal Kitchen is my go-to for bottled salad dressings. If not buying Primal Kitchen, study the ingredients lists to avoid dressings that use soybean oil or canola oil or add high-fructose corn syrup and other sugars.

***Precooked bacon is sold in the refrigerated sections of grocery stores. Or you can batch-cook bacon at home and freeze it for later!

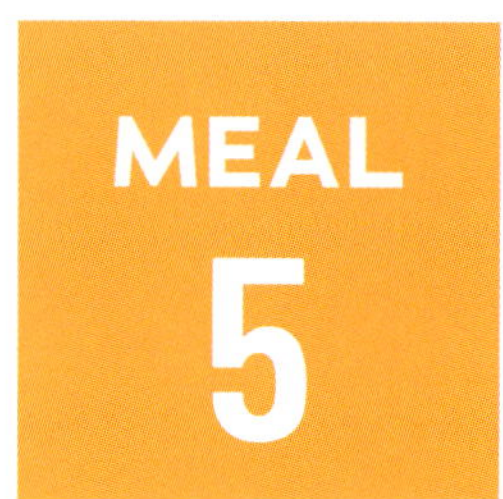

QUICK CHICKEN NOODLE SOUP

Rotisserie chicken

Chicken bone broth*

Frozen spinach

Low-carb noodles, such as egg white or shirataki**

SEASONINGS (OPTIONAL):

Fresh lemon juice

Minced garlic

Onion powder

Remove the meat from the bones of the rotisserie chicken, shredding it with your fingers as you go. Place in a large pot. One rotisserie chicken has about 1½ pounds of meat. Pour 4 cups of chicken bone broth into the pot and heat over medium heat. Remove the frozen spinach from the bag and add to the pot. Cover the pot and cook until the spinach is wilted, and the broth is steaming, about 10 minutes. Taste and add seasonings, if desired. Prepare the low-carb noodles following the package instructions. If using egg white or shirataki noodles, simply remove from the bag and drain. Put the prepared noodles in your serving bowl and ladle the hot soup on top, which will heat the noodles.

*My favorite brands of store-bought bone broth are EPIC, Fond, and Kettle & Fire.

**Egg white noodles are shelf-stable and can be purchased on Amazon. (I've yet to find them in grocery stores.) Shirataki noodles are another option; they're easily found in most grocery stores where the pastas are located.

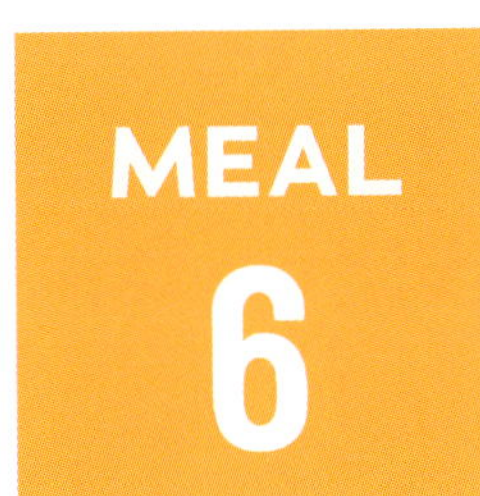

QUICK TACOS

Folios cheese wraps or Siete Foods grain-free taco shells*

Frozen ready-to-eat grilled chicken strips

Bagged shredded cheddar cheese

Jarred salsa

SUGGESTED TOPPINGS:

Sour cream

Avocado

Fresh cilantro

Prepare the Folio cheese wraps according to the heating instructions on the package. (The Siete Foods taco shells are ready to use as is.) Heat a small skillet over medium-high heat and add one serving of grilled chicken strips. Cover and allow to heat through for about 5 minutes. Uncover and top with shredded cheese. Cover for 1 minute to melt cheese. Once your cheese wraps are ready, place your chicken and cheese in the middle of the wrap and top with a serving of salsa. Add optional taco toppings, if desired.

*Folios cheese wraps are usually found in the deli section where cheeses are sold. Siete Foods taco shells can be found on the shelves with other taco shells.

CHAPTER 7

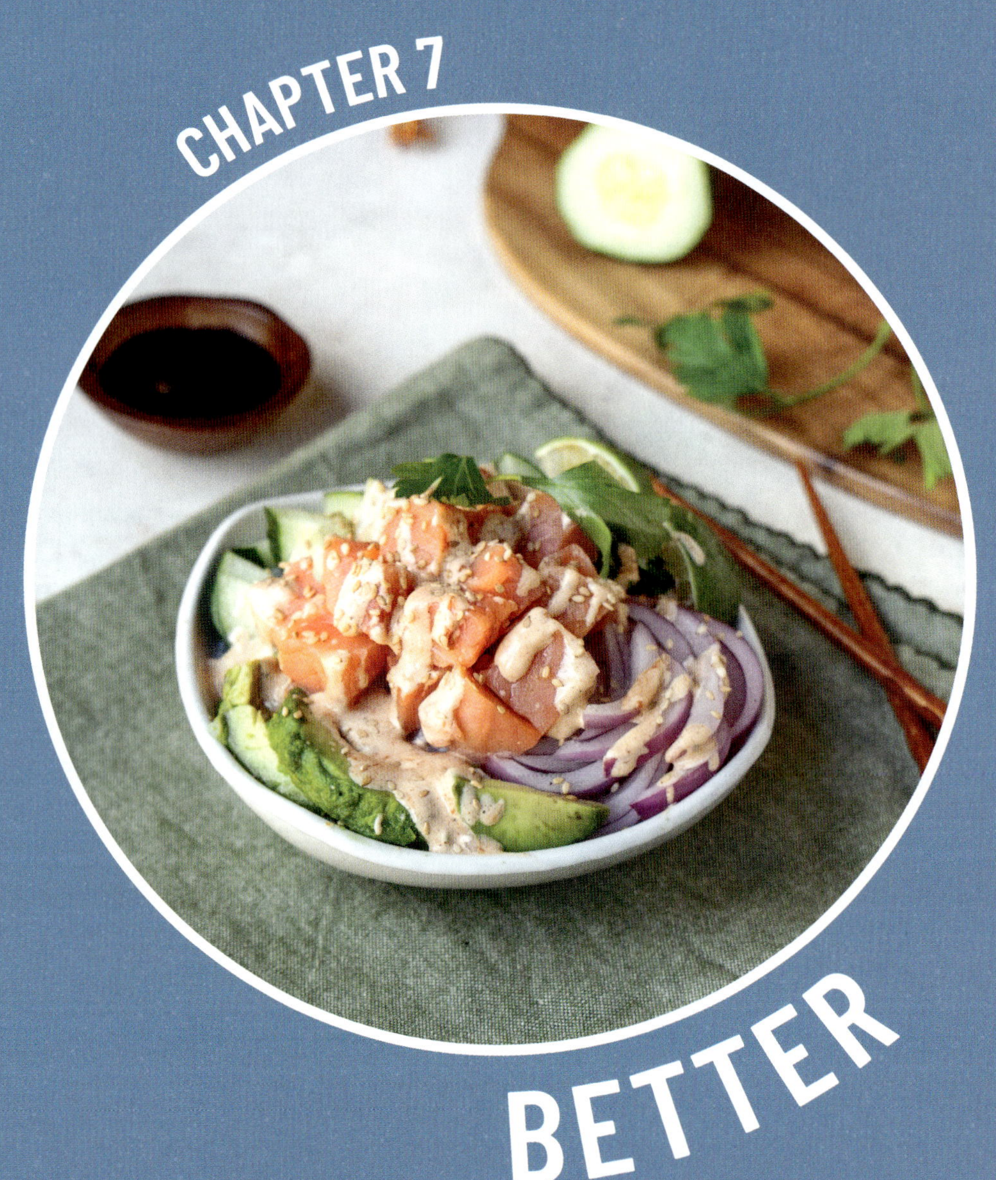

BETTER

BREAKFAST

LUNCH

DINNER & SIDES

DESSERTS

YIELD: 3 servings
PREP TIME: 2 minutes
COOK TIME: 35 minutes

HARD-BAKED EGGS

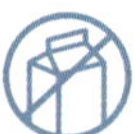 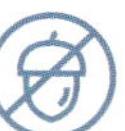 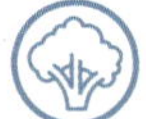

When you want hard-boiled eggs for egg salad, but don't want to spend time peeling eggs, try this easy alternative and make hard-baked eggs! This method is also ideal to use when your eggs are really fresh because fresh eggs when boiled are usually very hard to peel.

6 large eggs

¼ cup water

1. Preheat the oven to 350°F. Grease a 9 by 5-inch loaf pan (ceramic or metal) with cooking spray.
2. Crack the eggs into the loaf pan—no need to stir, and it doesn't matter if they crack. Pour in the water.
3. Bake for 30 to 35 minutes, until the whites and yolks are set.
4. Run a knife around the edge of the pan to loosen the cooked eggs, then flip the pan over to release the eggs onto a cutting board. Chop roughly or finely, according to your preference. Use in recipes that call for chopped hard-boiled eggs.

Calories	Fat	Protein	Total Carbs	Dietary Fiber	Net Carbs
143	10g	13g	1g	0g	1g

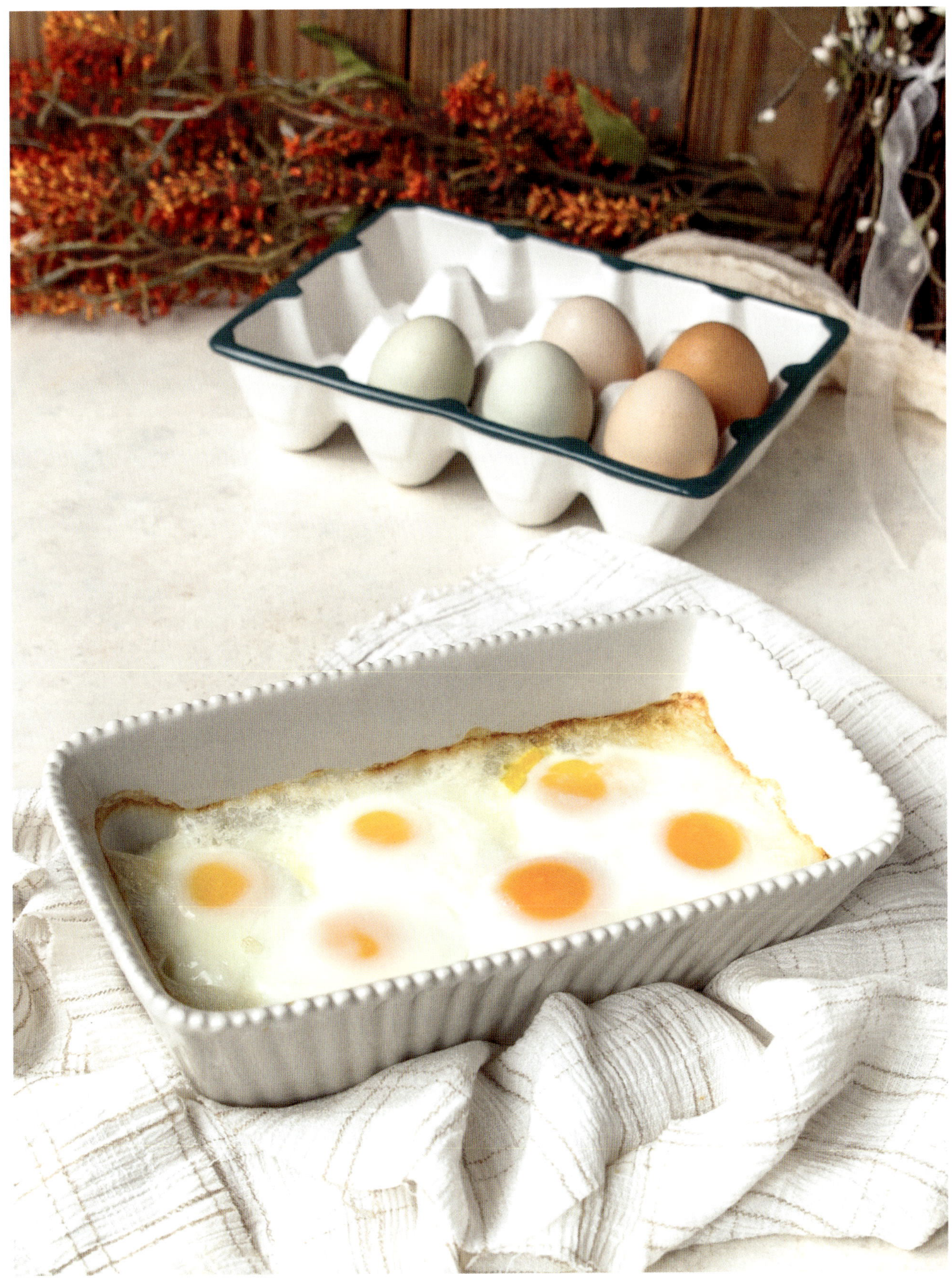

YIELD: 12 bars (1 per serving)
PREP TIME: 10 minutes
COOK TIME: 35 minutes

CHOCOLATE PROTEIN GRANOLA BARS

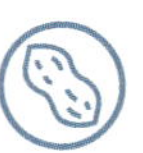

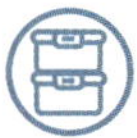

OPTION OPTION

No need to buy store-bought granola bars made with unhealthy oils and sweeteners when you can make this easy recipe at home. You can customize the ingredients to suit your tastes and needs. To make this peanut free, swap out the peanut butter for a nut butter or sunflower seed butter. To make this tree nut–free, omit the macadamia nuts and use more pumpkin and sunflower seeds.

1/2 cup raw macadamia nuts

1/2 cup hulled pumpkin seeds

1/2 cup hulled sunflower seeds

1/3 cup natural peanut butter or nut/seed butter of choice (see note)

2 tablespoons unsalted butter

1/3 cup liquid allulose

1/2 teaspoon vanilla extract

1 large egg

1/3 cup chocolate-flavored collagen peptides

Pinch of flaky sea salt

1/4 cup sugar-free chocolate chips

NOTE: Make sure the peanut butter or nut or sunflower seed butter you use for this recipe is unsweetened and unsalted.

1. Preheat the oven to 400°F. Line an 8-inch square baking dish with parchment paper, allowing the paper to hang over the sides for easy removal.
2. Place the nuts and seeds on a rimmed baking sheet and roast until slightly golden, about 10 minutes. Remove from the oven and allow to cool completely. Leave the oven on.
3. Meanwhile, heat the peanut butter and butter in a small saucepan over medium heat, whisking until completely melted. Remove the pan from the heat and allow the mixture to cool completely. Stir in the allulose and vanilla. Taste and adjust the sweetness to your liking, remembering you have the chocolate chips still to add.
4. Using a food processor or a cutting board and knife, chop the cooled nuts and seeds until you have a mix of some small and some chunky pieces.
5. Put the cooled peanut butter mixture, chopped nuts and seeds, egg, collagen, salt, and chocolate chips in a mixing bowl and stir to fully combine.
6. Press the mixture into the prepared baking dish until level. It will be sticky; use another piece of parchment on top to press the mixture down. Remove and discard the top piece of parchment.
7. Lower the oven temperature to 350°F and place the dish in the oven. Bake for 20 to 25 minutes, until the mixture is golden. Remove from the oven and allow to cool completely. As the mixture cools, it will firm up. Once set, slice into 12 bars.
8. Store in an airtight container in the refrigerator for up to 5 days or freeze for up to 3 months.

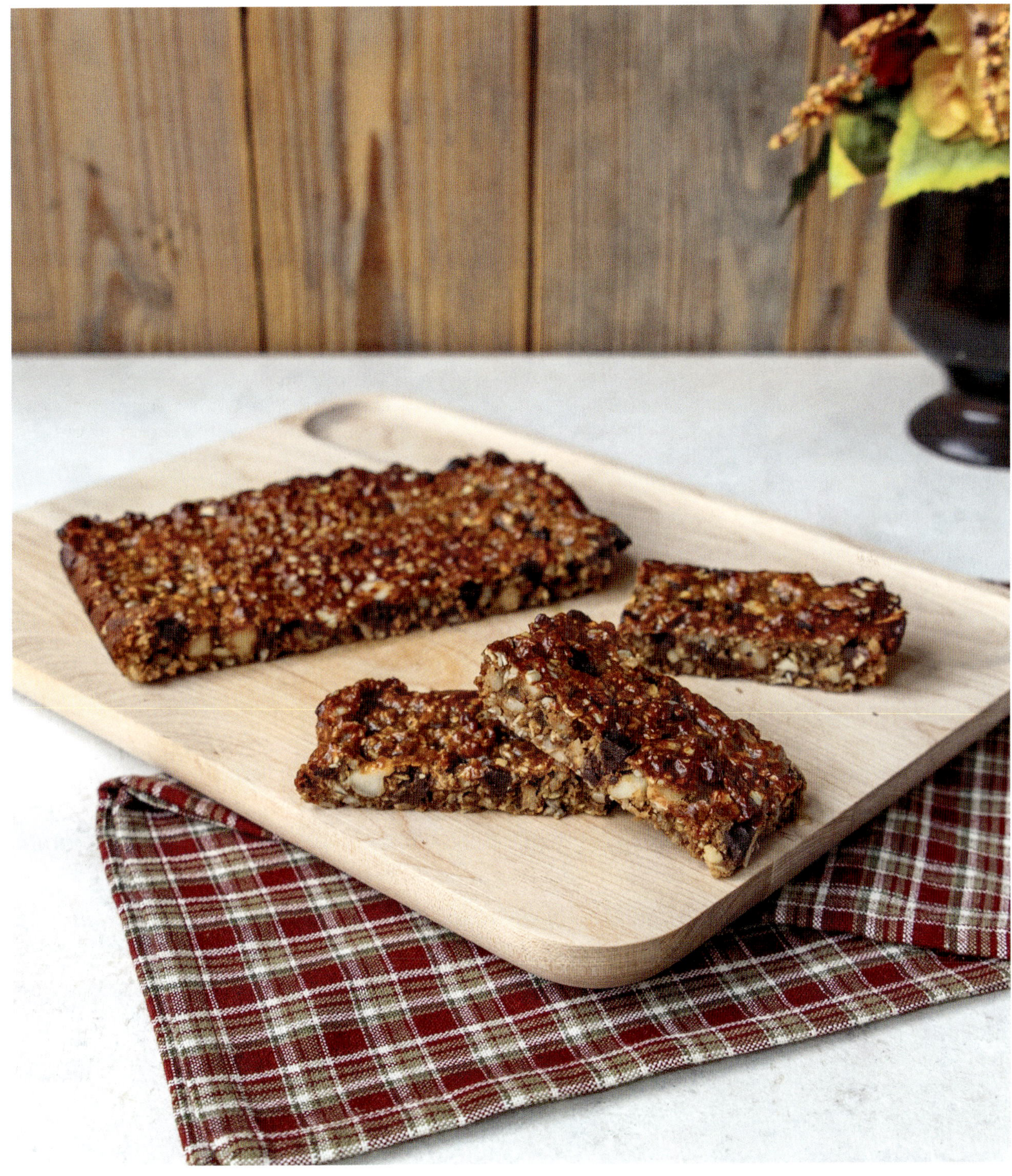

Calories	Fat	Protein	Total Carbs	Dietary Fiber	Net Carbs
182	16g	7g	5g	2g	3g

YIELD: 8 pancakes (2 pancakes per serving)
PREP TIME: 5 minutes
COOK TIME: 24 minutes

CINNAMON ROLL PROTEIN PANCAKES

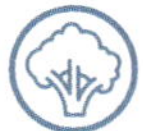
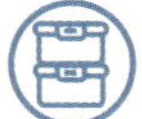

With 18 grams of protein in a serving, this is a great way to break your fast. These protein pancakes can be made ahead and frozen in individual servings for easy portion control.

FOR THE PANCAKES:

½ cup cottage cheese (4% milkfat)

4 large eggs

½ cup vanilla-flavored whey protein powder

½ cup blanched almond flour

½ teaspoon vanilla extract

½ teaspoon ground cinnamon

1 teaspoon cinnamon-flavored liquid stevia or liquid monk fruit

½ teaspoon baking powder

4 tablespoons avocado oil, coconut oil, or bacon grease, divided, for the pan

FOR THE CINNAMON ROLL TOPPING:

¼ cup low-carb brown sugar–style sweetener

2 teaspoons unsalted butter, softened

1½ teaspoons ground cinnamon

Pinch of fine sea salt

1. Place all the ingredients for the pancakes in a blender and blend until smooth, or mix well by hand. If mixing by hand, you will not get the batter completely smooth, but that's okay for this recipe.
2. In a small bowl, mix the cinnamon roll topping ingredients until combined, then transfer the mixture to a pastry bag fitted with a piping tip or a plastic bag. If using a plastic bag, snip off the tip of one corner of the bag. Set the bag aside on a plate.
3. Heat 2 tablespoons of the oil in a large nonstick skillet over medium heat.
4. Using a ¼-cup measuring cup, scoop up a portion of the batter and pour it into the skillet. Repeat to make a total of 4 pancakes. Once the pancakes look set on top (they will be matte, not glossy), 1 to 2 minutes, pipe a little less than 2 teaspoons of the topping onto each pancake, starting at the center and swirling twice around. Then flip the pancakes over and cook for another minute, or until the bottoms are browned. Place on a plate.
5. Heat the remaining 2 tablespoons of oil in the pan. Spoon in the rest of the batter, making 4 more pancakes, and add the cinnamon roll topping as described above.
6. Store leftovers in an airtight container in the fridge for up to 5 days. Pancakes can also be stored in the freezer for up to 1 month; place a piece of parchment paper between the pancakes to keep them from sticking together. Thaw before reheating. Reheat in the microwave for 1 to 2 minutes or in a small skillet on the stovetop over medium heat.

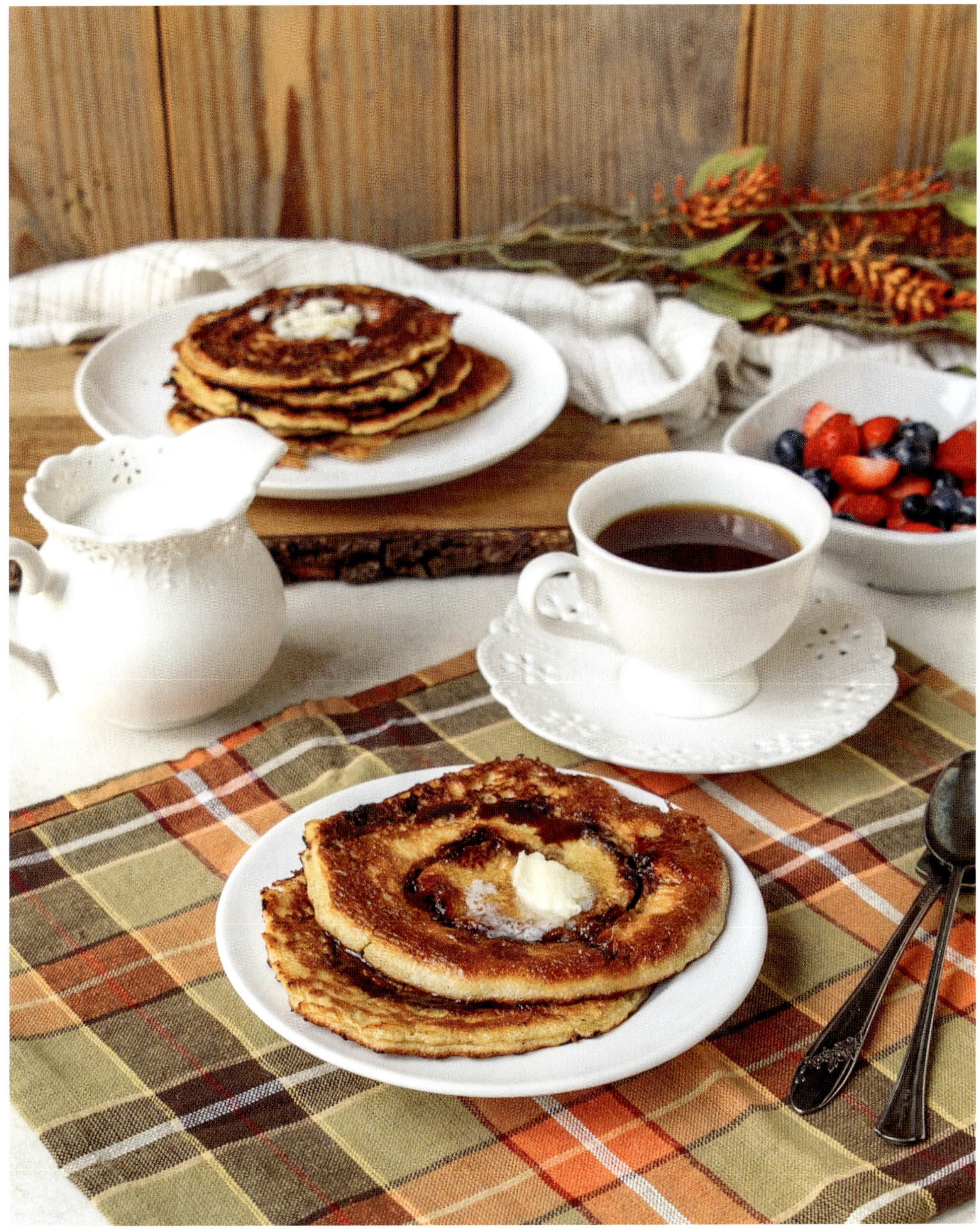

Calories	Fat	Protein	Total Carbs	Dietary Fiber	Net Carbs
226	15g	18g	6g	2g	4g

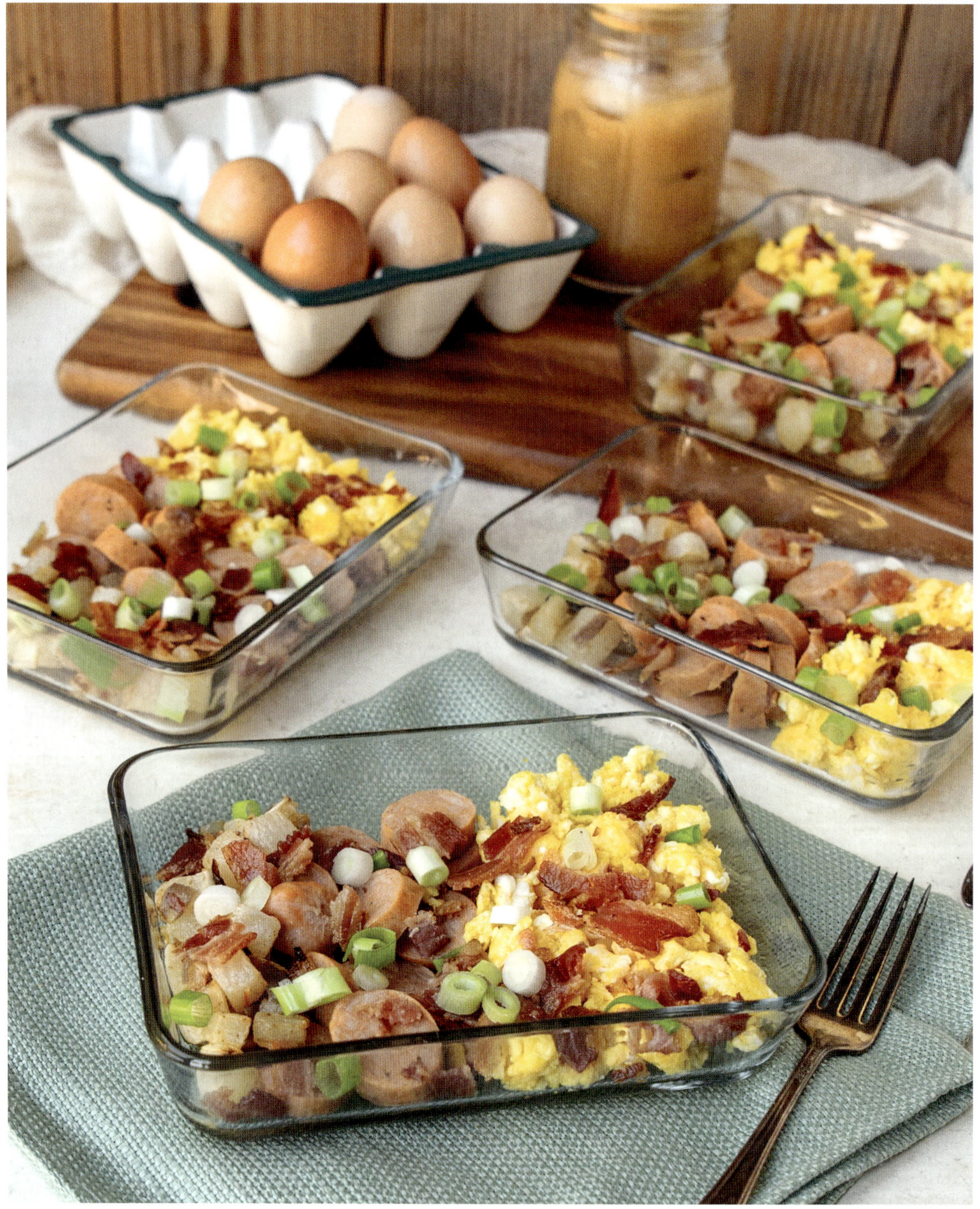

Calories	Fat	Protein	Total Carbs	Dietary Fiber	Net Carbs
375	24g	31g	7g	1g	6g

YIELD: 4 servings
PREP TIME: 15 minutes
COOK TIME: 30 minutes

ON-THE-GO HIGH-PROTEIN BREAKFASTS

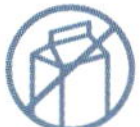 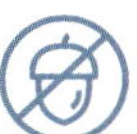 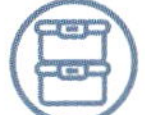

While this high-protein breakfast may take a bit longer to prep and cook, it's an ideal recipe to make ahead when you have time to devote to meal prep. Once cooked and cooled, store individual servings in the fridge or freezer.

2 cups diced daikon radishes or red radishes

½ cup diced red onions

1 tablespoon avocado oil

¼ teaspoon salt

¼ teaspoon pepper

8 slices regular-cut bacon

8 large eggs

2 tablespoons bacon grease or avocado oil

4 fully cooked chicken sausage links (see note)

1 tablespoon sliced scallions, for garnish

NOTE: For convenience, I buy fully cooked chicken sausages, ready to use without the need for cooking at home.

1. Preheat the oven to 425°F.
2. Place the radishes and onions on a rimmed baking sheet and toss with the avocado oil, salt, and pepper.
3. Bake for 15 minutes, then reduce the oven temperature to 400°F and add the bacon to one side of the pan. Bake for another 15 minutes, or until the bacon is crisp and the vegetables are fork-tender.
4. Meanwhile, cook the eggs: Whisk the eggs in a medium bowl. Heat the bacon grease in a large nonstick skillet over medium heat, then pour in the eggs and cook, stirring often to scramble the eggs, until the eggs are set and cooked to your liking. Remove the pan from the heat and set aside.
5. When the vegetables and bacon are done, transfer the bacon to a paper towel–lined plate to absorb the grease. Divide the radish and onion mixture among 4 (3¾-cup) microwave-safe meal prep containers. Divide the scrambled eggs evenly among the containers.
6. Slice the precooked sausages one at a time and add to each container.
7. Crumble 2 slices of bacon into each container, then garnish with the sliced scallions.
8. Store in the fridge for up to 4 days or in the freezer for up to 3 months. Reheat in the microwave for 2 to 3 minutes, until heated through.

YIELD: 6 servings
PREP TIME: 10 minutes
COOK TIME: 20 minutes

SHEET PAN OMELET

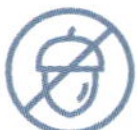
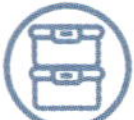

This is an easy meal prep recipe that makes delicious eggs without the hassle of cooking them on the stovetop. Cook, cool, and pack in individual serving containers for an easy grab-and-go meal. The omelet will keep up to 3 days in the refrigerator or up to 1 month in the freezer. To reheat, microwave for 1 to 2 minutes until hot.

12 large eggs

1/3 cup heavy cream

1 cup shredded cheddar cheese

1/2 teaspoon fine sea salt

1/4 teaspoon ground black pepper

SUGGESTED TOPPINGS:

3 ounces mushrooms of choice, sliced

1/3 cup chopped scallions

6 slices regular-cut bacon, baked (see page 76) and chopped

1. Preheat the oven to 375°F. Grease a rimmed baking sheet with cooking spray.
2. In a large bowl, whisk together the eggs, cream, and cheese. Pour the mixture onto the prepared pan.
3. Sprinkle on the toppings, if using. Bake for 10 minutes. Rotate the pan and bake for another 5 to 10 minutes, until the eggs are set.

Calories	Fat	Protein	Total Carbs	Dietary Fiber	Net Carbs
264	20g	17g	1g	0g	1g

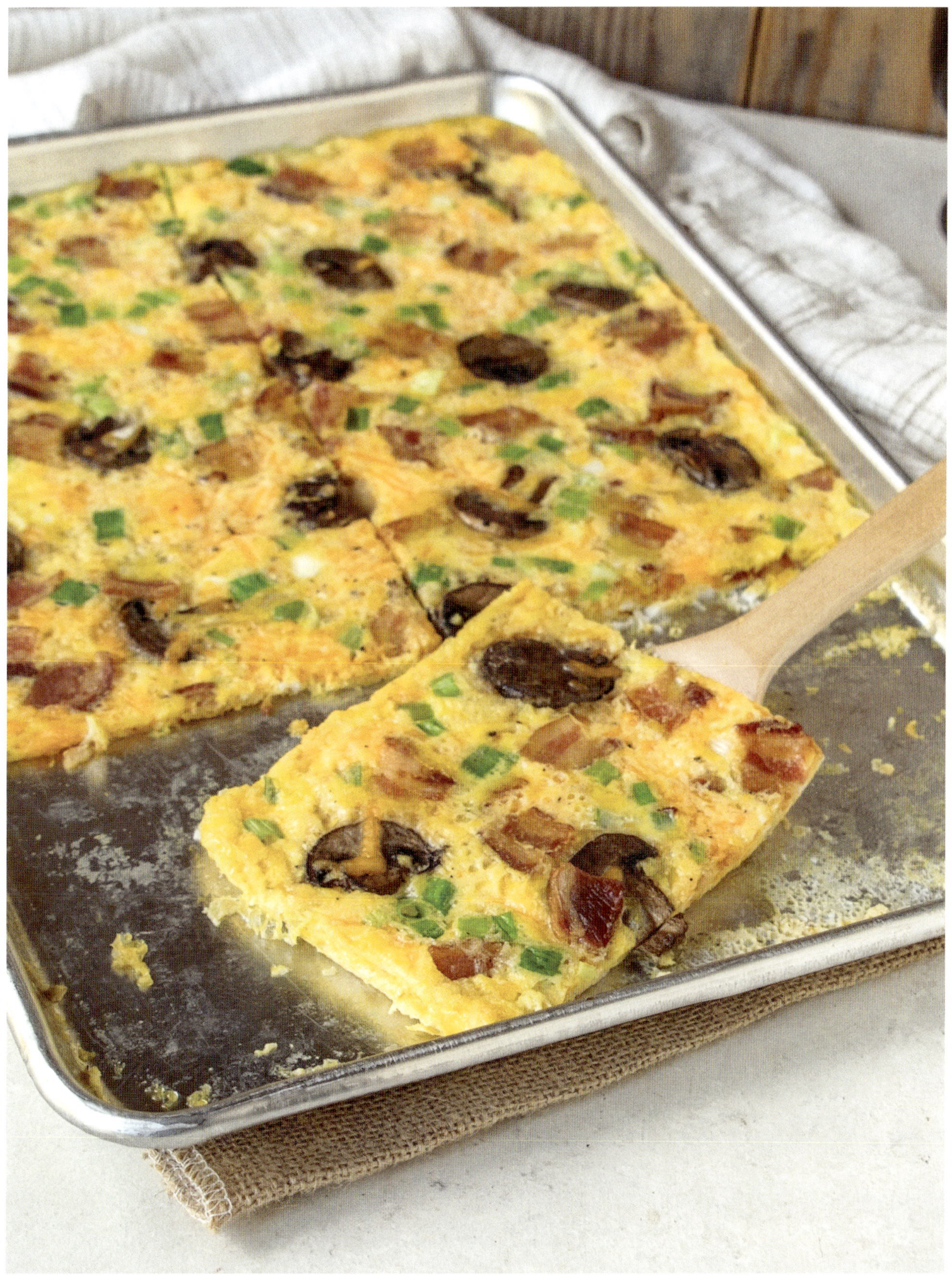

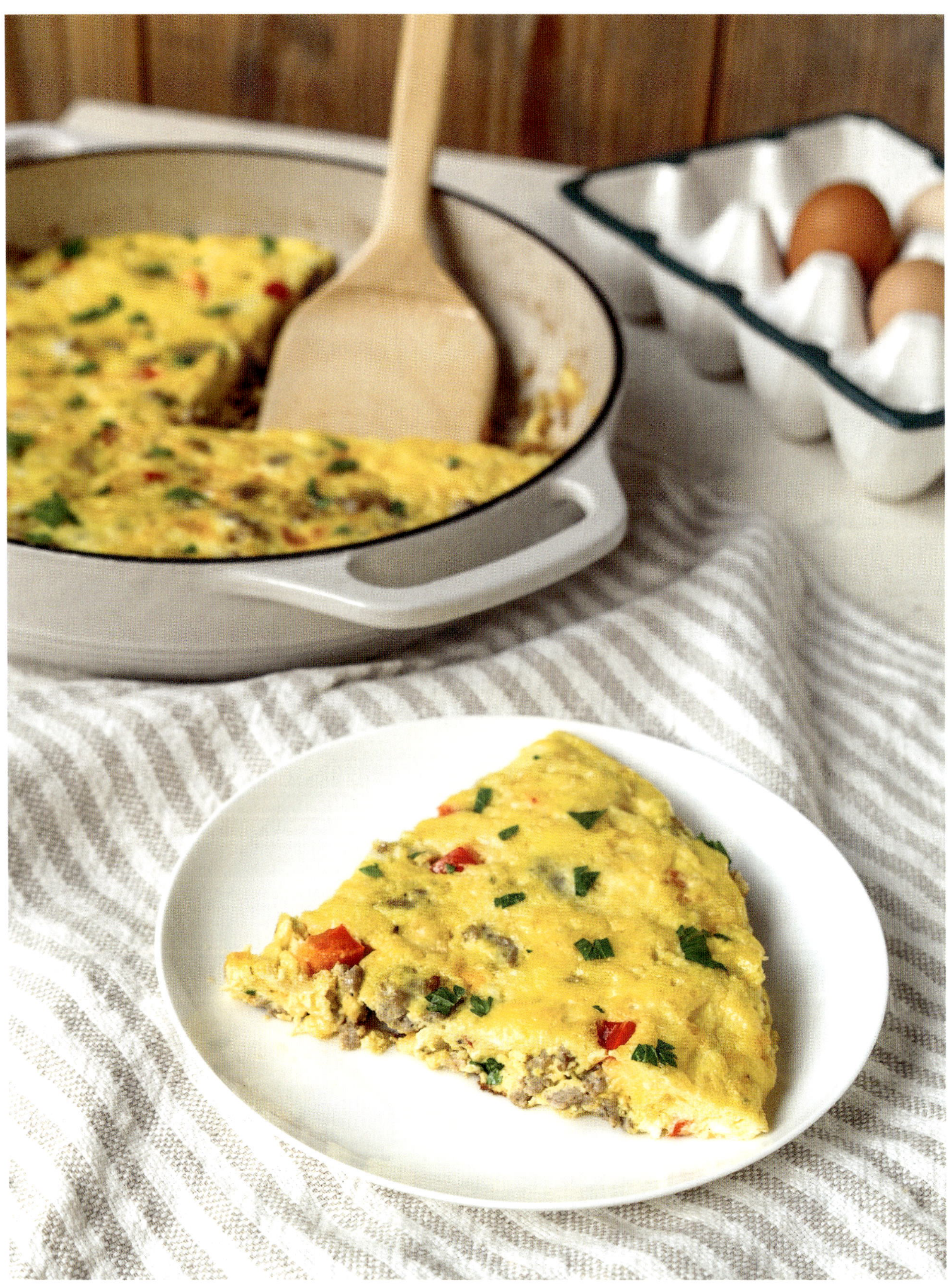

YIELD: 4 servings
PREP TIME: 5 minutes
COOK TIME: 15 minutes

BREAKFAST FRITTATA

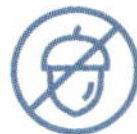

This is an easy recipe to make ahead. Cook, cool, slice into four pieces, and pack in airtight containers in the fridge for up to 5 days to enjoy for breakfast or lunch. To reheat, place on a microwave-safe plate and microwave for 1 to 2 minutes or place on a small rimmed baking sheet and warm in a preheated 350°F oven for 5 minutes.

- **1 pound ground pork**
- **½ cup chopped red bell peppers**
- **½ cup chopped yellow onions**
- **8 large eggs**
- **1 cup heavy cream**
- **½ cup shredded cheddar cheese (optional)**
- **½ teaspoon fine sea salt**
- **¼ teaspoon seasoning blend of choice (see note)**
- **¼ teaspoon ground black pepper**

NOTE: I like to use Bell's seasoning in this frittata, but feel free to use your favorite savory blend. If you'd like to make this Good (Enough), omit the bell peppers and onions

1. Have an oven rack placed in the top position.
2. Brown the pork in a 10-inch ovenproof skillet or braiser over medium-high heat, 5 to 6 minutes, stirring often to crumble it as it cooks. Drain off some of the fat, leaving about 2 tablespoons in the pan.
3. Add the bell peppers and onions to the skillet, reduce the heat to medium, and cook until the vegetables begin to soften.
4. Whisk together the eggs, cream, cheese (if using), and seasonings, then pour the mixture over the cooked pork and vegetables in the skillet.
5. Cover the pan and reduce the heat to medium-low. Cook for 10 minutes, or until the edges are set but the middle is still slightly jiggly. Set the oven to the broil setting.
6. Uncover, place the pan in the oven, and broil for 2 to 4 minutes, until golden brown. Allow to cool for about 5 minutes. Slice into 4 pieces and enjoy.

Calories	Fat	Protein	Total Carbs	Dietary Fiber	Net Carbs
642	54g	32g	1g	0g	1g

YIELD: 4 servings
PREP TIME: 10 minutes
(not including time to cook bacon or eggs)

BETTER BLT SALAD

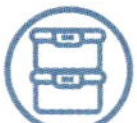

While a bacon, lettuce, and tomato salad is tasty as is, increasing the protein with hard-cooked eggs makes it even better. To save time peeling the eggs, try my recipe for Hard-Baked Eggs on page 166.

2 romaine lettuce hearts (about 11 ounces)

8 ounces bacon, baked (see page 76)

2 large Roma tomatoes (about 6 ounces)

1 small red onion (about 1¾ ounces)

4 large hard-boiled eggs, peeled and halved or chopped, or 1 cup chopped Hard-Baked Eggs (page 166)

FOR THE DRESSING:

¼ cup avocado oil mayonnaise

¼ cup sour cream

1 tablespoon extra-virgin olive oil

1 clove garlic, minced

¼ teaspoon fine sea salt

¼ teaspoon ground black pepper

2 tablespoons sliced scallions

1. Chop the lettuce and place in a large serving bowl or divide it evenly among 4 individual storage containers if meal prepping. Chop the bacon, tomatoes, and onion and toss with the lettuce.
2. Whisk together the dressing ingredients in a small bowl.
3. Just before serving, toss the salad with the dressing. If meal prepping, store the dressing and salad in separate containers. When stored separately, the salad and dressing will keep for up to 3 days.

Calories	Fat	Protein	Total Carbs	Dietary Fiber	Net Carbs
265	24g	8g	7g	2g	5g

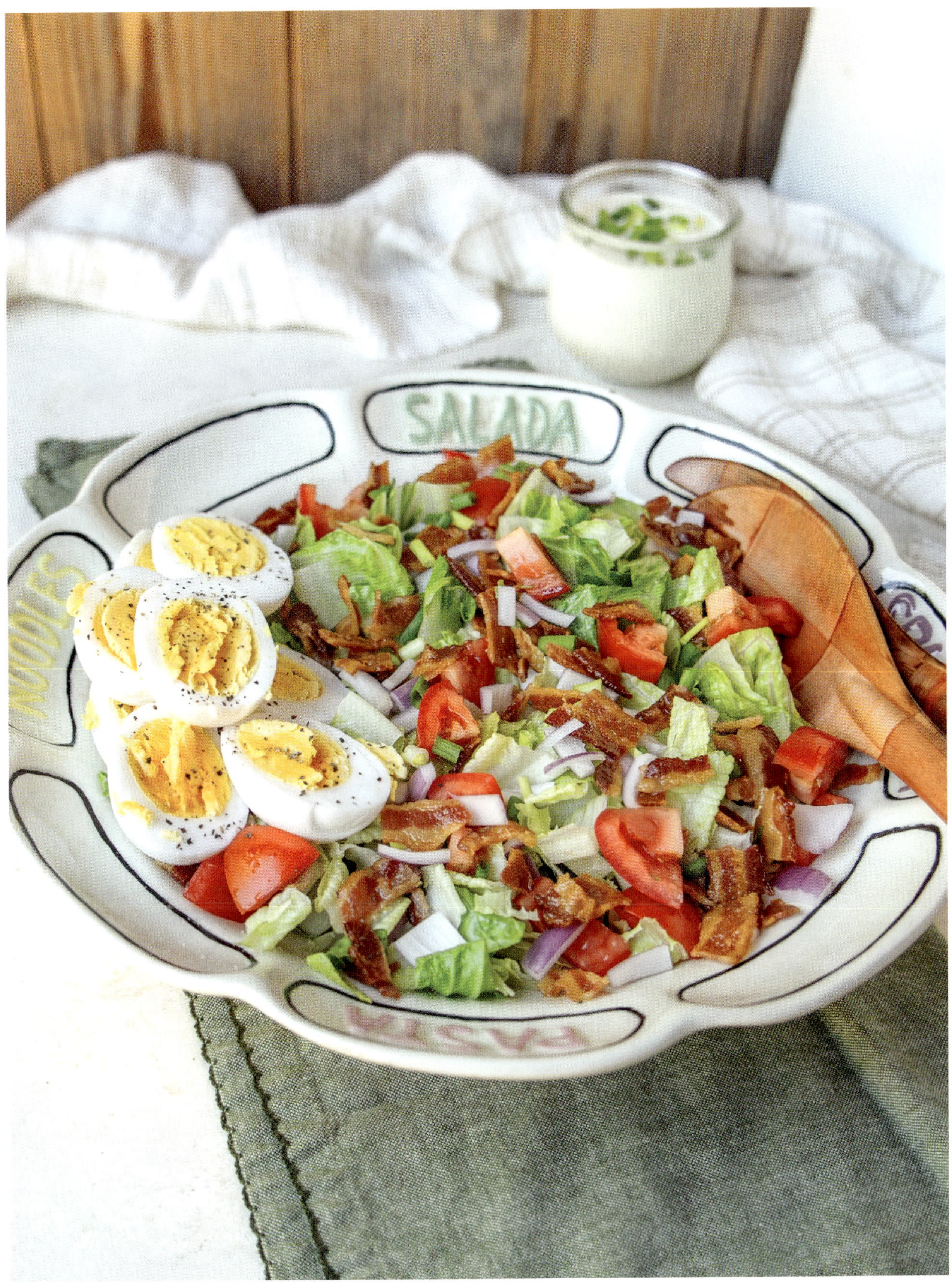
SALADA
NOODLES
PASTA

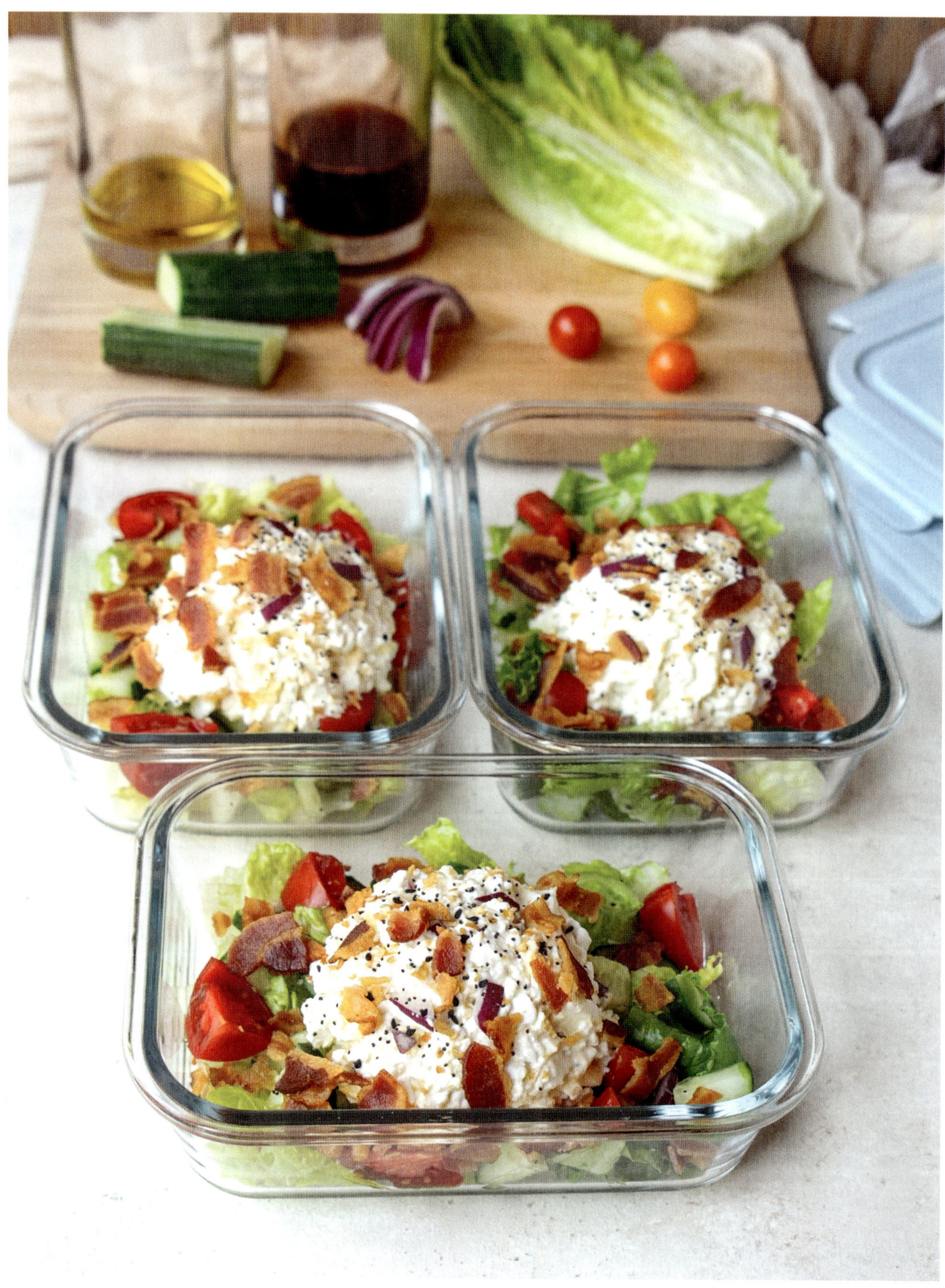

YIELD: 3 servings
PREP TIME: 10 minutes (not including time to cook eggs and bacon)

ON-THE-GO COTTAGE CHEESE EGG SALADS

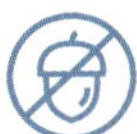
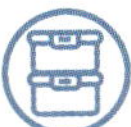

I know that cottage cheese isn't often mixed with egg for egg salad, but don't knock it till you try it! Plus, it increases your protein and will keep you quite satisfied!

- 3 cups chopped romaine lettuce
- 1½ cups cottage cheese (4% milkfat)
- 6 large hard-boiled eggs, peeled and chopped, or 1 batch Hard-Baked Eggs (page 166), chopped
- ¾ cup sliced cucumbers
- ¾ cup chopped tomatoes (or quartered if small)
- 3 tablespoons chopped red onions
- 6 slices regular-cut bacon, baked (see page 76)
- Dressing of choice, for serving (optional)
- Everything bagel seasoning, for garnish (optional)

1. Evenly divide the chopped lettuce among 3 (4-cup) storage containers, putting 1 cup in each.
2. In a medium bowl, gently mix together the cottage cheese and chopped egg, then evenly divide the mixture among the containers, scooping it into a mound for a pretty presentation, if desired.
3. Add ¼ cup cucumbers, ¼ cup chopped tomatoes, and 1 tablespoon chopped onions to each container. Cover with the lid.
4. Place 2 slices of cooked bacon in each of 3 zip-top bags or wrap in parchment paper. Place 1 bag with each container.
5. Store in the fridge for up to 3 days. Just before serving, crumble the bacon over the salad, drizzle with dressing, if using, and garnish with everything bagel seasoning, if desired.

Calories	Fat	Protein	Total Carbs	Dietary Fiber	Net Carbs
329	18g	29g	9g	2g	7g

YIELD: 3 servings
PREP TIME: 10 minutes
(not including time to cook eggs or optional bacon)

DILL PICKLE EGG SALAD

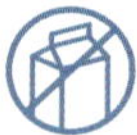
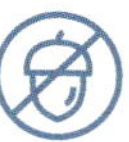
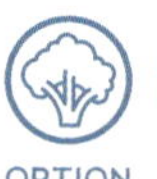

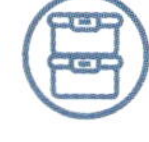

Enjoy in a bowl, on a bed of lettuce, or on my Cottage Cheese Cloud Bread Rolls (page 88). Just like the On-the-Go Cottage Cheese Egg Salads on page 181, you could easily make this a meal prep recipe. Simply store any additional serving components, such as lettuce or rolls, separately.

6 hard-boiled eggs, peeled and chopped, or 1 batch Hard-Baked Eggs (page 166), chopped

1 tablespoon finely diced red onions or scallions

1 medium dill pickle (about 1 ounce), diced

¼ cup avocado oil mayonnaise

1 tablespoon dill pickle juice (from the pickle jar)

1½ teaspoons Dijon mustard or prepared yellow mustard

¼ teaspoon fine sea salt

Ground black pepper, to taste

FOR GARNISH (OPTIONAL):

Diced cooked bacon

Dill pickle slices

1. Stir together the chopped eggs, onions, and pickle in a medium bowl.
2. In a small bowl, whisk together the remaining ingredients. Taste and adjust the seasoning if needed. Pour this mixture over the eggs, onions, and pickle and stir to coat.
3. Store in an airtight container in the fridge for up to 3 days. If serving topped with bacon and/or dill pickle slices, add them right before serving.

Calories	Fat	Protein	Total Carbs	Dietary Fiber	Net Carbs
293	27g	13g	2g	1g	1g

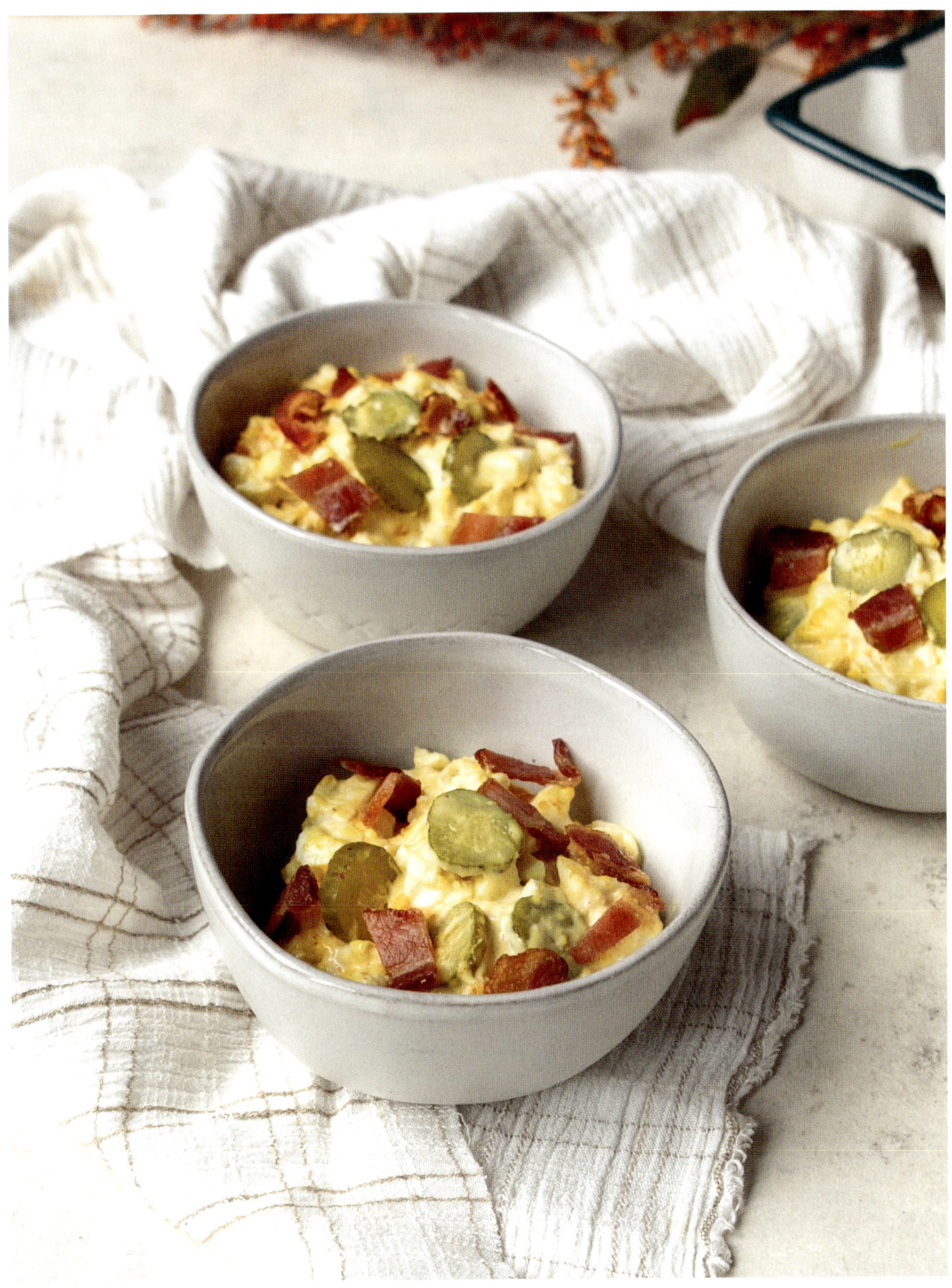

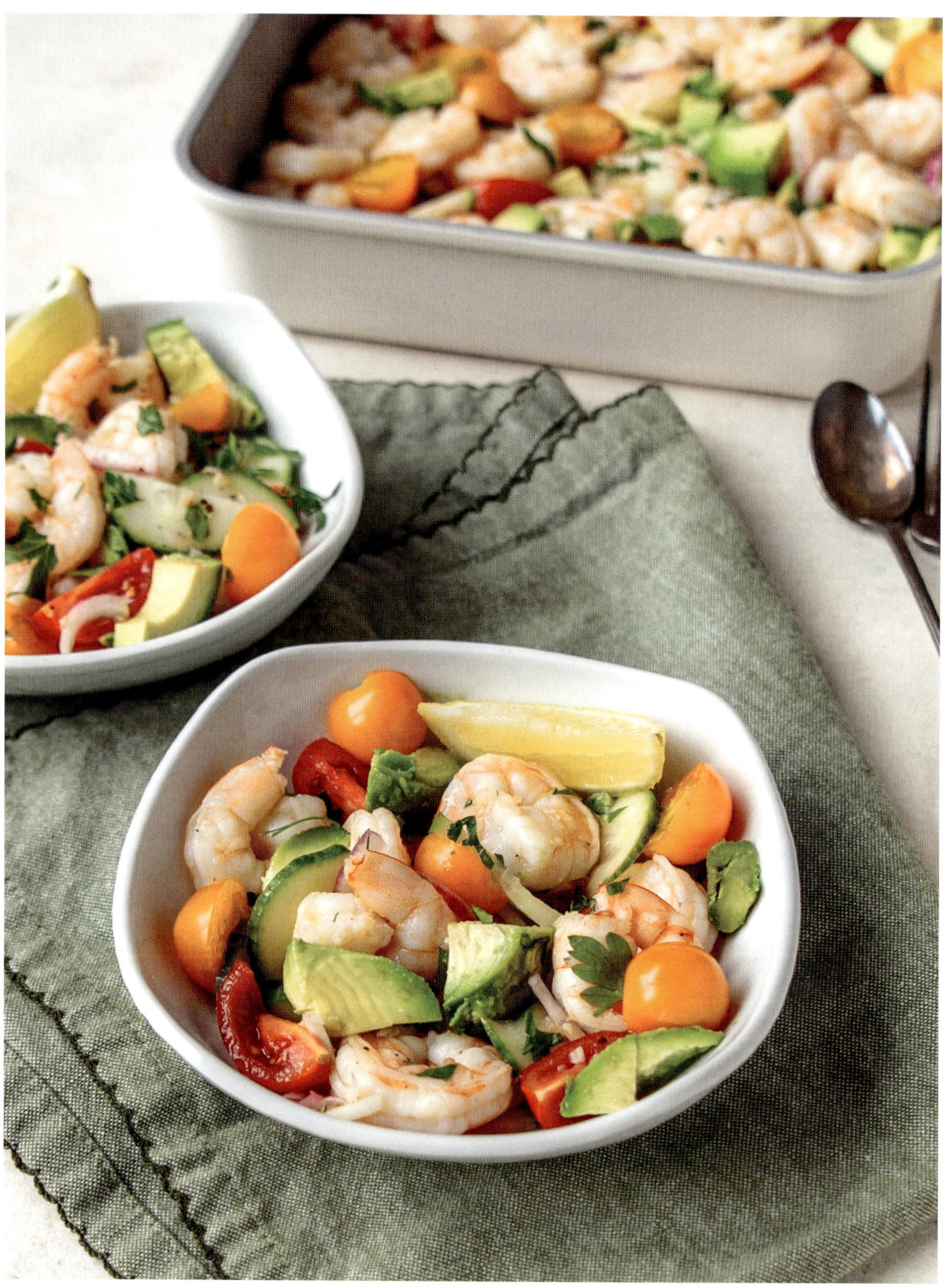

YIELD: 4 servings
PREP TIME: 10 minutes, plus 4 to 6 hours to chill
COOK TIME: 6 minutes

SHRIMP ESCABECHE

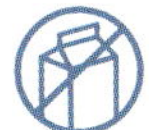  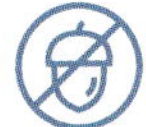

On a recent trip to New Orleans, I enjoyed a delicious shrimp escabeche. It's slightly different than ceviche because the shrimp are cooked instead of tossed raw in citrus juices. Fresh, tasty, and full of protein, it makes a fantastic meal.

- 1 teaspoon fine sea salt
- 1 pound large shrimp, peeled and deveined
- ¼ cup extra-virgin olive oil
- 2 cloves garlic, minced
- ½ cup white wine vinegar
- ½ cup thinly sliced red onions
- ½ cup diced tomatoes (quartered or halved if small)
- ½ cup sliced cucumbers
- ½ teaspoon ground black pepper
- ½ cup diced avocado (optional)
- Chopped fresh cilantro, for garnish (optional)
- Lemon wedges, for serving (optional)

1. Bring a large pot of water to a boil. Add the salt, then the shrimp. Cook the shrimp just until pink and cooked through, about 5 minutes. Drain and set aside.
2. Heat the olive oil in a small skillet over medium heat. Add the garlic and cook for about 1 minute, until fragrant, then add the shrimp. Turn off the heat and toss together.
3. Pour the vinegar into an 8-inch square ceramic or glass dish, then add the onions, tomatoes, cucumbers, pepper, and shrimp along with the cooking oil from the pan. Toss to evenly coat all the ingredients in the oil and vinegar, cover, and refrigerate for 4 to 6 hours to chill and develop the flavor.
4. If using avocado, gently stir it in just before serving. If desired, garnish with cilantro and serve with lemon wedges. Store in an airtight container in the fridge for up to 2 days.

Calories	Fat	Protein	Total Carbs	Dietary Fiber	Net Carbs
444	29g	33g	9g	2g	7g

YIELD: 1 serving
PREP TIME: 10 minutes

SALMON POKE BOWL

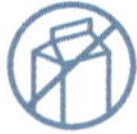  

A super simple but quick way to enjoy a fresh seafood dish without much effort. I like to drizzle a little bit of coconut aminos over the top before serving. If you don't care for or can't find sushi-grade salmon, you can swap in the same quantity of sushi-grade tuna.

FOR THE POKE BOWL:

⅓ cup chopped romaine lettuce

½ cup drained shirataki rice or cooked cauliflower rice

4 ounces raw sushi-grade salmon (aka sashimi), cut into ½-inch cubes

⅓ cup chopped cucumbers

¼ cup thinly sliced red onions

½ small Hass avocado (about 2 ounces), sliced

FOR GARNISH/SERVING:

Sesame seeds (optional)

Fresh parsley sprigs and/or chopped fresh parsley (optional)

2 small lime wedges

Coconut aminos (optional)

FOR THE DRESSING:

2 tablespoons avocado oil mayonnaise

1 teaspoon Sriracha

1 teaspoon lime juice

Fine sea salt, to taste (see note)

1. Arrange the poke bowl ingredients in a serving bowl, starting with the rice and lettuce to create a bed for the rest of the ingredients. Garnish with sesame seeds and/or parsley, if desired.
2. In a small bowl, whisk together the dressing ingredients. Drizzle the dressing over the poke bowl and serve with lime wedges and coconut aminos, if desired.
3. The poke bowl can be refrigerated for up to 2 days. If making it ahead, wait to add the avocado and drizzle the dressing until just before serving.

NOTE: If you plan to enjoy this bowl with coconut aminos, go light on the salt in the dressing or omit it altogether.

Calories	Fat	Protein	Total Carbs	Dietary Fiber	Net Carbs
490	41g	24g	11g	1g	10g

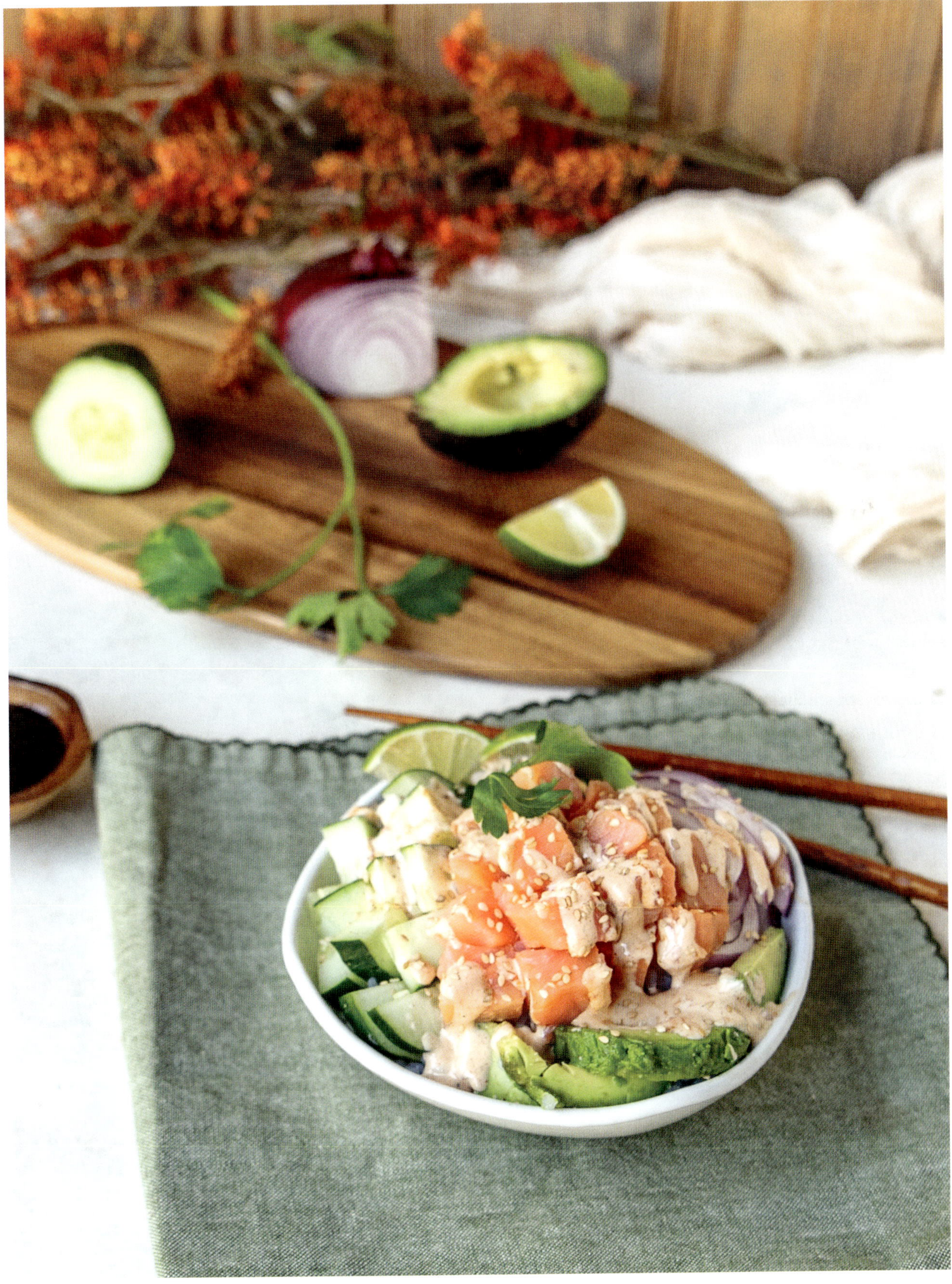

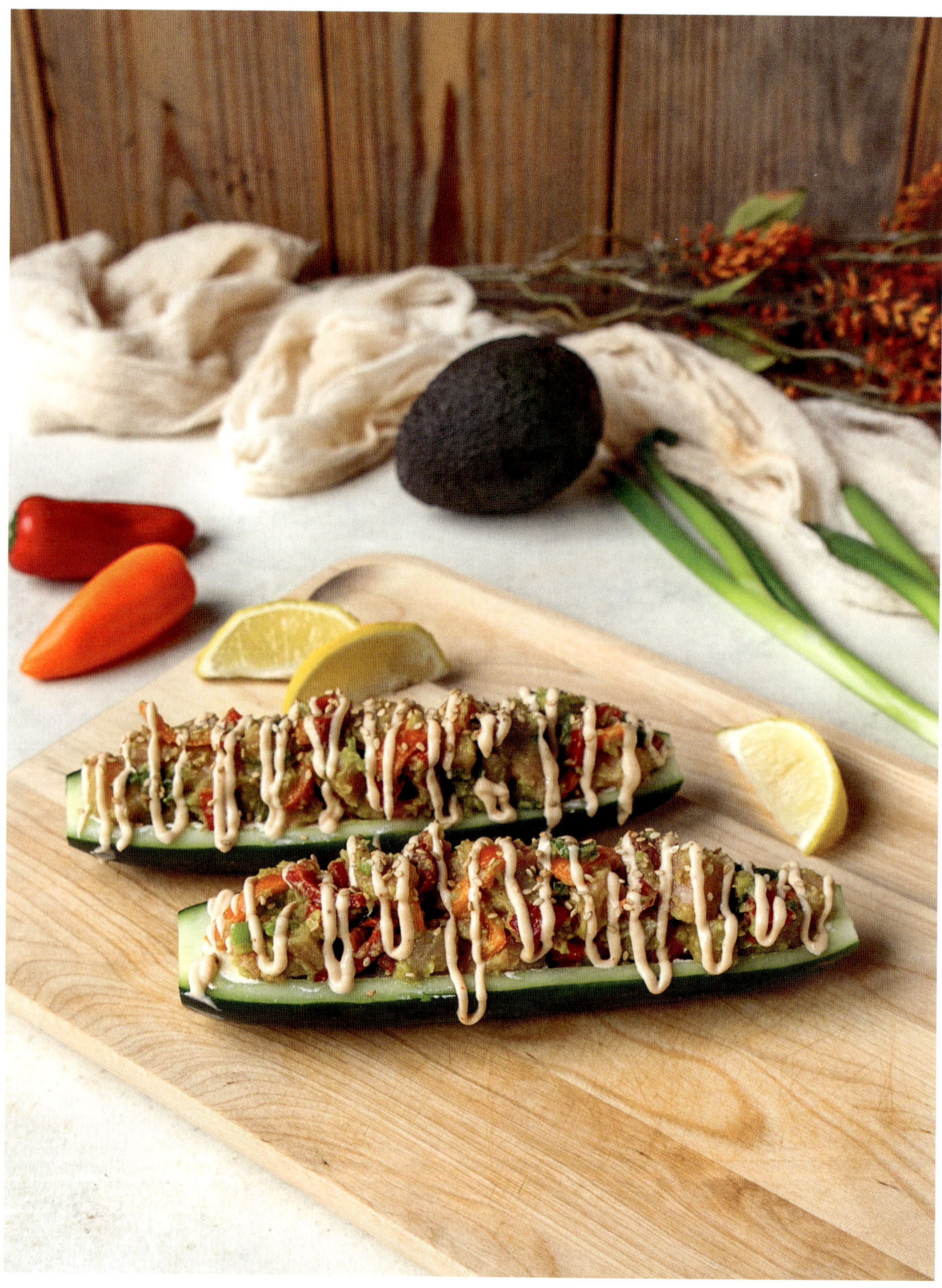

YIELD: 2 servings
PREP TIME: 10 minutes

SALMON SUSHI BOATS

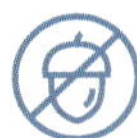

A halved and scooped-out cucumber forms the boats for this refreshing meal.

FOR THE BOATS:

1 medium cucumber (about 7 ounces)

1 ounce (2 tablespoons) cream cheese

6 ounces raw sushi-grade salmon (aka sashimi), chopped

¼ cup mashed avocado

½ cup chopped red bell peppers

2 tablespoons chopped scallions

1 tablespoon fresh lemon juice

FOR THE DRESSING:

1 tablespoon avocado oil mayonnaise

½ teaspoon Sriracha

½ teaspoon fresh lemon juice

Fine sea salt, to taste

Sesame seeds, for garnish (optional)

Lemon wedges, for serving (optional)

1. Cut the ends off the cucumber, then slice it in half lengthwise. Scoop out the seeds. Dry the insides of the scooped-out halves with a paper towel.
2. Spread 1 tablespoon of cream cheese onto each cucumber boat.
3. Put the salmon, avocado, bell peppers, scallions, and lemon juice in a medium bowl and gently stir to combine. Evenly spoon the salmon mixture into the cucumber boats. Set aside.
4. In a small bowl, whisk together the dressing ingredients. Drizzle the dressing over the stuffed cucumber boats or, for a prettier presentation, transfer the dressing to a small plastic bag, snip off one corner, and pipe it over the boats.
5. Enjoy immediately or store covered tightly with cling wrap in the refrigerator for up to 1 day.

Calories	Fat	Protein	Total Carbs	Dietary Fiber	Net Carbs
362	28g	21g	10g	2g	8g

YIELD: 4 servings
PREP TIME: 10 minutes
COOK TIME: 10 minutes

BAKED BREADED PORK CHOPS

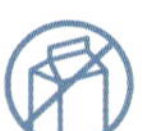 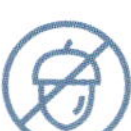 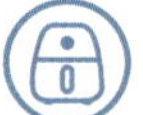

For this recipe, you have the choice of using the oven or air fryer. Both methods work well, though the air fryer gives the chops a crispier exterior that my family enjoys. I like to pair these chops with a side of Garlic Parmesan Broccoli (page 137).

2 large eggs

1 cup pork rind panko

1 teaspoon Italian seasoning

1/2 teaspoon sea salt

1/4 teaspoon ground black pepper

1/4 teaspoon garlic powder

1/4 teaspoon onion powder

4 (5-ounce) bone-in pork chops (about 1/2 inch thick; see note)

FOR THE MUSTARD SAUCE (OPTIONAL):

1/4 cup avocado oil mayonnaise

2 tablespoons prepared yellow mustard

Pinch of fine sea salt

1. Preheat the oven or air fryer to 400°F. Line a rimmed baking sheet or the air fryer basket with parchment paper.
2. Whisk the eggs in a shallow bowl. Place the pork rind panko in another shallow bowl and stir in the seasonings.
3. Dip one pork chop at a time in the beaten eggs, then dredge both sides in the seasoned panko and set on the prepared pan or basket.
4. Bake in the oven for 10 minutes or air-fry for 5 minutes, then flip over and bake for another 10 minutes in the oven or another 5 minutes in the air fryer, or until the internal temperature registers 145°F.
5. While the pork chops are cooking, prepare the mustard sauce, if using: In a small bowl, whisk together the ingredients until combined. Cover and refrigerate until ready to serve.
6. Serve the chops with mustard sauce, if desired.

NOTE: If you prefer, you can use thicker chops for this recipe. However, the cook time will increase. If using 1-inch-thick chops, you will need to add another 10 to 15 minutes.

Calories	Fat	Protein	Total Carbs	Dietary Fiber	Net Carbs
378	20g	49g	1g	0.3g	0.7g

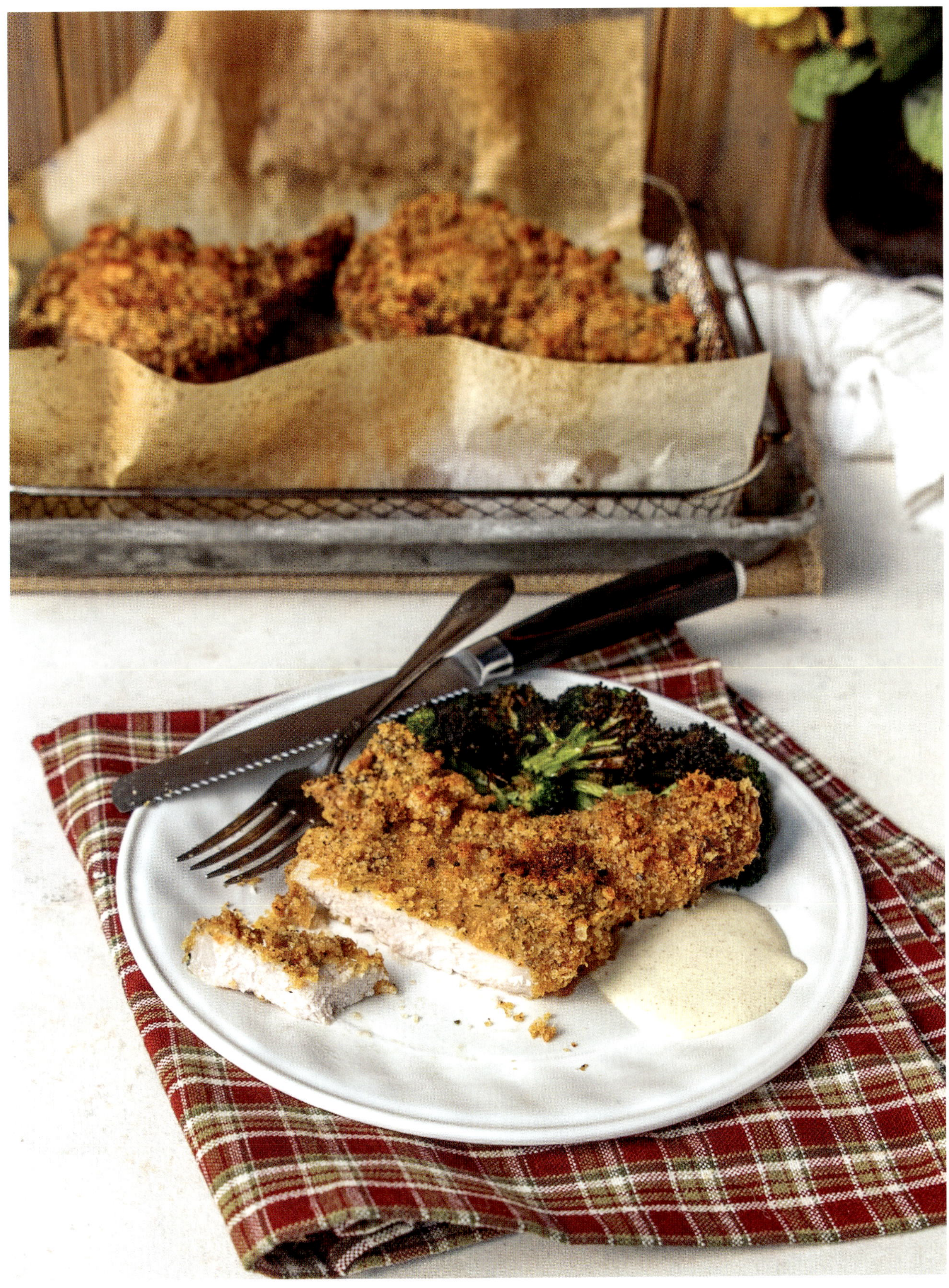

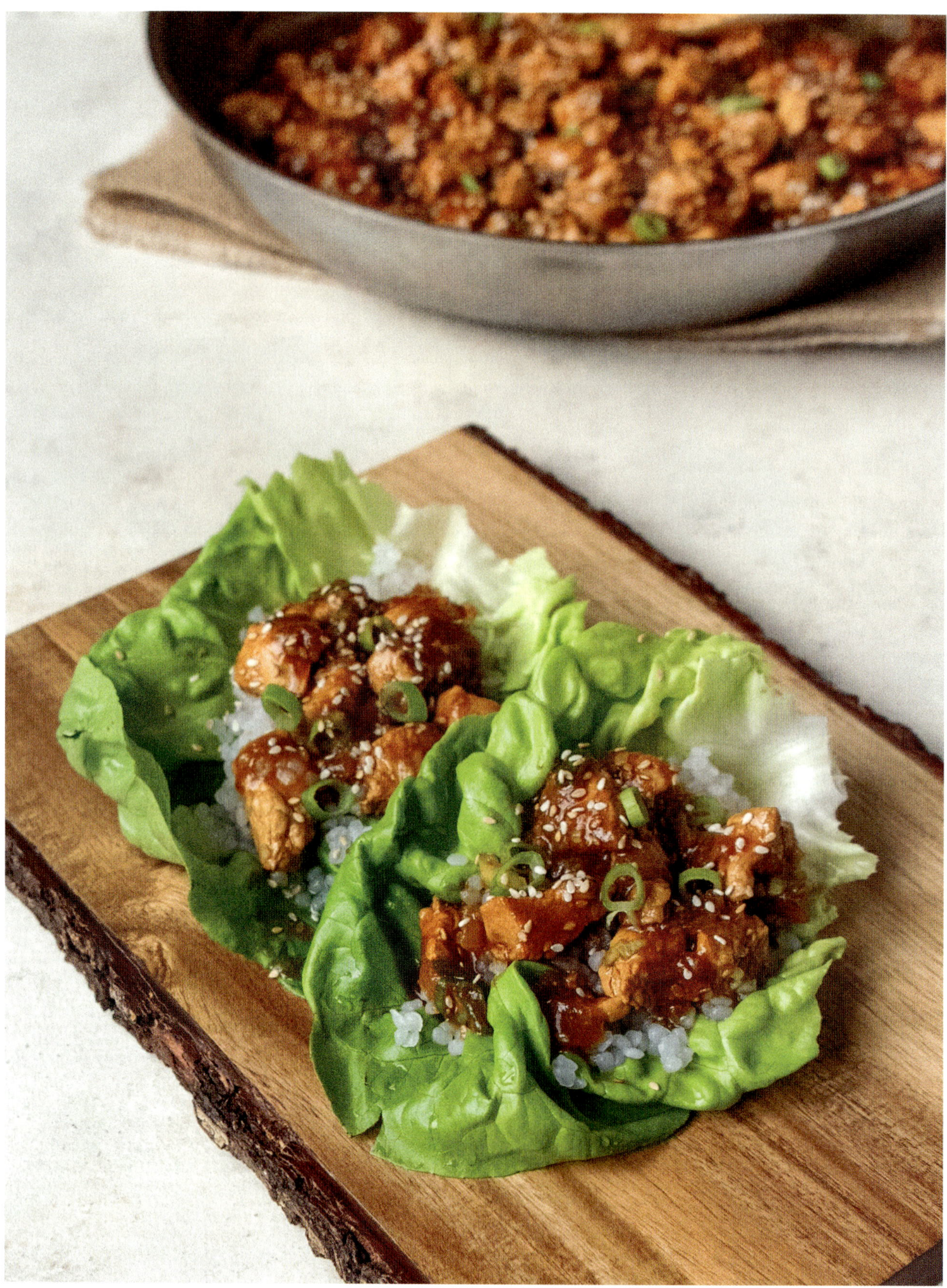

YIELD: 4 servings
PREP TIME: 10 minutes
COOK TIME: 18 minutes

BOURBON CHICKEN LETTUCE WRAPS

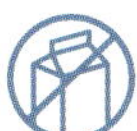  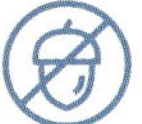

Bourbon chicken is a perfect balance of sweet, savory, tangy, and umami flavors. The sauce typically combines brown sugar, soy sauce, garlic, ginger, and bourbon, creating a rich, slightly smoky, and caramelized glaze. You can easily omit the bourbon if you don't have any or don't care to use it.

FOR THE BOURBON CHICKEN:

2 tablespoons avocado oil

1 cup chopped yellow onions

1 pound boneless, skinless chicken breasts, cut into 1-inch cubes

⅓ cup coconut aminos

1 tablespoon minced garlic

1 tablespoon low-carb brown sugar–style sweetener

1 tablespoon bourbon

2 teaspoons Sriracha

1 teaspoon red pepper flakes

1 cup chicken bone broth

1 teaspoon glucomannan or xanthan gum

FOR SERVING/GARNISH:

8 large Boston lettuce leaves

Shirataki rice, drained and warmed (optional)

Sesame seeds (optional)

Chopped scallions (optional)

1. Heat the avocado oil in a large skillet over medium-high heat. Add the onions and cook for 4 to 5 minutes, until tender. Add the chicken and cook for 5 minutes, or until cooked through (no longer pink in the center).
2. In a small bowl, whisk together the coconut aminos, garlic, brown sugar sweetener, bourbon, Sriracha, and red pepper flakes. Pour over the chicken in the skillet.
3. Add the broth to the skillet, then sprinkle the glucomannan over the mixture. Continue to cook, stirring continuously, over medium-low heat for 5 to 8 minutes, until the sauce thickens.
4. To serve, place two lettuce leaves each on four serving plates. If using shirataki rice, spoon it into the lettuce leaves, then top with the bourbon chicken. Garnish with sesame seeds and/or scallions, if desired.

Calories	Fat	Protein	Total Carbs	Dietary Fiber	Net Carbs
253	10g	25g	10g	1g	9g

YIELD: 8 servings
PREP TIME: 15 minutes
COOK TIME: 20 minutes

CHICKEN CAPRESE CASSEROLE

When you use rotisserie chicken, this hearty meal comes together quickly. You could also use cooked chicken leftovers (1½ to 1¾ pounds cooked meat should do it). Serve over zucchini noodles, egg white noodles, shirataki noodles, or cauliflower rice.

- Meat from 1 (2- to 2¼-pound) rotisserie chicken, chopped
- ½ cup pesto sauce
- ½ cup avocado oil mayonnaise
- ½ cup sour cream
- 2 cups shredded mozzarella cheese (part skim), divided
- ½ cup grated Parmesan cheese
- 1 cup halved grape tomatoes, divided
- ½ cup roughly chopped fresh basil, for garnish

1. Preheat the oven to 375°F. Grease a 9 by 13-inch baking dish.
2. In a large bowl, stir together the chicken, pesto, mayonnaise, sour cream, 1 cup of the mozzarella, and the Parmesan cheese.
3. Spread the chicken mixture in the prepared baking dish. Top with the remaining cup of mozzarella cheese and ½ cup of the tomatoes.
4. Cover with aluminum foil and bake for 20 minutes, or until the cheese is melted. As soon as the casserole comes out of the oven, top with the remaining tomatoes and the basil.
5. Store leftovers in an airtight container in the fridge (or simply cover with plastic wrap) for up to 3 days. Alternatively, you can portion it into individual containers for easy lunches or cool the casserole completely and cover it to freeze for up to 3 months.

BASED ON USING A 2-POUND ROTISSERIE CHICKEN

Calories	Fat	Protein	Total Carbs	Dietary Fiber	Net Carbs
429	32g	32g	4g	0.5g	3.5g

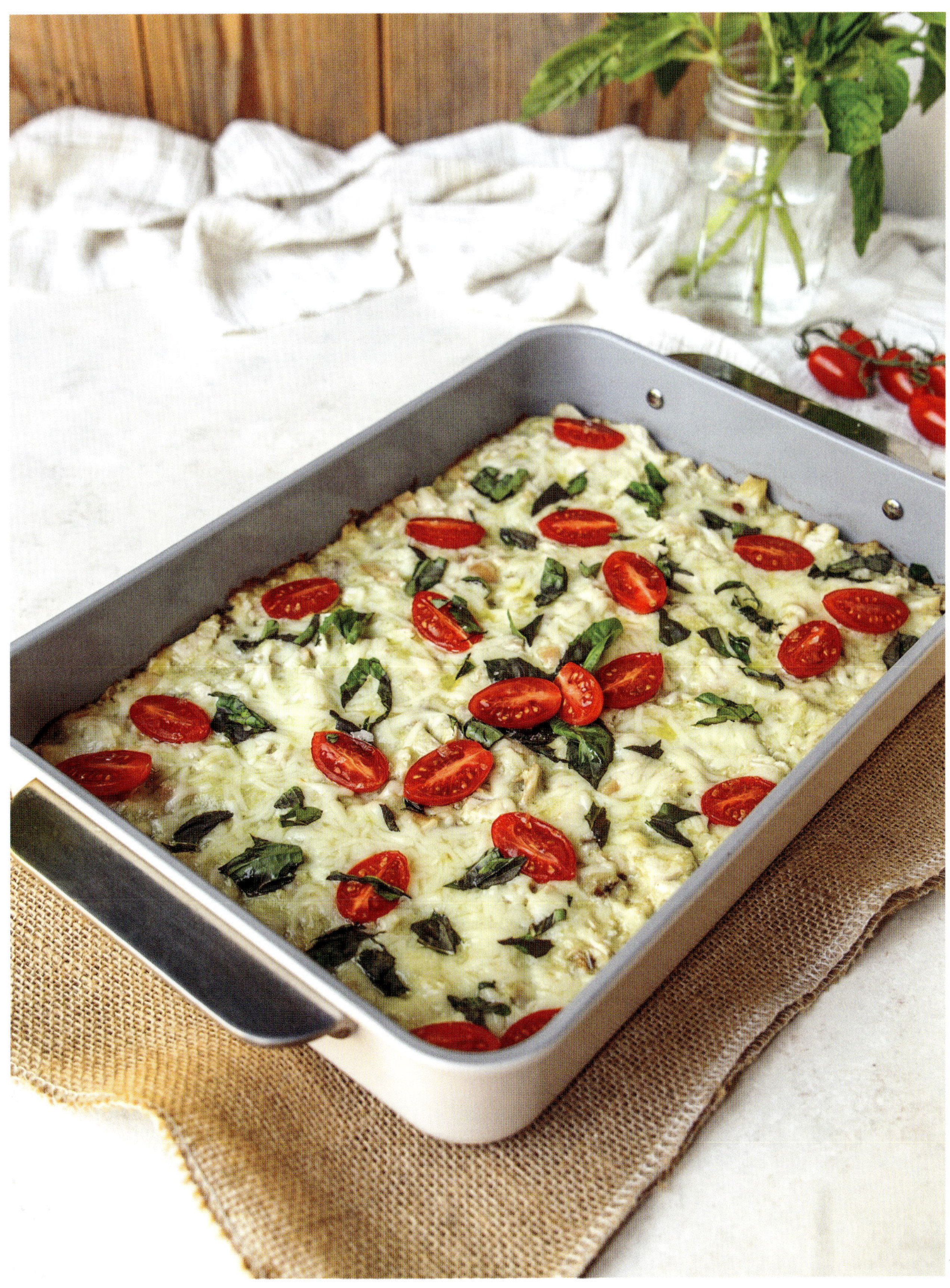

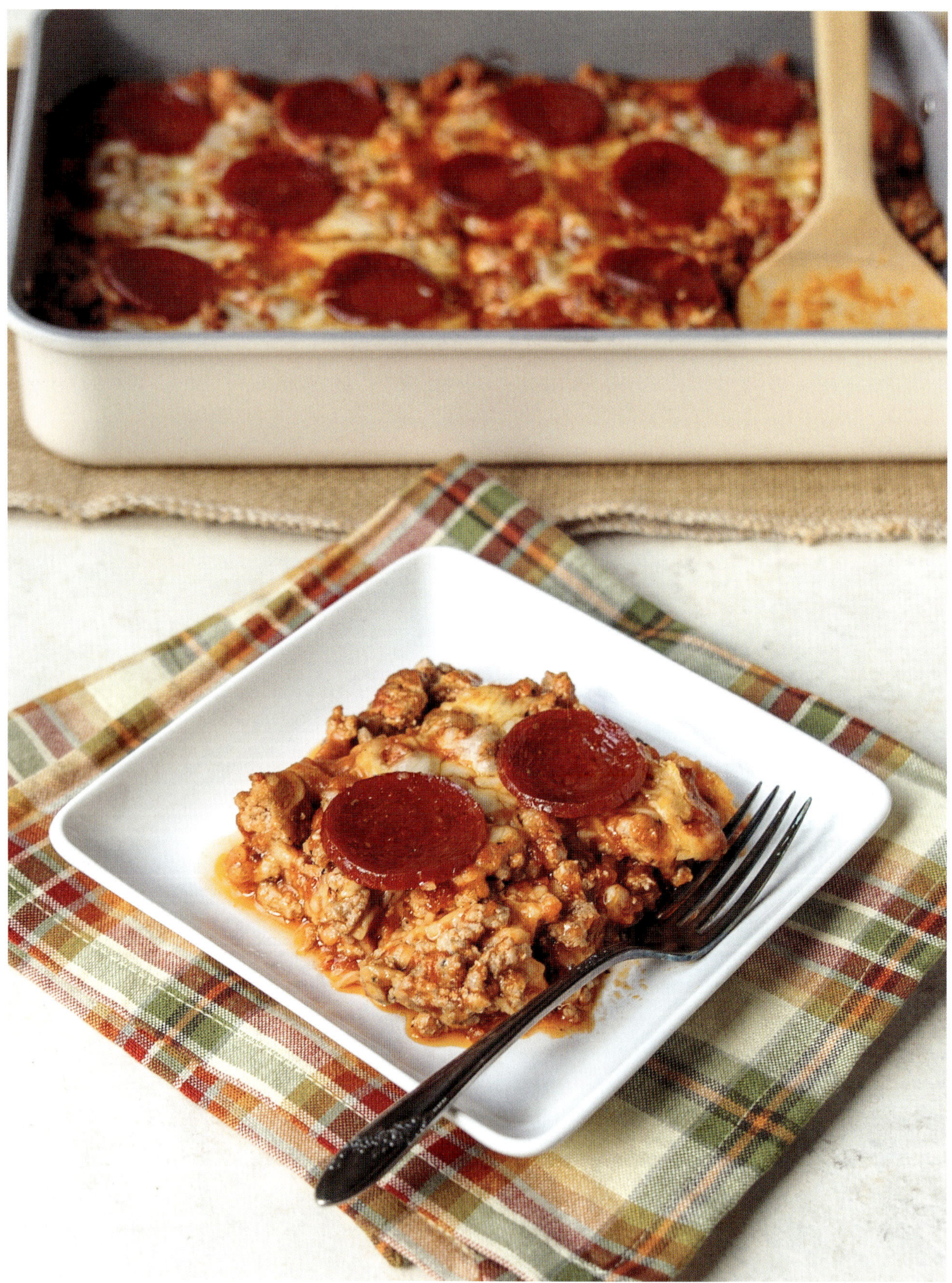

YIELD: 8 servings
PREP TIME: 10 minutes
COOK TIME: 30 minutes

CRUSTLESS PEPPERONI PIZZA BAKE

 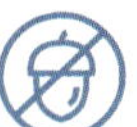 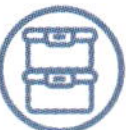 

This recipe is a cross between pizza and lasagna. It has all the great flavors of pizza, built up in delicious layers. This "pizza" is crustless, but you won't miss the crust, and it keeps it low carb! For meals on the go, you can also bake, portion into individual servings in airtight containers, cool completely, and freeze for up to 3 months.

2 pounds ground pork

1 tablespoon extra-virgin olive oil

2 cups low-carb marinara sauce

6 Folios cheddar cheese wraps, or 8 ounces sliced or shredded cheddar cheese

2 cups shredded mozzarella cheese (part skim)

1½ ounces pepperoni (about 25 slices)

1. Preheat the oven to 425°F. Spray a 9 by 13-inch baking pan with cooking spray.
2. Brown the pork in the olive oil in a large skillet over medium-high heat, crumbling it as it cooks. Add the marinara sauce and stir to combine. Simmer for 5 minutes, then remove the pan from the heat and set aside.
3. Lay two of the cheese wraps in the prepared baking pan. Slice a third wrap in half to cover the bottom of the pan with none overlapping. If using sliced or shredded cheddar, spread half of it evenly across the bottom of the prepared pan.
4. Spread 1 cup of the mozzarella over the cheese wraps or cheddar cheese in the pan. Top with half of the pepperoni. Place the remaining cheese wraps or cheddar cheese in an even layer over the pepperoni. Evenly top with the meat sauce. Cover with the remaining cup of mozzarella and then the rest of the pepperoni slices.
5. Bake uncovered for 20 minutes, or until bubbling around the edges and the cheese is melted.

Calories	Fat	Protein	Total Carbs	Dietary Fiber	Net Carbs
482	49g	36g	3g	1g	2g

YIELD: 8 servings
PREP TIME: 8 minutes
COOK TIME: 40 minutes

CHEESEBURGER PIE

When you're feeling like a cheeseburger but don't want to make individual patties and grill or fry them on the stove, try this easy meat pie. It's like a giant cheeseburger, and it takes less than 50 minutes from start to finish!

2 pounds 80/20 or 90/10 ground beef

1 cup chopped yellow onions

1 tablespoon extra-virgin olive oil or avocado oil (if using 90/10 ground beef)

1/2 teaspoon fine sea salt

1/4 teaspoon ground black pepper

4 large eggs

1 1/2 cups heavy cream

1 teaspoon baking powder

1 1/2 cups shredded cheddar cheese, divided

SUGGESTED TOPPINGS:

Chopped or crumbled cooked bacon

Sliced or chopped dill pickles

Diced tomatoes

1. Preheat the oven to 350°F.
2. Put the ground beef, onions, and oil (if using lean beef) in a 12-inch cast-iron skillet or other ovenproof pan, such as a braiser or casserole. Cook over medium-high heat, crumbling the meat as it cooks, until the beef is browned and the onions are tender, 6 to 8 minutes. Drain off the excess fat, leaving about 2 tablespoons in the pan. Sprinkle with the salt and pepper, then turn off the heat and allow to cool slightly before adding the egg mixture.
3. In a mixing bowl, whisk together the eggs, cream, baking powder, and 1 cup of the cheddar cheese. Pour this mixture into the skillet and stir until nicely combined with the beef. Sprinkle the remaining 1/2 cup of cheddar over the top and place the skillet in the oven.
4. Bake for 30 to 35 minutes, until the pie is browned around the edges, the center is puffed and golden, and a knife inserted in the center comes out clean. Allow to cool for about 10 minutes, then slice and enjoy with the toppings of your choice.
5. Store covered in the fridge for up to 3 days or freeze for up to 3 months. Thaw it the night before you want to enjoy it. Reheat uncovered in a 350°F oven for 15 to 20 minutes.

Calories	Fat	Protein	Total Carbs	Dietary Fiber	Net Carbs
584	49g	28g	3g	0.4g	1.6g

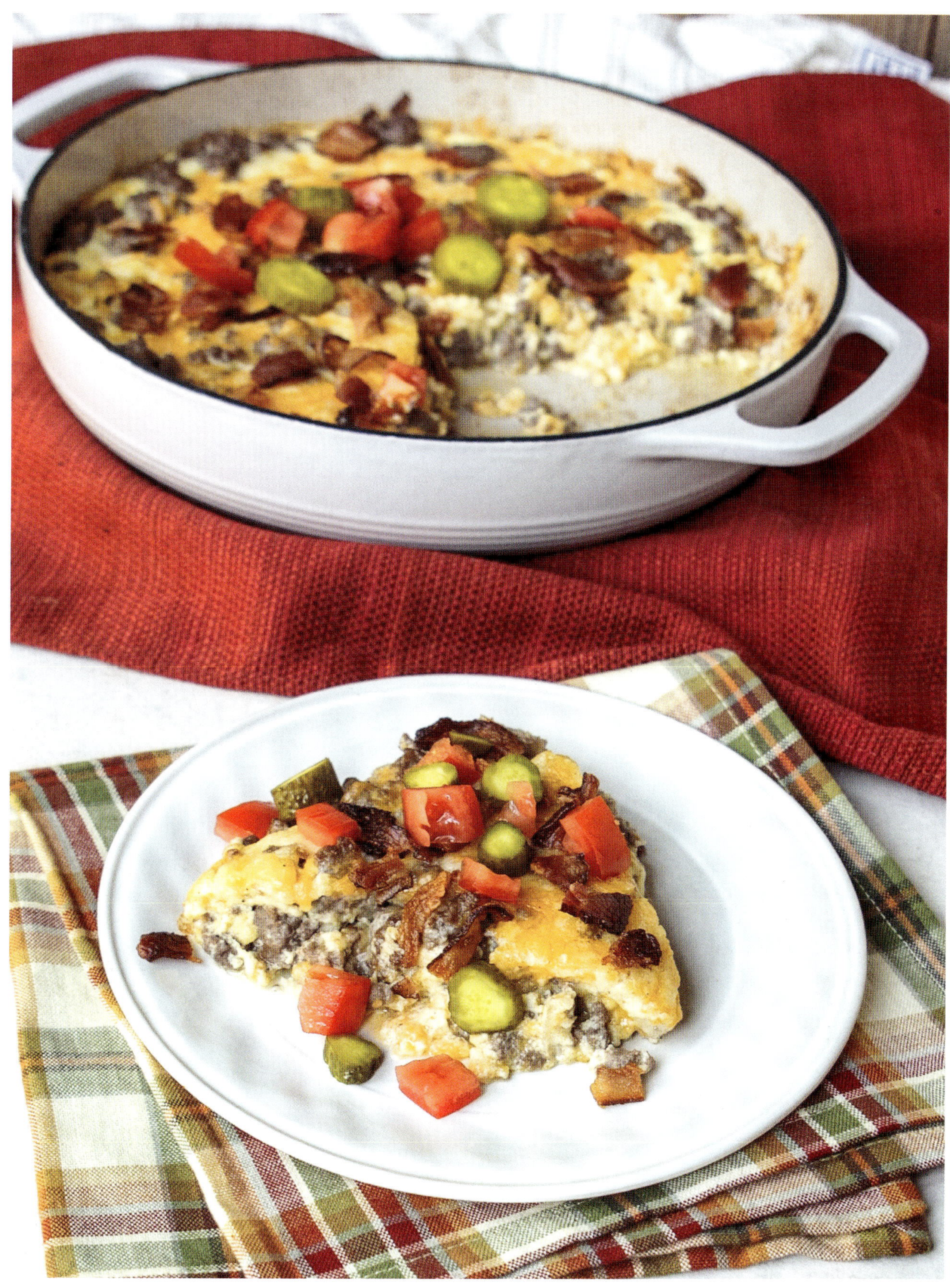

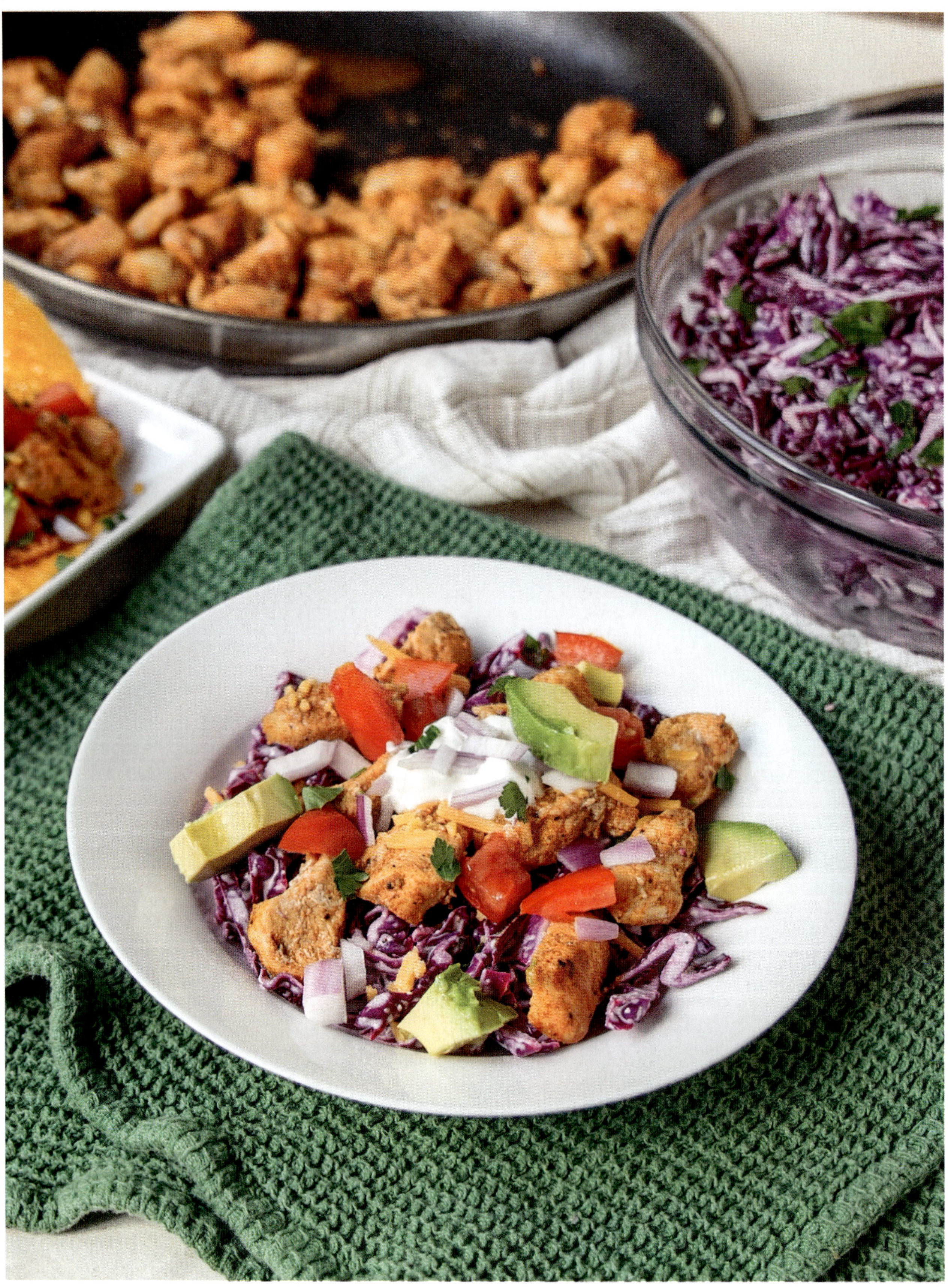

YIELD: 4 servings
PREP TIME: 5 minutes (not including time to prepare slaw)
COOK TIME: 6 minutes

CHICKEN TACO BOWLS

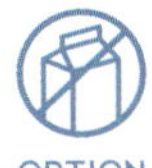
OPTION

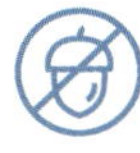

This is a better version of the super simple chicken taco recipe on page 131. Here you will cook up some fresh chicken breast instead of using precooked, and you replace the store-bought taco shells with a bed of delicious homemade slaw. If you've made the slaw ahead, this meal comes together very quickly; if not, count on about 25 minutes of prep time.

1½ pounds boneless, skinless chicken breasts

1 teaspoon paprika

½ teaspoon chili powder

½ teaspoon garlic powder

½ teaspoon onion powder

½ teaspoon fine sea salt

¼ teaspoon ground black pepper

¼ teaspoon cayenne pepper

2 tablespoons extra-virgin olive oil, for the pan

4 cups Red Cabbage Slaw (page 217), for serving

SUGGESTED TOPPINGS:

Sour cream

Finely chopped red onion

Diced tomato

Diced avocado

Shredded cheese of choice

Chopped fresh cilantro

Squeeze of lime juice

1. Chop the chicken into bite-sized pieces, about 1 inch. Place the chicken pieces in a large bowl. Add the seasonings and stir to coat.
2. Pour the olive oil into a large skillet and set over medium-high heat.
3. When the oil is hot, add the chicken to the skillet and cook for 5 to 6 minutes, until cooked through (with no pink remaining in the center).
4. To serve, divide the slaw evenly among four serving bowls, then top with the chicken. Add the toppings of your choice.

Calories	Fat	Protein	Total Carbs	Dietary Fiber	Net Carbs
260	12g	36g	1g	0.4g	0.6g

YIELD: one 9-inch crust (2 servings)
PREP TIME: 10 minutes (not including time to cook chicken)
COOK TIME: 25 minutes

COTTAGE CHEESE CHICKEN CRUST

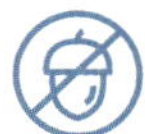

A sturdy high-protein crust that can hold up to toppings. If using rotisserie chicken for this recipe, one breast should give you the 5 ounces of meat you need.

5 ounces cooked chicken breast

3/4 cup cottage cheese (4% milkfat)

1 large egg

1/4 cup grated Parmesan cheese

1/4 cup shredded mozzarella cheese (part skim)

1/4 teaspoon Italian seasoning

1/4 teaspoon onion powder

1/4 teaspoon garlic powder

1/4 teaspoon fine sea salt

1. Preheat the oven to 400°F. Line two rimmed baking sheets with parchment paper.
2. Put all the ingredients in a food processor and chop until smooth. The mixture will be thick. If you don't have a food processor, be sure to very finely shred or mince the cooked chicken before combining it with the rest of the ingredients in a large bowl.
3. Scoop the dough onto the center of one of the prepared baking sheets. Using the back of a spoon, spread the mixture out into a round 9-inch circle about 1/4 inch thick.
4. Bake for 15 minutes, then remove from the oven and flip the par-baked crust over onto the second lined baking sheet. The easiest way to do this is to take hold of the ends of the parchment paper under the crust, lift it up, and flip it over onto the other pan. Slowly and gently pull off the parchment that is now on top of the crust, using a metal spatula to help you peel it off. Return the crust to the oven and bake for another 5 to 10 minutes, until golden brown.
5. Use as the base for your favorite pizza toppings.
6. Store in an airtight container in the fridge for up to 3 days or let cool completely and freeze for up to 6 months.

Calories	Fat	Protein	Total Carbs	Dietary Fiber	Net Carbs
321	15g	40g	5g	0.2g	4.8g

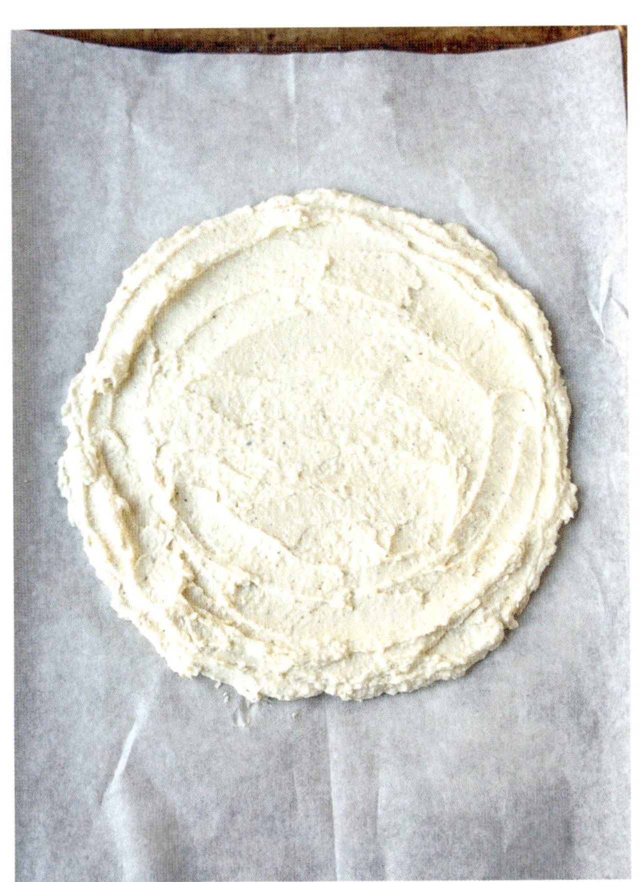

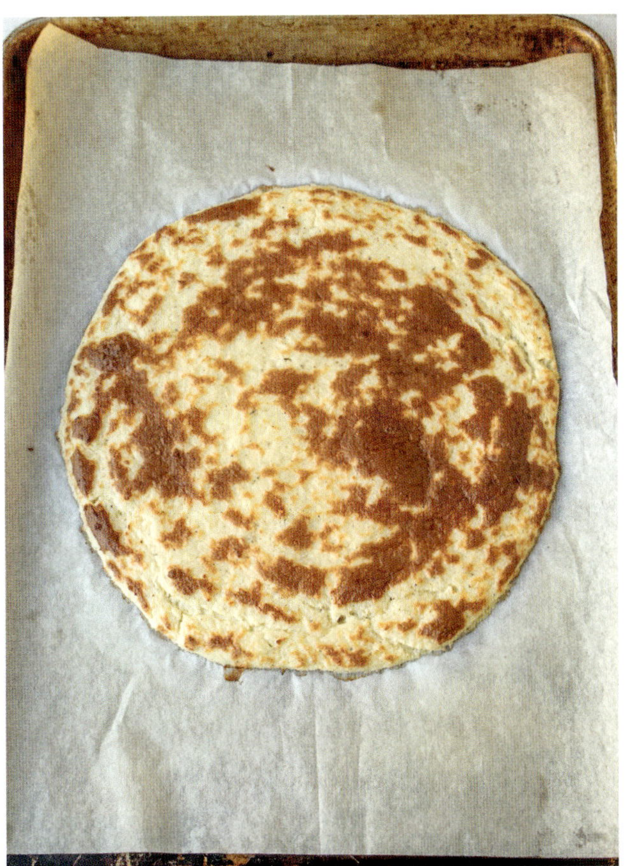

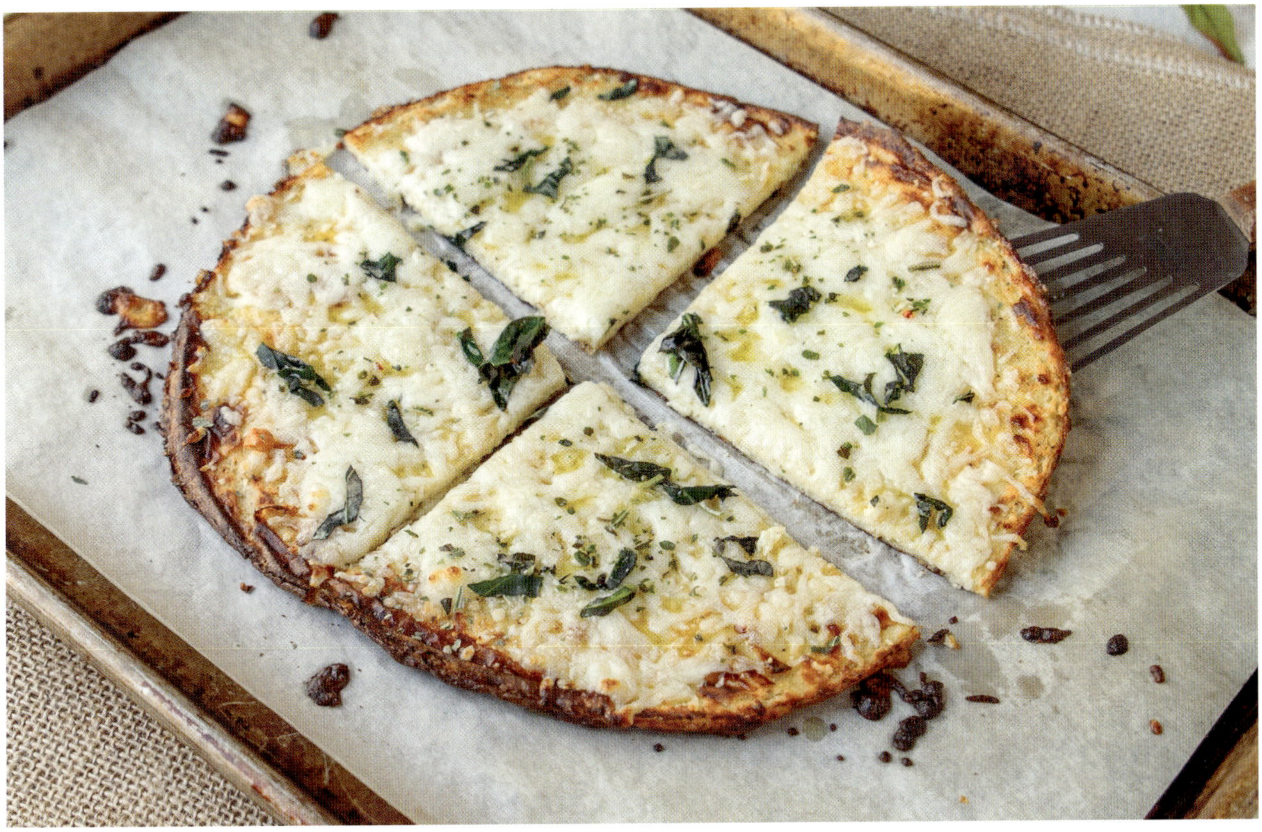

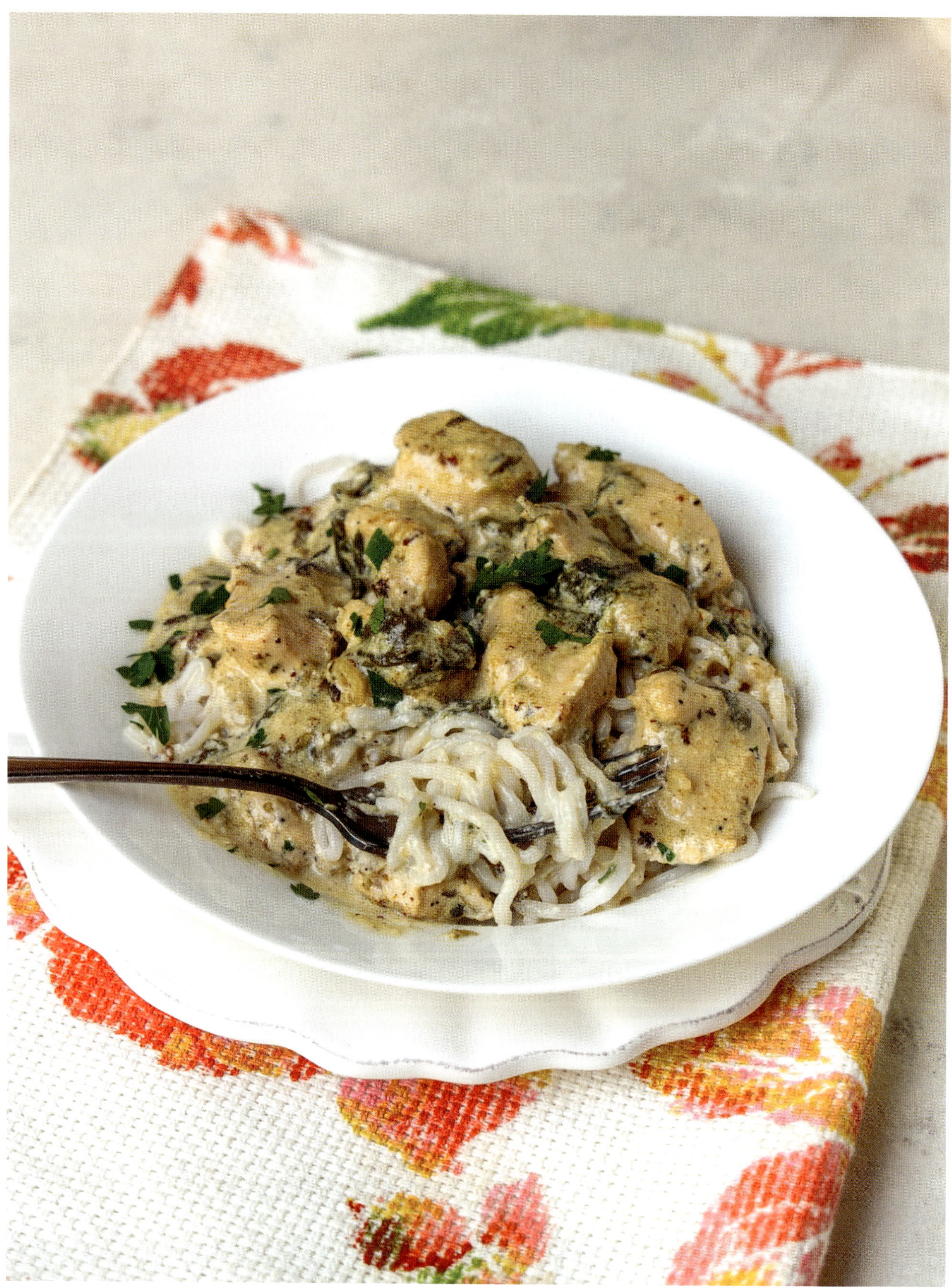

YIELD: 4 servings
PREP TIME: 15 minutes
COOK TIME: 25 minutes

CHICKEN SPINACH ALFREDO

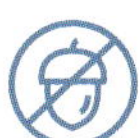

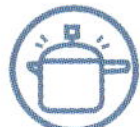

This is one of the easiest meals to freezer prep because everything gets dumped into a gallon-size freezer bag. Thanks to the Instant Pot, this meal can also be on the table from start to finish in less than 45 minutes, and even more quickly if you're freezer prepping. So either way is a win! If you don't have an Instant Pot, you can cook this recipe in a slow cooker (see variation below); however, it will take significantly longer. If you love the flavors of this dish and are looking for a batch-cooked version that will leave you with lots of leftovers, try my recipe for Chicken Spinach Alfredo Casserole (page 254) in the Best chapter.

2 pounds boneless, skinless chicken breasts, cut into 1-inch pieces

3 cups heavy cream

4 cloves garlic, minced

1½ cups grated Parmesan cheese

2 teaspoons dried parsley

½ teaspoon fine sea salt

½ teaspoon ground black pepper

8 ounces fresh baby spinach

1 teaspoon glucomannan or xanthan gum (optional, to thicken)

Chopped fresh parsley, for garnish (optional)

1. If freezer prepping, put all the ingredients, except the glucomannan, in a gallon-size zip-top bag and freeze for up to 3 months. Thaw overnight in the refrigerator before cooking.
2. Put all the ingredients, except the glucomannan, in an Instant Pot. (If freezer prepping, simply pour the thawed contents of the freezer bag into the Instant Pot.) Seal the lid and cook on manual mode at high pressure for 25 minutes. Press cancel to end cooking and allow the Instant Pot to naturally release pressure. After the pressure releases, carefully open the lid. If desired, sprinkle on the glucomannan and mix to thicken the sauce. Serve garnished with chopped parsley, if desired.

VARIATION: Slow Cooker Chicken Spinach Alfredo. Put the thawed contents of the freezer bag in an 8-quart slow cooker. Cover and cook on low for 4 to 6 hours, until the chicken is fork-tender and no longer pink. If desired, sprinkle on the glucomannan and mix to thicken the sauce. Serve garnished with chopped parsley, if desired

Calories	Fat	Protein	Total Carbs	Dietary Fiber	Net Carbs
424	76g	63g	6g	1g	5g

YIELD: 6 servings
(5 meatballs per serving)
PREP TIME: 20 minutes
COOK TIME: 30 minutes

RICOTTA MEATBALLS IN MARINARA SAUCE

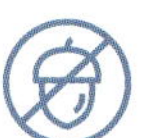
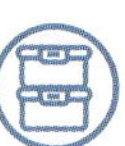
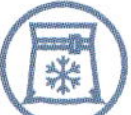

These meatballs in sauce have many possibilities. You can enjoy them as is or serve them over a bed of zucchini noodles, palmini noodles, shirataki noodles, or egg white noodles. Or try a meatball sub using cloud bread rolls (see recipe on page 88 for homemade rolls)!

2 cups ricotta cheese (part skim)

2 large eggs, beaten

4 cloves garlic, minced

1 cup grated Parmesan cheese

1/4 cup chopped fresh parsley, plus more for garnish if desired

1/4 cup chopped fresh basil

1 1/2 cups pork rind panko

1/2 teaspoon onion powder

1/4 teaspoon garlic powder

1/2 teaspoon fine sea salt

1/4 teaspoon ground black pepper

2 pounds 85/15 ground beef

2 tablespoons extra-virgin olive oil, for the pan

24 ounces low-carb marinara sauce

1. In a large bowl, stir the ricotta, eggs, garlic, and Parmesan until combined.
2. Add the parsley, basil, pork rind panko, onion powder, garlic powder, salt, and pepper. Stir to combine.
3. Stir in the ground beef just until combined; don't overmix. Form into thirty 1 1/2-inch meatballs.
4. If freezer prepping, place the raw meatballs in an airtight container and freeze for up to 3 months. Thaw overnight in the refrigerator before cooking.
5. When ready to cook the meatballs, heat 1 tablespoon of the olive oil in a large skillet over medium-high heat. Once the oil is hot, brown half of the meatballs. Remove from the pan and repeat with the remaining tablespoon of oil and meatballs.
6. Return the first batch of browned meatballs to the skillet, add the marinara sauce, and reduce the heat to low. Cover the pan and simmer until the meatballs are cooked through, 15 to 20 minutes. The meatballs are done when the internal temperature reaches 160°F. Garnish with fresh parsley, if desired.

Calories	Fat	Protein	Total Carbs	Dietary Fiber	Net Carbs
784	61g	49g	9g	1g	8g

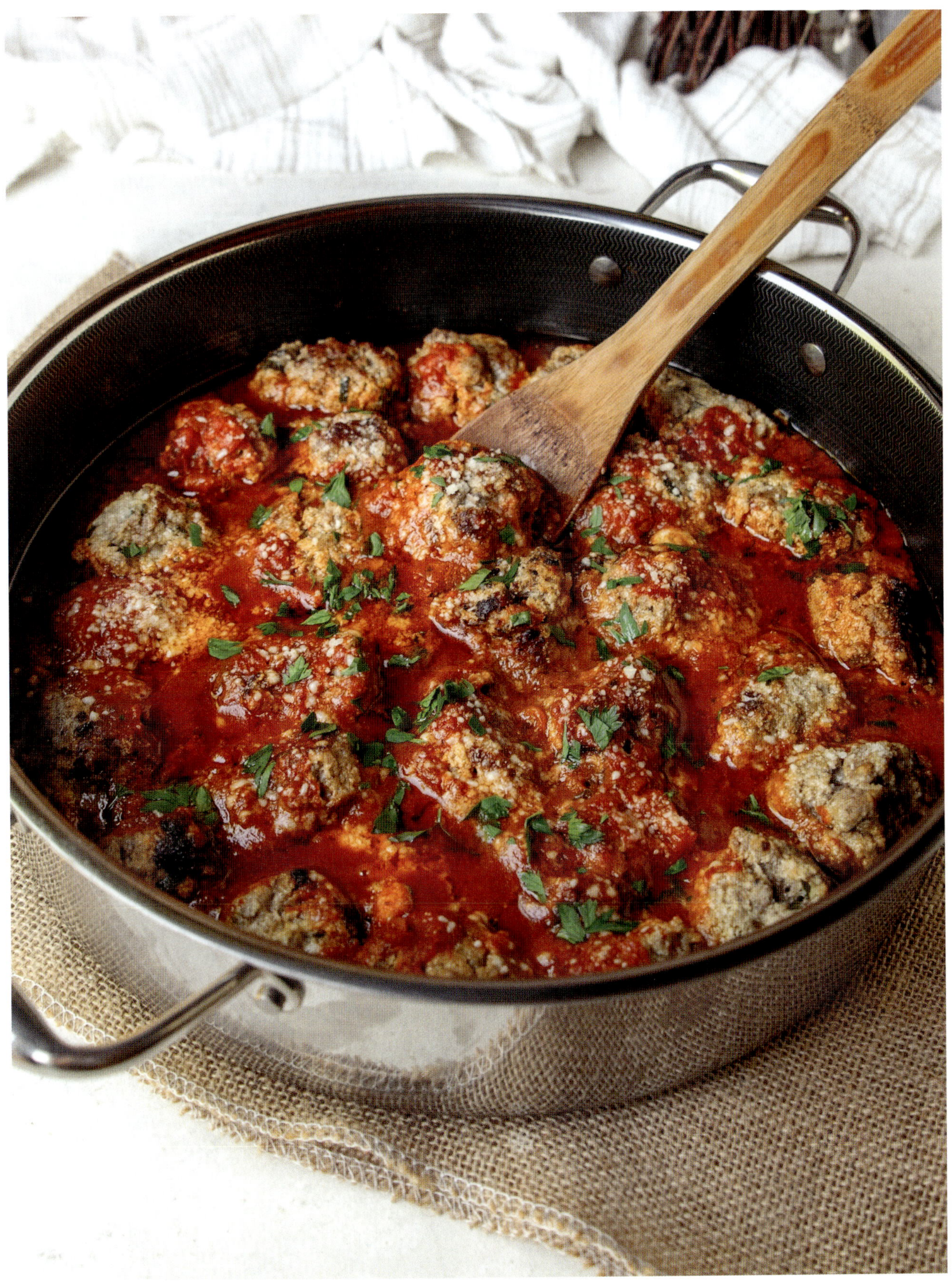

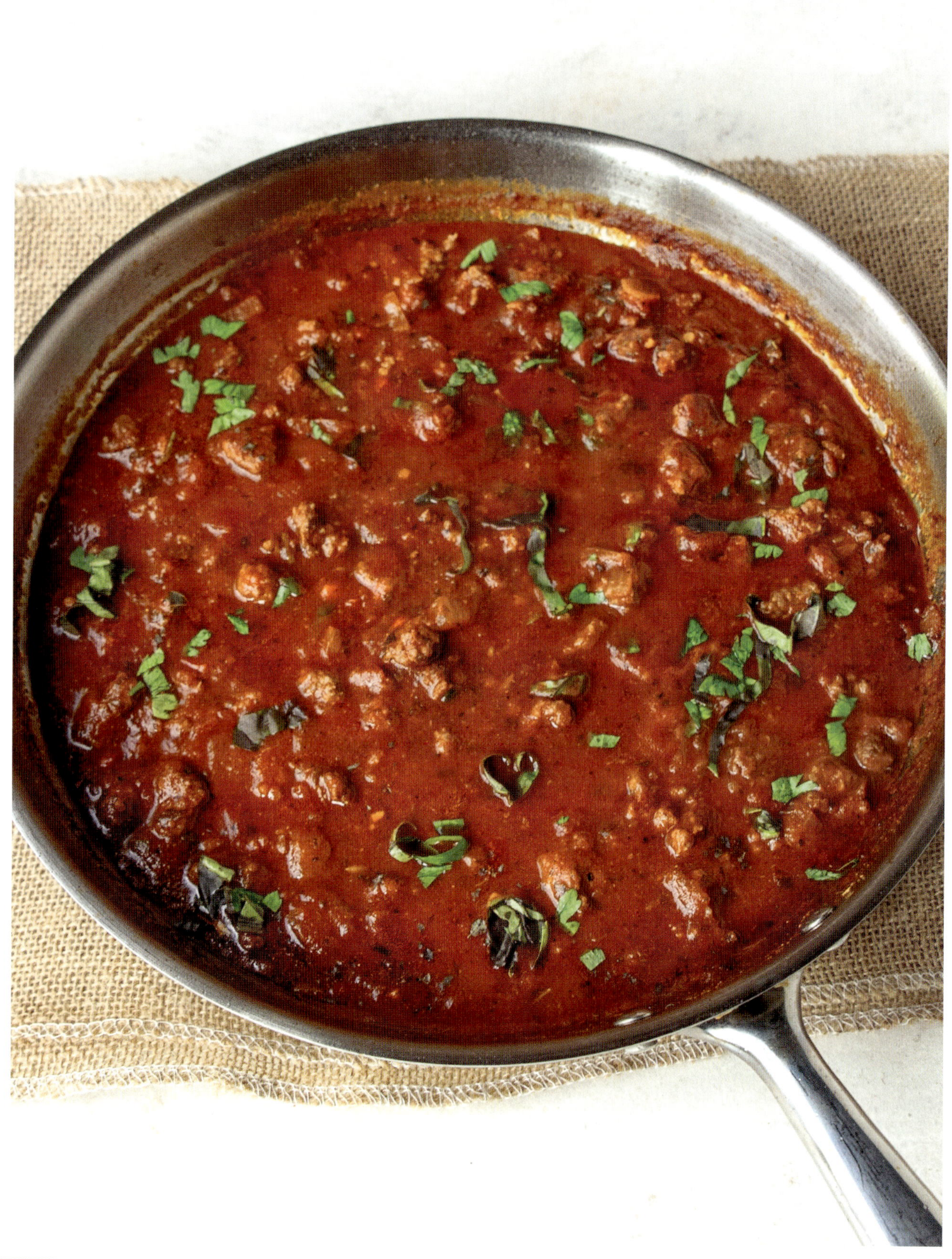

YIELD: 10 servings (1/2 cup per serving)
PREP TIME: 10 minutes
COOK TIME: 30 minutes

PORK RAGU

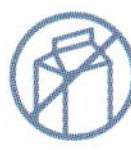 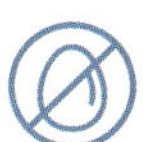 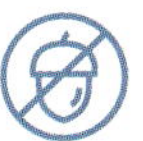 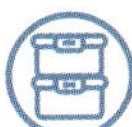

Enjoy this ragu over shirataki noodles, egg white noodles, or my cabbage fettuccine (page 221). You can also make this dish with 85/25 ground beef, to make more of a Bolognese style sauce, minus the milk used in a traditional Bolognese sauce.

- 2 tablespoons extra-virgin olive oil or avocado oil
- 1 cup chopped yellow onions
- 3 cloves garlic, minced
- 1 pound ground pork
- 2 teaspoons fennel seeds, crushed
- 1/2 cup chicken bone broth
- 1/2 cup red wine or more chicken broth
- 2 tablespoons tomato paste
- 1 (14-ounce) can crushed tomatoes
- 2 teaspoons Italian seasoning
- 1 teaspoon fine sea salt
- 1/2 teaspoon ground black pepper
- Red pepper flakes, to taste (optional)
- 1/4 cup chopped fresh parsley or basil, for garnish

1. Heat the oil in a large skillet over medium heat. Sauté the onion and garlic just until fragrant.
2. Turn the heat to high and add the ground pork and fennel seeds. Cook, breaking the meat up as best you can, until browned, 6 to 8 minutes. Add the broth, wine, and tomato paste and stir to combine. Simmer until reduced by half, 2 to 3 minutes.
3. Stir in the remaining ingredients and bring to a boil. Cover and reduce the heat to medium-low. Simmer for 20 to 25 minutes, until the sauce is reduced by half.
4. Taste and adjust the seasonings if needed. Garnish with fresh parsley or basil before serving.
5. Use immediately or let cool completely before storing in an airtight container in the refrigerator for up to 5 days or in the freezer for up to 3 months.

Calories	Fat	Protein	Total Carbs	Dietary Fiber	Net Carbs
181	13g	9g	6g	2g	4g

YIELD: 6 servings (4 meatballs per serving)
PREP TIME: 15 minutes
COOK TIME: 20 minutes

GENERAL TSO'S CHICKEN MEATBALLS

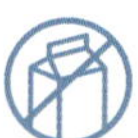  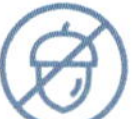

A family favorite! Tender chicken meatballs are coated in a rich and tangy sauce with a gentle kick from red pepper flakes. No need to add a thickener if you take the time to let the sauce slowly reduce. Enjoy the meatballs as is or serve them with a low-carb side like egg white noodles, cauliflower rice, or cooked broccoli.

FOR THE MEATBALLS:

2 pounds ground chicken

2 teaspoons minced garlic

1/2 teaspoon onion powder

1 tablespoon grated fresh ginger

1/2 cup pork rind panko

1/4 cup coconut aminos or gluten-free soy sauce

1/4 teaspoon fine sea salt

1/4 teaspoon ground black pepper

FOR THE SAUCE:

2 tablespoons avocado oil

2 tablespoons grated fresh ginger

2 teaspoons minced garlic

1 1/2 cups chicken bone broth

1/4 cup coconut aminos or gluten-free soy sauce

2 tablespoons apple cider vinegar

2 tablespoons unsweetened tomato puree

1/2 teaspoon red pepper flakes

FOR GARNISH:

1/2 teaspoon sesame seeds

2 scallions, finely sliced

1. Preheat the oven to 425°F. Line a rimmed baking sheet with parchment paper.
2. Put the meatball ingredients in a large bowl and, using your hands, mix to combine.
3. Roll the meat mixture into 2-inch balls, making a total of 24 meatballs. Place on the prepared pan and bake for 20 minutes, or until the internal temperature registers 165°F. While the meatballs are baking, prepare the sauce.
4. In a small bowl, mix together all the sauce ingredients. Pour the sauce into a large skillet and set over medium heat. Bring to a low simmer and cook until it reduces down and is fairly thick, about 10 minutes.
5. Once the meatballs are done, add them to the sauce and toss to coat. Serve garnished with the sesame seeds and sliced green onions.
6. Store leftovers in an airtight container in the fridge for up to 3 days or freeze for up to 3 months. Thaw before reheating in a skillet over medium heat to warm through.

Calories	Fat	Protein	Total Carbs	Dietary Fiber	Net Carbs
310	18g	29g	7g	0.4g	6.3g

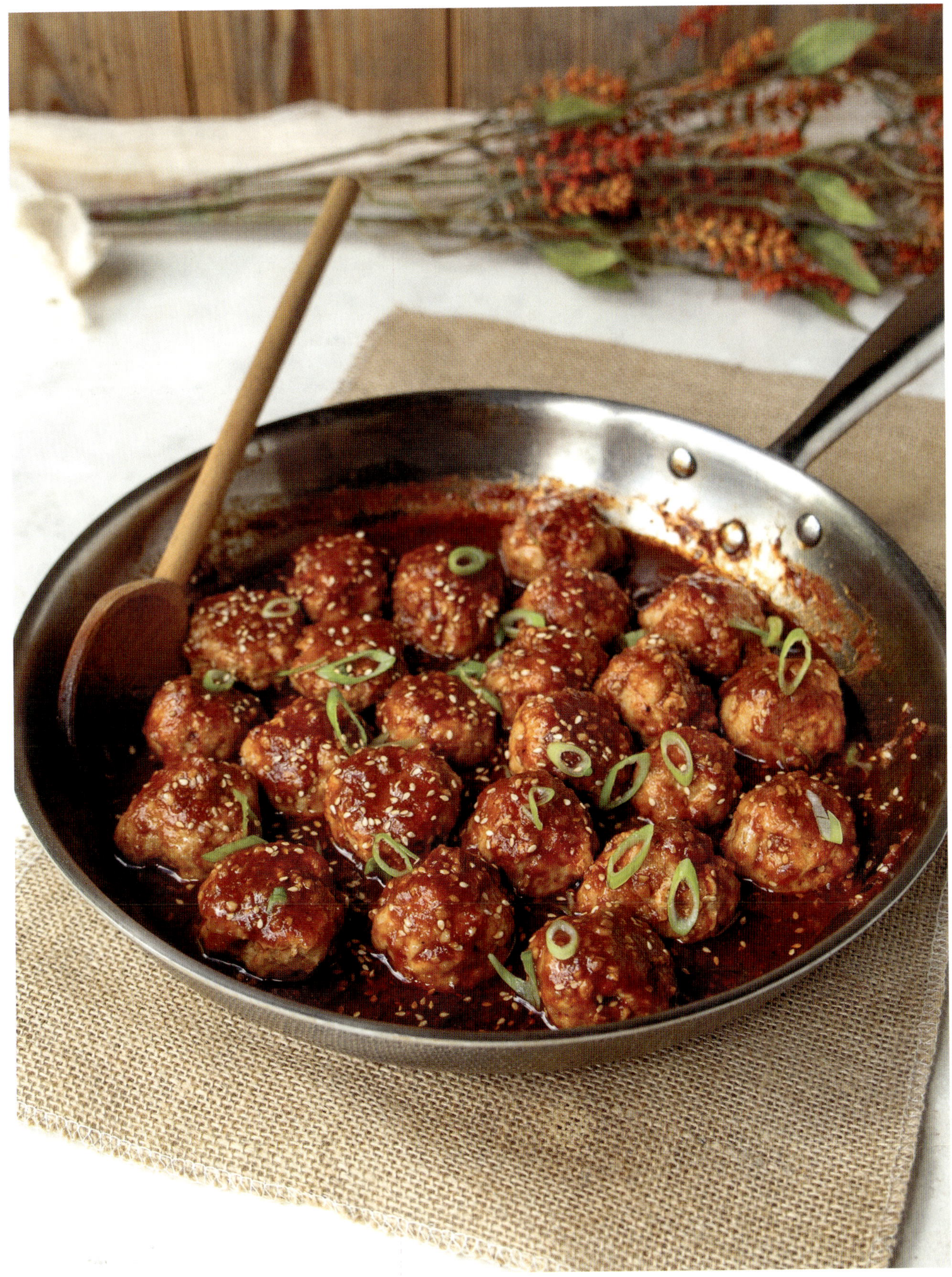

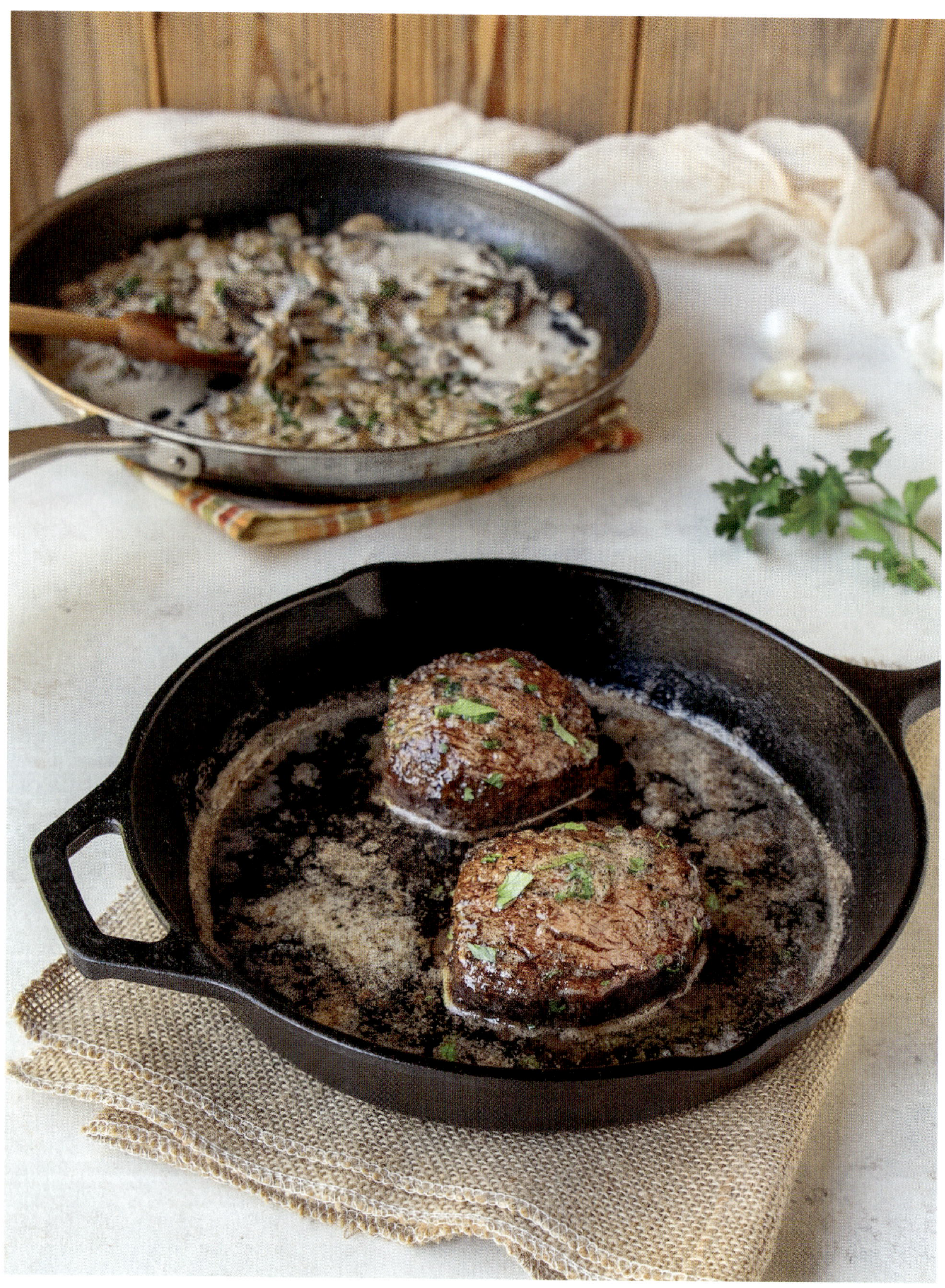

YIELD: 2 servings

PREP TIME: 5 minutes, plus 30 minutes to temper steaks

COOK TIME: 10 to 14 minutes, depending on preferred doneness

BUTTERY FILET MIGNON

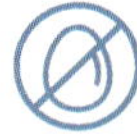 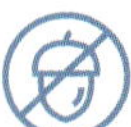

Date nights at home require a little bit of indulgence, and this filet mignon hits the spot!

- 2 (8-ounce) filet mignons (about 1½ inches thick)
- 1 teaspoon fine sea salt
- ½ teaspoon ground black pepper
- ¼ cup (½ stick) salted butter
- Pan drippings, or 1 cup Creamy Mushroom Sauce (page 214), for serving (optional)

1. Take the filets out of the fridge 30 minutes prior to cooking. Preheat the oven to 400°F.
2. Pat the steaks dry and season both sides with the salt and pepper.
3. Preheat a medium cast-iron or other ovenproof skillet over medium-high heat. Put the butter in the hot pan; when the butter has melted and the foaming has subsided, place the steaks in the pan.
4. Sear for 2 to 3 minutes while continuously spooning the butter over the tops of the steaks and tilting the pan to move the butter around so it doesn't burn.
5. When the steaks release easily from the pan, flip them over and sear for 2 to 3 minutes more while spooning the butter over them. When the steaks are nicely seared on both sides, transfer the pan to the oven.
6. Cook the filets until a thermometer inserted in the center of a steak registers 125°F to 130°F for medium, 6 to 8 minutes. If you're looking for medium rare, remove the steaks from the oven at 120°F.
7. Remove the steaks to a cutting board (if left in the pan, they will continue to cook). Let rest for 5 minutes before slicing.
8. Serve with pan drippings or, if desired, creamy mushroom sauce.

NOTE: If you'd like to make a double batch of this recipe for a family dinner instead of date night, simply use a large skillet.

Calories	Fat	Protein	Total Carbs	Dietary Fiber	Net Carbs
540	36g	50g	0.3g	0.1g	0.2g

YIELD: 2 cups
(1/2 cup per serving)
PREP TIME: 10 minutes
COOK TIME: 15 minutes

CREAMY MUSHROOM SAUCE

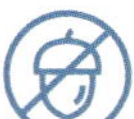

This mushroom sauce partners with steak exceptionally well, but really, it's an easy side for most any entrée. My baked pork chops (page 190) or ricotta meatballs (page 206) would be fantastic served with this sauce, especially over cauliflower rice.

- 2 tablespoons extra-virgin olive oil
- 8 ounces sliced white mushrooms
- 1/2 cup sliced yellow onions
- 4 cloves garlic, minced
- 1 teaspoon Italian seasoning
- 1 teaspoon Dijon mustard
- 1 teaspoon fresh lemon juice
- 1/2 cup chicken bone broth
- 1/2 cup heavy cream
- Salt and pepper
- 1 tablespoon chopped fresh parsley

1. Heat the olive oil in a medium skillet over medium-high heat. Add the mushrooms and onion and sauté until the mushrooms have released their water, it has cooked off, and the mushrooms and onions are browned, about 10 minutes.
2. Reduce the heat to medium and stir in the garlic, Italian seasoning, mustard, and lemon juice. Cook for 1 minute, then stir in the broth to deglaze the pan. Cook for 1 minute more to reduce slightly.
3. Pour in the cream, bring to a simmer, and cook for 3 to 4 minutes, or until the sauce has thickened.
4. Season with salt and pepper to taste and stir in the parsley just before serving.

Calories	Fat	Protein	Total Carbs	Dietary Fiber	Net Carbs
191	17g	2g	6g	1g	5g

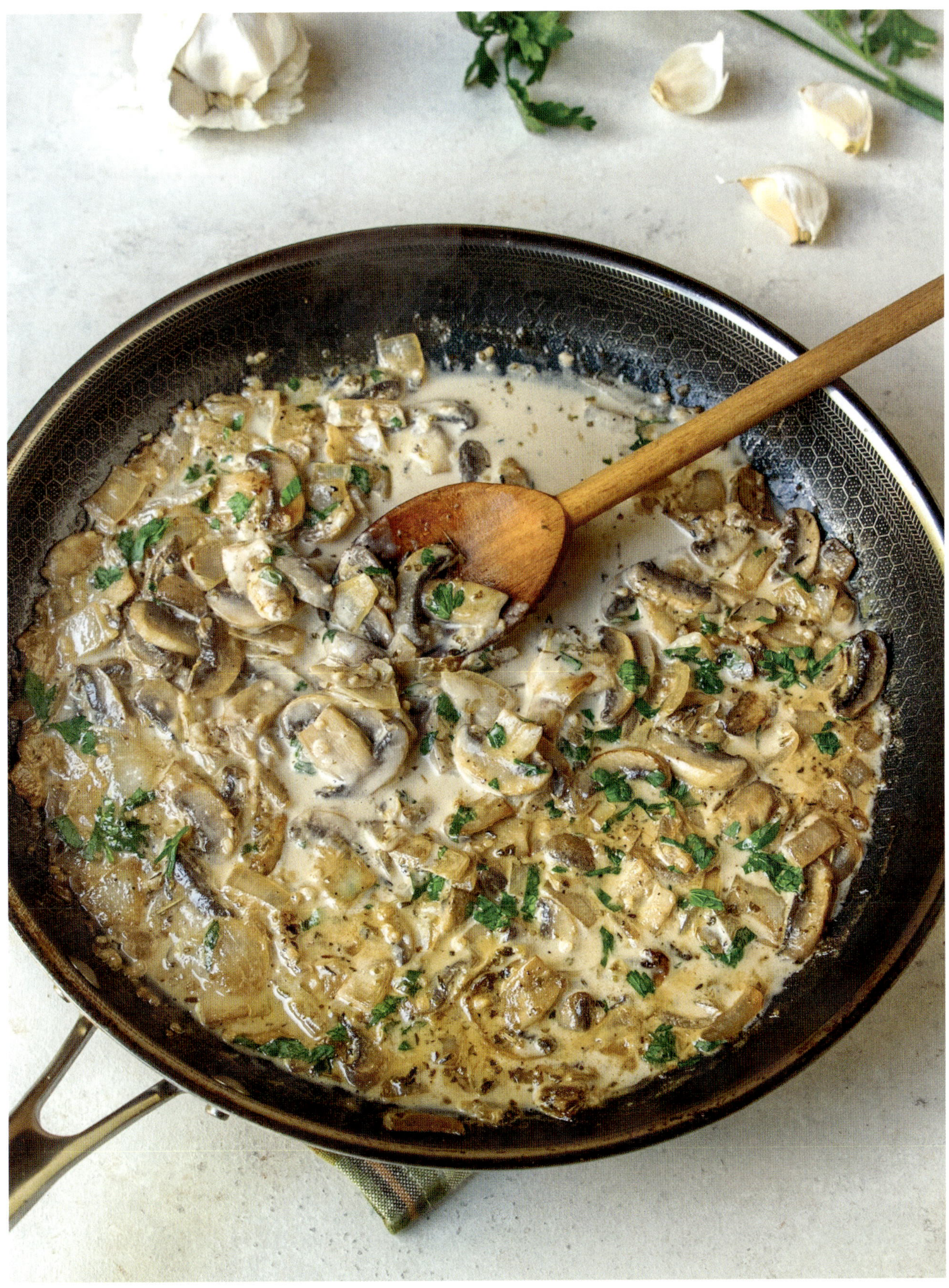

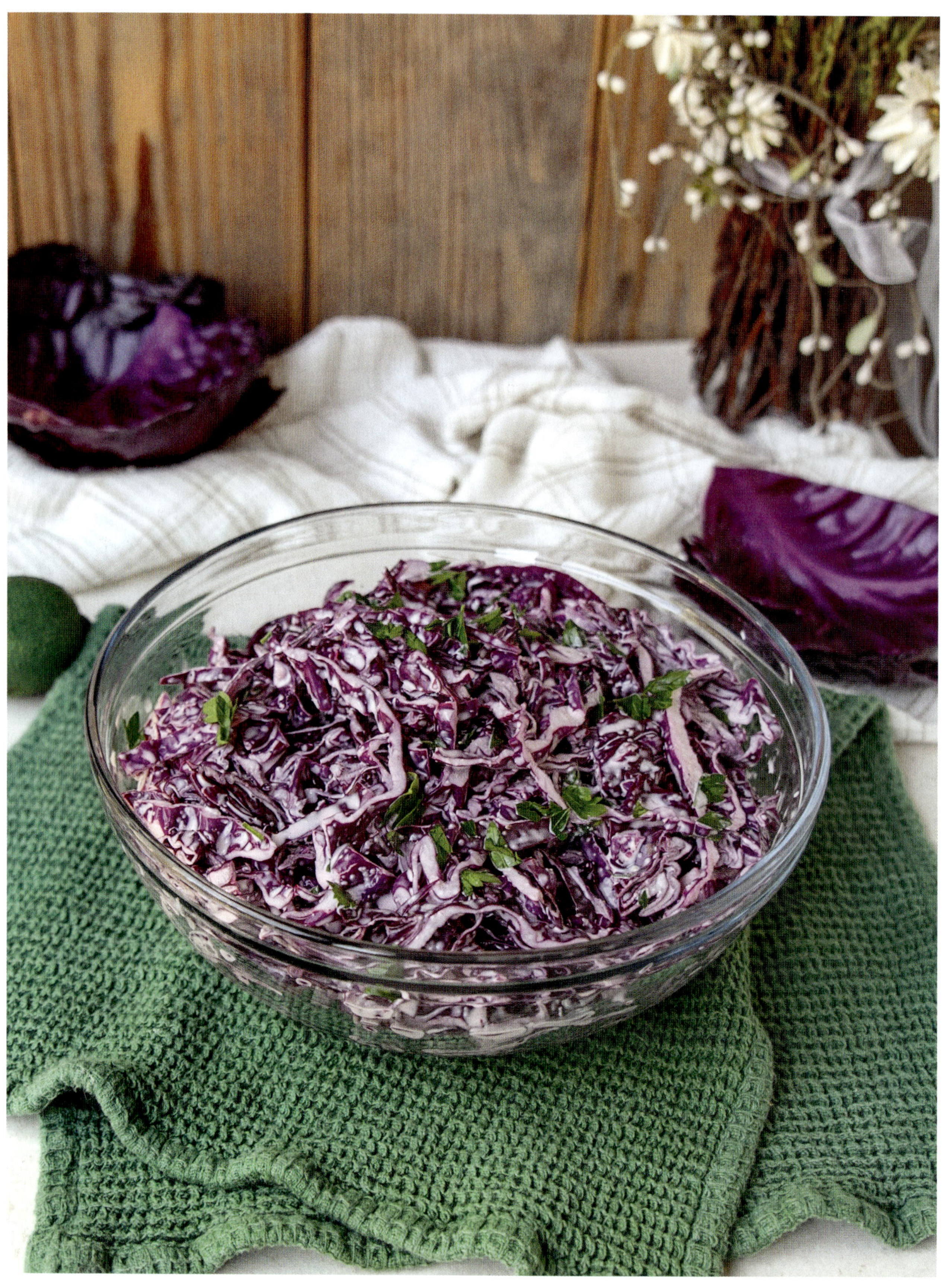

YIELD: 4 servings
(1 loosely packed cup per serving)
PREP TIME: 20 minutes

RED CABBAGE SLAW

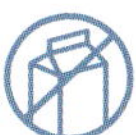
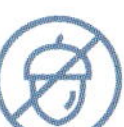
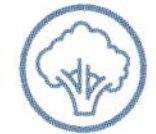

Having a delicious fresh slaw recipe to accompany any main entrée is always a smart idea for adding freshness, color, and crunch. This is our favorite slaw, and it goes well with many proteins, especially my chicken taco bowls (page 201) or breaded pork chops (page 190).

½ medium head red cabbage (about 15 ounces), cored, outer leaves removed

FOR THE DRESSING:

½ cup avocado oil mayonnaise

⅓ cup fresh lime juice

1 tablespoon extra-virgin olive oil

½ cup chopped fresh cilantro

½ teaspoon fine sea salt

¼ teaspoon onion powder

¼ teaspoon garlic powder

Ground black pepper, to taste

2 tablespoons chopped fresh parsley, for garnish (optional)

1. Finely slice or shred the cabbage and place in a large serving bowl.
2. In a small bowl, whisk together the dressing ingredients. Pour the dressing over the cabbage and toss to coat. Garnish with fresh parsley, if desired, and enjoy.
3. Store leftovers in an airtight container in the fridge for up to 5 days.

Calories	Fat	Protein	Total Carbs	Dietary Fiber	Net Carbs
107	11g	1g	4g	1g	3g

YIELD: 8 servings
PREP TIME: 10 minutes
(not including time to cook bacon)
COOK TIME: 15 minutes

BRUSSELS SPROUTS IN CARBONARA SAUCE

Even if you've never been a fan of Brussels sprouts, I think this recipe with creamy carbonara sauce will win you over.

1½ pounds Brussels sprouts

2 tablespoons extra-virgin olive oil

¼ teaspoon fine sea salt

¼ teaspoon ground black pepper

2 cloves garlic, minced

½ cup chicken bone broth

1 cup heavy cream

½ cup grated Parmesan cheese

½ cup shredded mozzarella cheese (part skim)

8 slices thick-cut bacon, baked (see page 76) and chopped

1. Trim the ends off the Brussels sprouts. Remove the outer layers and slice the sprouts in half.
2. Heat the olive oil in a medium skillet over medium-high heat. Add the Brussels sprouts and cook for 3 to 4 minutes, stirring occasionally, until the cut sides are nicely browned.
3. Add the salt, pepper, garlic, and broth to the skillet. Lower the heat to medium and simmer for 4 to 5 minutes, until the sprouts are almost cooked through. (You should be able to slide a knife into the sprouts but with some resistance, particularly at the center.)
4. Pour in the cream and simmer for 2 minutes to reduce slightly. Add the cheeses and continue to simmer until the sauce thickens and coats the back of a spoon and the Brussels sprouts are cooked all the way through. Sprinkle the bacon over the top and enjoy!
5. Store leftovers in an airtight container in the fridge for up to 3 days.

Calories	Fat	Protein	Total Carbs	Dietary Fiber	Net Carbs
204	15g	8g	9g	3g	6g

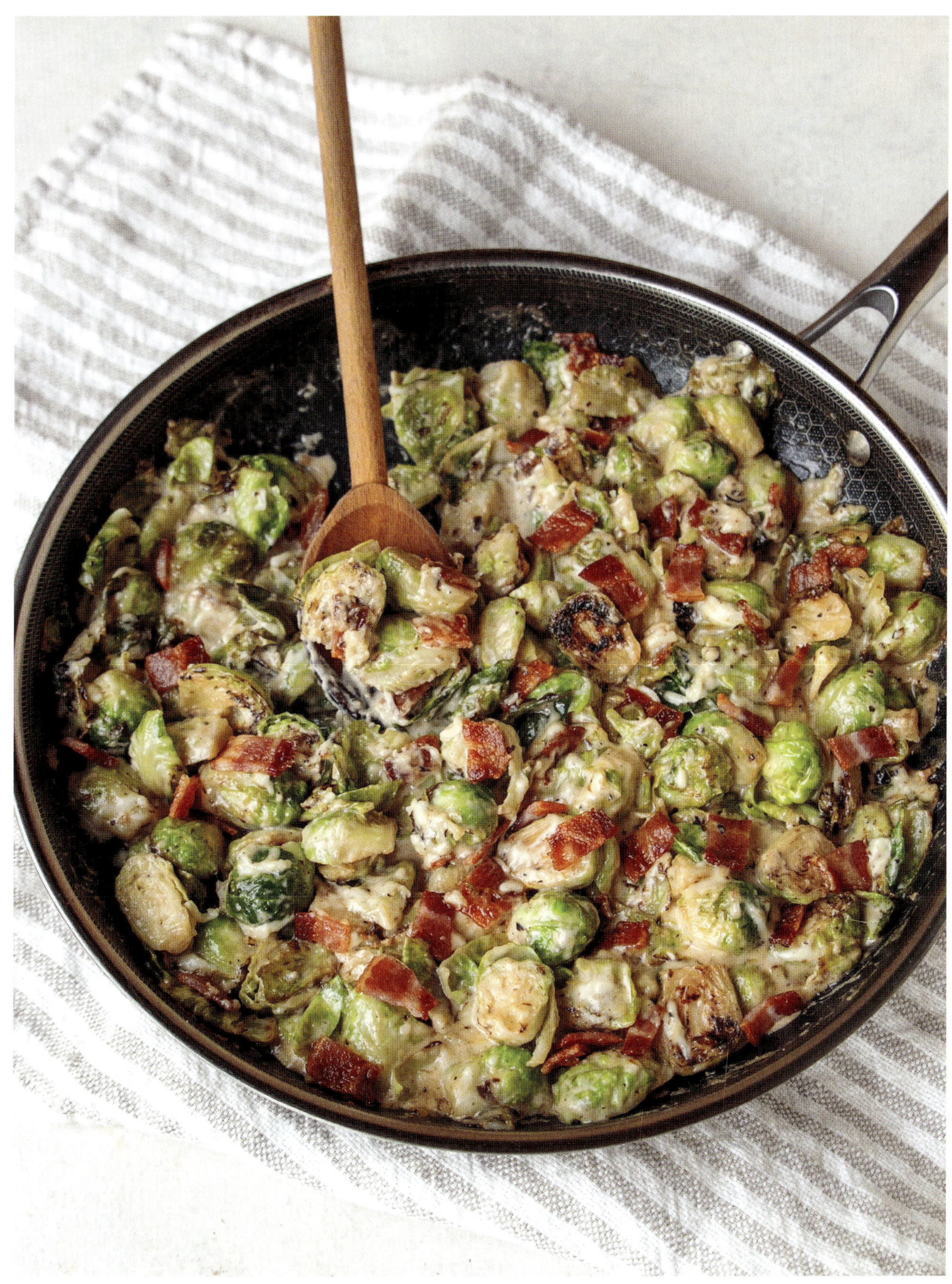

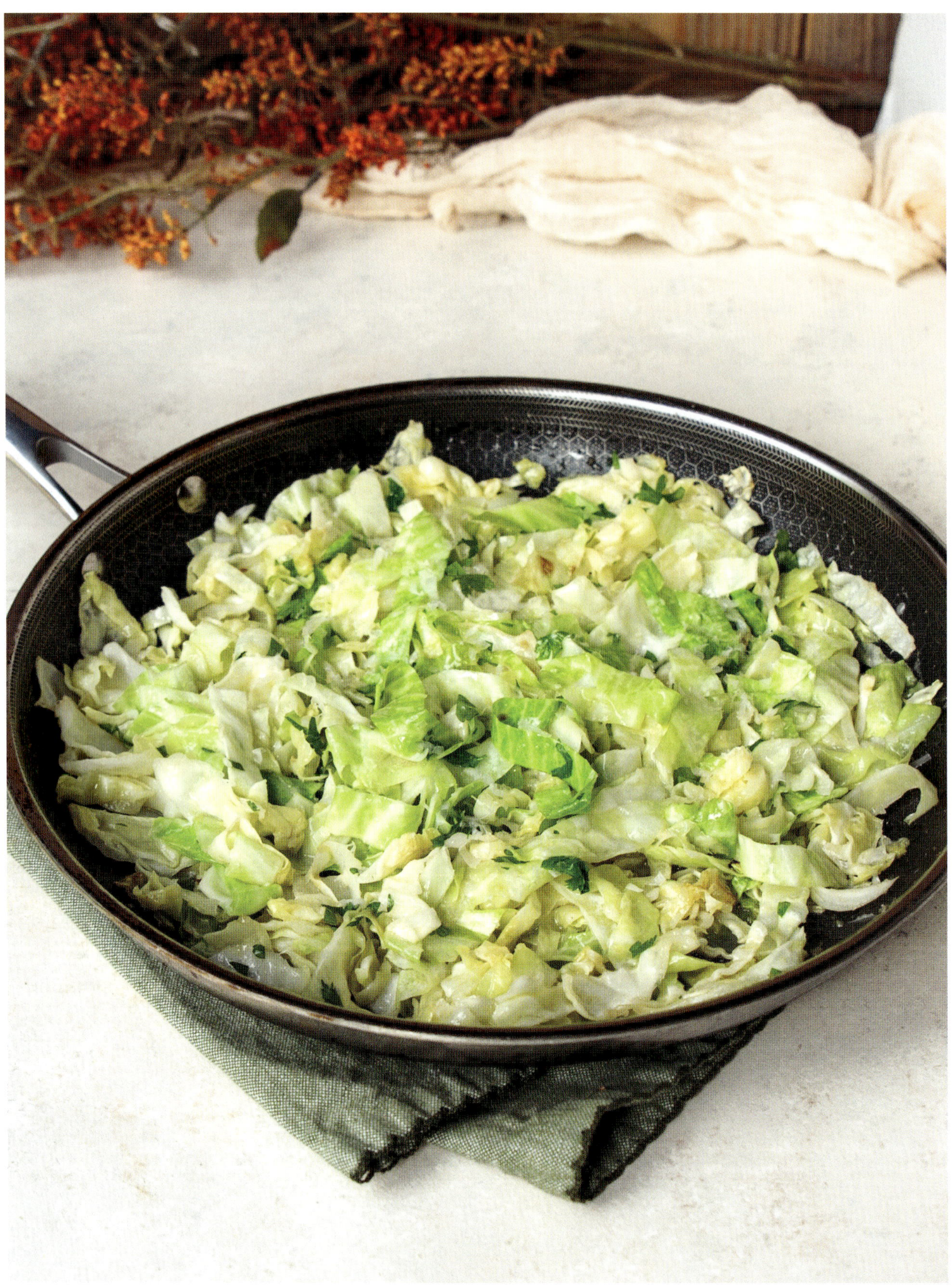

YIELD: 4 servings
PREP TIME: 10 minutes
COOK TIME: 10 minutes

SIMPLE CABBAGE FETTUCCINE

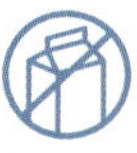
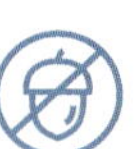

OPTION

Here's a low-carb swap to enjoy with any dish that calls for pasta. It's a quick way to mimic the idea of fettuccine.

- 1 small head green cabbage (about 1 pound), cored and outer leaves removed
- 2 tablespoons extra-virgin olive oil
- ½ teaspoon fine sea salt
- ¼ teaspoon ground black pepper
- ½ teaspoon garlic powder
- ½ teaspoon onion powder

SUGGESTED TOPPINGS:

- Grated Parmesan cheese
- Chopped fresh parsley
- Fresh lemon juice
- Red pepper flakes

1. Carefully remove the leaves from the head of cabbage, then cut off and discard the center stem of each leaf. Stack the leaves and cut lengthwise into ½-inch-wide strips.
2. Heat the olive oil in a large skillet over medium heat. Place the "fettuccine" cabbage noodles in the skillet and sauté until tender, about 10 minutes. Season with the salt, pepper, garlic powder, and onion powder and toss to combine. Garnish with toppings of your choice, if desired.

Calories	Fat	Protein	Total Carbs	Dietary Fiber	Net Carbs
93	7g	2g	7g	3g	4g

YIELD: 16 bars (1 per serving)
PREP TIME: 10 minutes, plus 1 hour to chill
COOK TIME: 5 minutes (for the ganache)

NO-BAKE COOKIE DOUGH BARS

I love having easy no-bake recipes when I need a treat for unexpected guests. This cookie dough is perfect to make ahead and keep in the fridge for up to a week or freeze in individual servings for whenever you need a little treat. Make it nut free by swapping the almond flour with sunflower seed meal.

3½ cups blanched almond flour

¾ cup (1½ sticks) unsalted butter, softened

3 scoops vanilla-flavored collagen peptides (45 grams)

1 teaspoon vanilla-flavored liquid stevia

1 teaspoon vanilla extract

½ cup monk fruit/allulose blend

¼ teaspoon fine sea salt

1 cup sugar-free chocolate chips

1 batch Ganache (page 84), freshly made

1. Place all the cookie dough ingredients, except the chocolate chips, in a food processor and process until smooth. Taste and add additional sweetener if desired. Scoop the dough into a large mixing bowl and stir in the chocolate chips.
2. Line an 8-inch square baking dish or pan with parchment paper, allowing the paper to overhang the sides. Spread the cookie dough into the dish as level as you can. I use another piece of parchment on top of the cookie dough to press down with my hands and then use the base of a dry measuring cup to press and level the dough. Chill in the fridge for at least 30 minutes or up to 24 hours before topping with the ganache.
3. When the cookie dough is almost ready to come out of the fridge, make the ganache. Pour the ganache over the chilled cookie dough and refrigerate for 30 minutes to set the ganache.
4. Slice into 16 bars. Keep refrigerated until ready to serve. Store in an airtight container in the fridge for up to 1 week or freeze for up to 3 months.

Calories	Fat	Protein	Total Carbs	Dietary Fiber	Net Carbs
350	33g	8g	8g	3g	5g

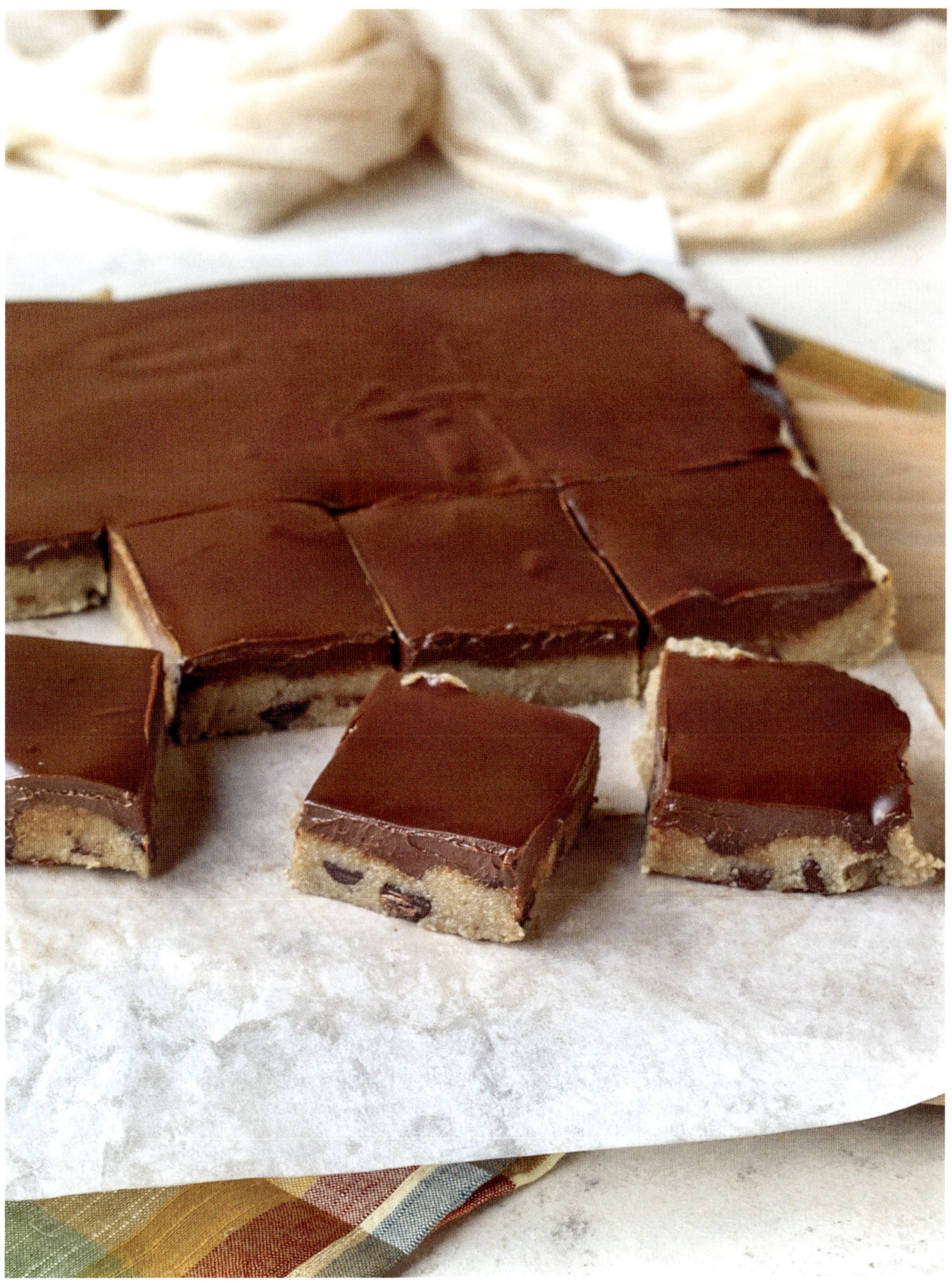

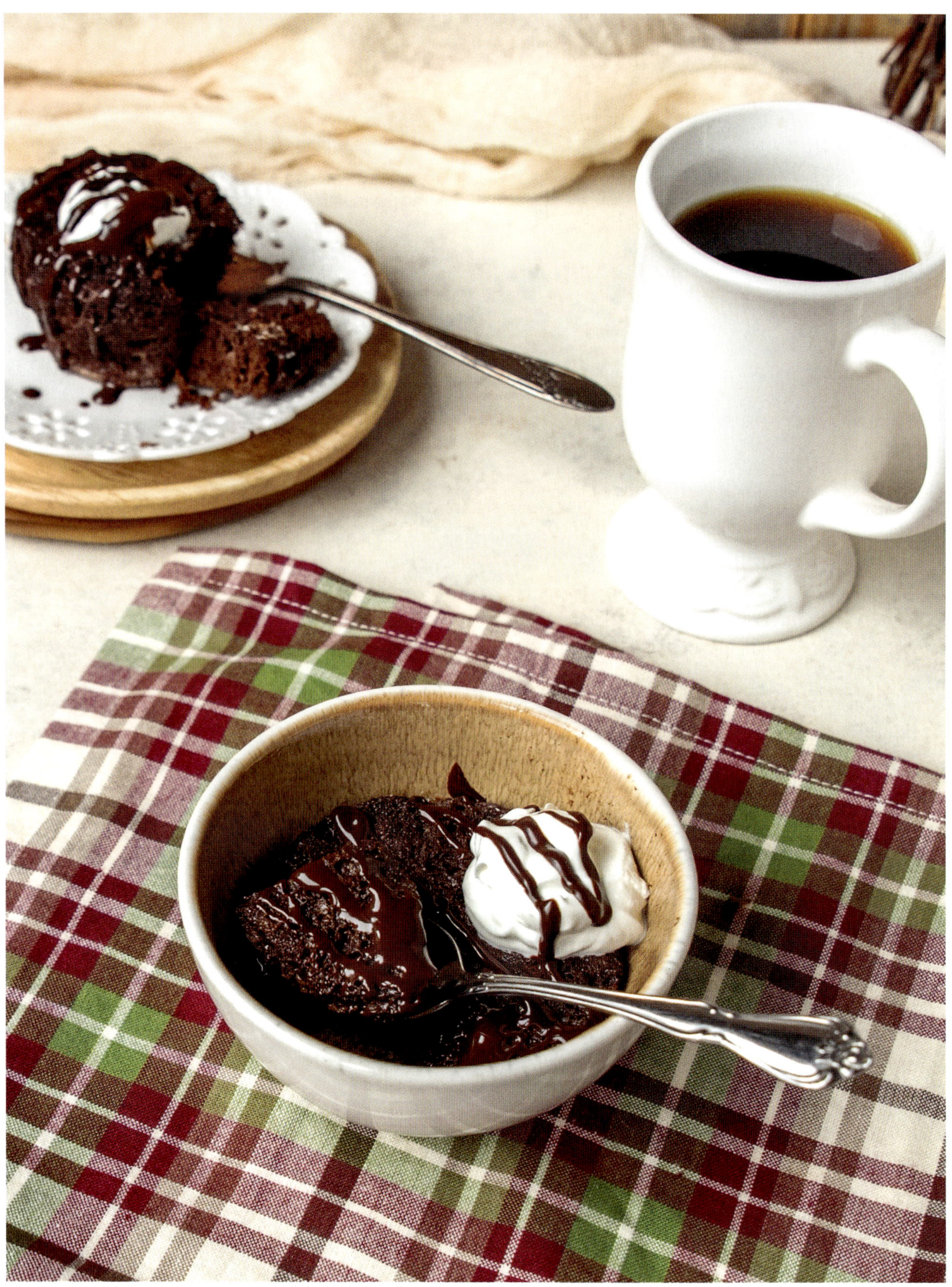

YIELD: 1 serving
PREP TIME: 7 minutes
COOK TIME: 6 or 20 minutes, depending on method used for cake

CHOCOLATE PROTEIN CAKE WITH GANACHE

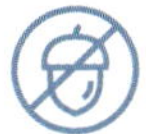
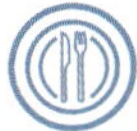

When chocolate cake isn't quite indulgent enough, ganache comes to the rescue.

1 Chocolate Protein Cake (page 141)

2 tablespoons Ganache (page 84), freshly made

Whipped cream (optional)

Make the cake and ganache following the recipes on pages 141 and 84. After the cake is done, drizzle it with the ganache. Serve with a dollop of whipped cream, if desired.

Calories	Fat	Protein	Total Carbs	Dietary Fiber	Net Carbs
243	17g	16g	9g	3g	6g

YIELD: 4 servings
PREP TIME: 10 minutes
COOK TIME: 30 minutes

DAIRY-FREE LEMON SOUFFLES

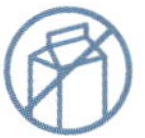
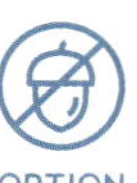
OPTION
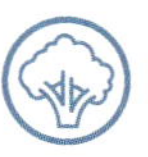
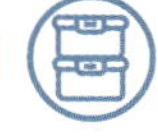

This easy souffle recipe is a quick dessert, perfect for when you want something for yourself as a meal prep option for the week ahead or as a weeknight dessert for your family.

4 large eggs, separated

⅓ cup confectioners'-style low-carb sweetener

3 tablespoons sunflower seed meal or blanched almond flour

1 teaspoon grated lemon zest

3 tablespoons fresh lemon juice

½ teaspoon lemon-flavored liquid stevia

Pinch of fine sea salt

1. Preheat the oven to 375°F with a rack in the lower third of the oven. Grease 4 (8-ounce) ramekins with cooking spray and place on a rimmed baking sheet. Set aside.
2. Put the egg whites in the bowl of a stand mixer fitted with the whisk attachment or in a medium mixing bowl. Using the stand mixer or a handheld electric mixer, whip the whites until stiff peaks form.
3. In another large mixing bowl, whisk the egg yolks, confectioners'-style sweetener, and sunflower seed meal by hand until combined. Add the lemon zest and juice, stevia, and salt and whisk to combine.
4. Fold the whipped egg whites into the egg yolk mixture in small increments until all is incorporated. Evenly distribute among the ramekins, filling each one completely so the mixture is slightly mounded on top.
5. Bake for 25 to 30 minutes, until the souffles have risen and are puffed and browned. Remove from the oven and allow to cool for about 5 minutes before serving. Refrigerate leftovers for up to 5 days to be enjoyed cold, straight from the fridge.

Calories	Fat	Protein	Total Carbs	Dietary Fiber	Net Carbs
108	7g	8g	2g	1g	1g

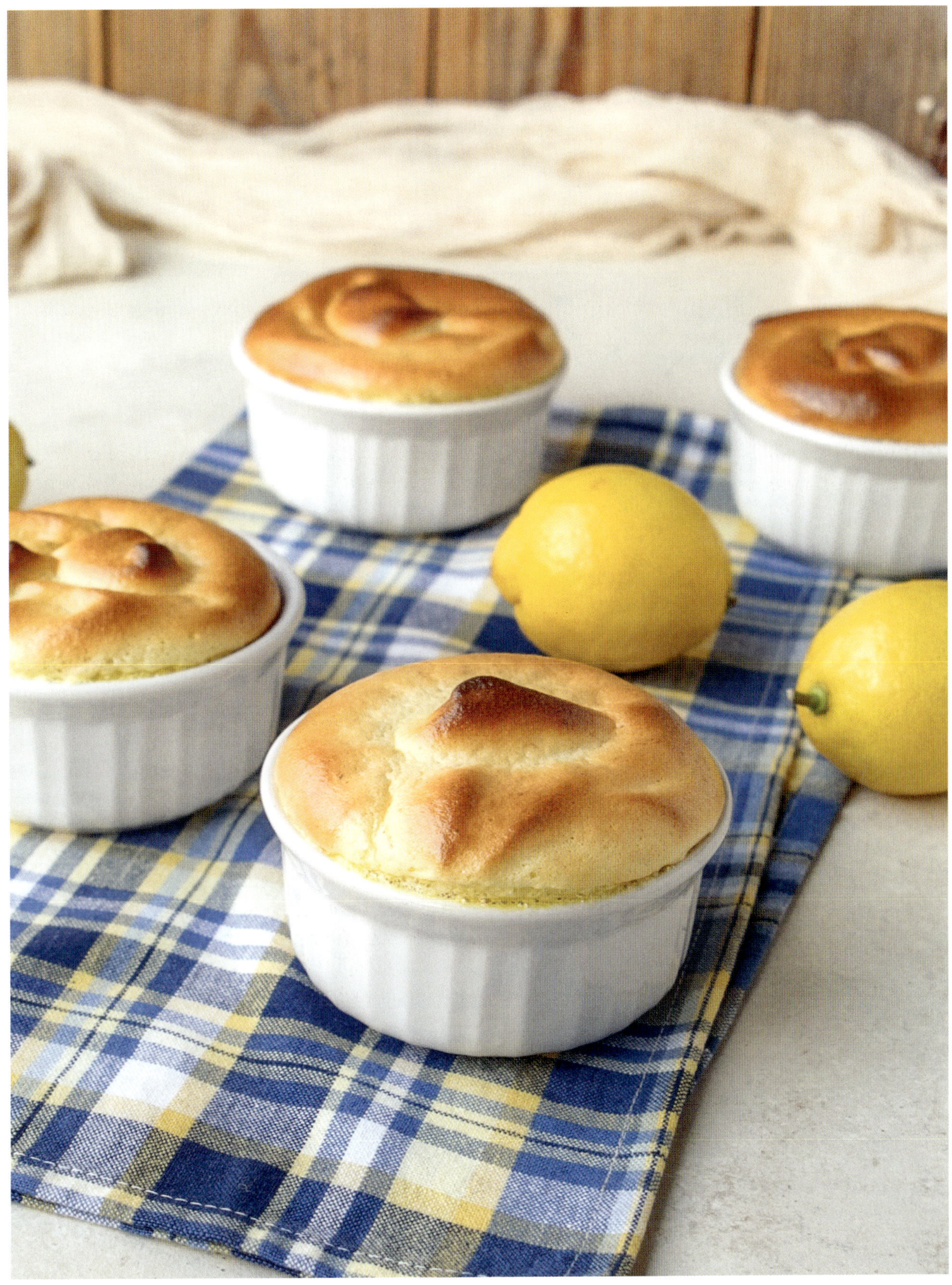

CHAPTER 8

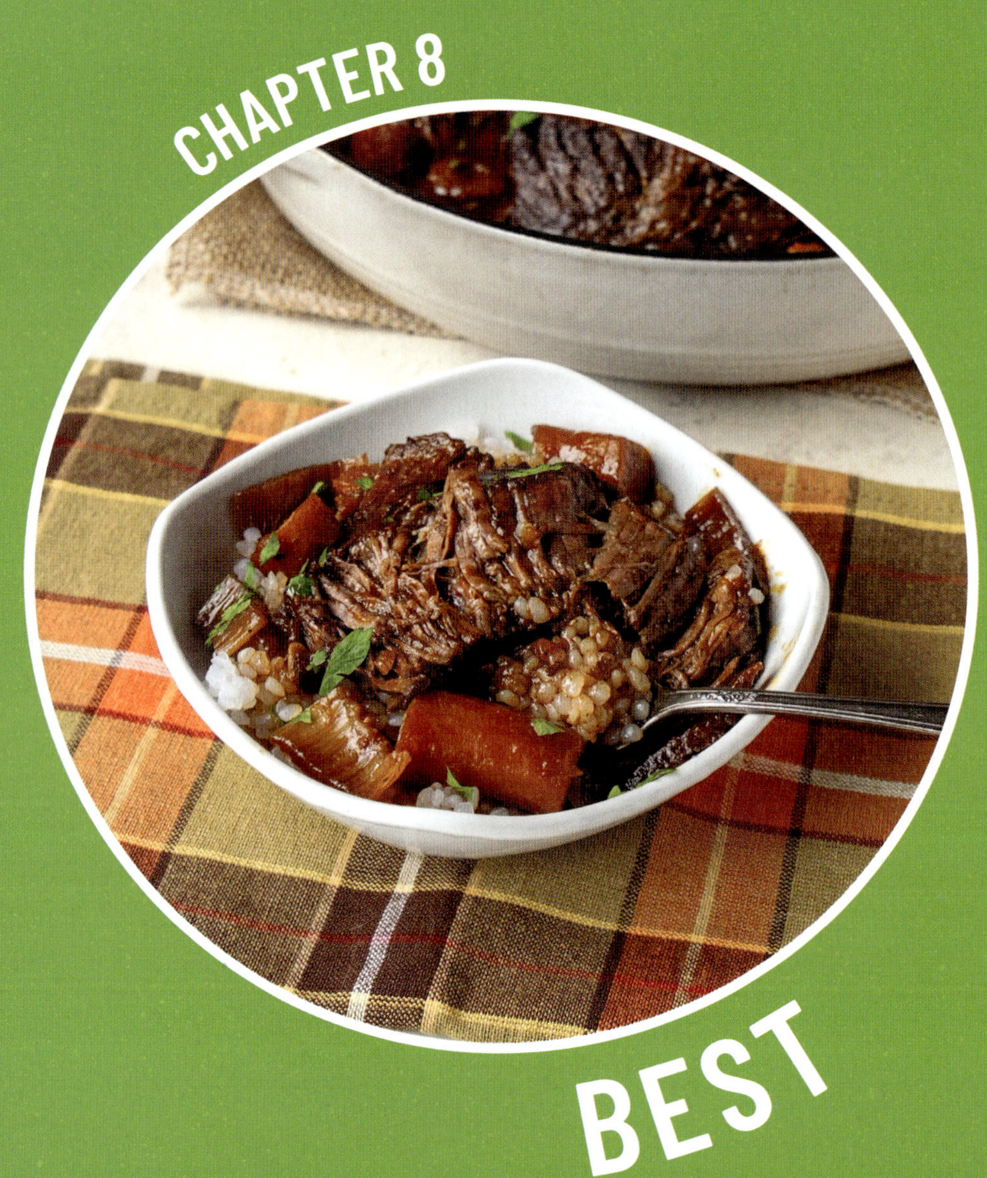

BEST

BREAKFAST

LUNCH

DINNER & SIDES

DESSERTS

YIELD: 6 scones (1 per serving)
PREP TIME: 10 minutes
COOK TIME: 25 minutes

CARAMEL APPLE SCONES

 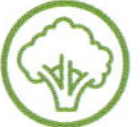

These are lovely when apple season comes around. To enjoy all the flavors of a caramel apple in a delicious low-carb scone, you can optionally drizzle the scones with caramel sauce before serving.

- 1 cup sunflower seed meal
- 6 tablespoons coconut flour, plus 1 tablespoon for the pan
- 1/4 cup low-carb brown sugar–style sweetener
- 1/2 teaspoon baking powder
- 1/2 teaspoon glucomannan or xanthan gum
- 1/4 teaspoon fine sea salt
- 1/4 cup heavy cream
- 1/2 cup chopped apple
- 2 tablespoons cold unsalted butter
- 1 large egg
- 1 tablespoon apple pie spice
- 1 teaspoon apple extract
- Keto Caramel Sauce (page 83), for serving (optional)

1. Preheat the oven to 325°F and line a baking sheet with parchment paper or a silicone baking mat.
2. In a large bowl, stir together all the ingredients until combined. Form into a ball.
3. Sprinkle a tablespoon of coconut flour on the prepared pan, then place the ball of dough in the center of the pan. Using your hands, press the dough into a circle about 6 inches in diameter and 3/4 inch thick. Cut into 6 triangles and move them 1/4 inch apart.
4. Bake for 25 minutes, or until a toothpick inserted in the center of a scone comes out clean. Let cool on the pan for about 5 minutes before carefully transferring to a cooling rack. Allow to cool for another 10 minutes before serving. If desired, drizzle with caramel sauce.
5. Store in a lidded container at room temperature for up to 3 days or in the freezer for up to 3 months. If planning to freeze the scones, omit the caramel sauce.

Calories	Fat	Protein	Total Carbs	Dietary Fiber	Net Carbs
174	15g	5g	8g	4g	4g

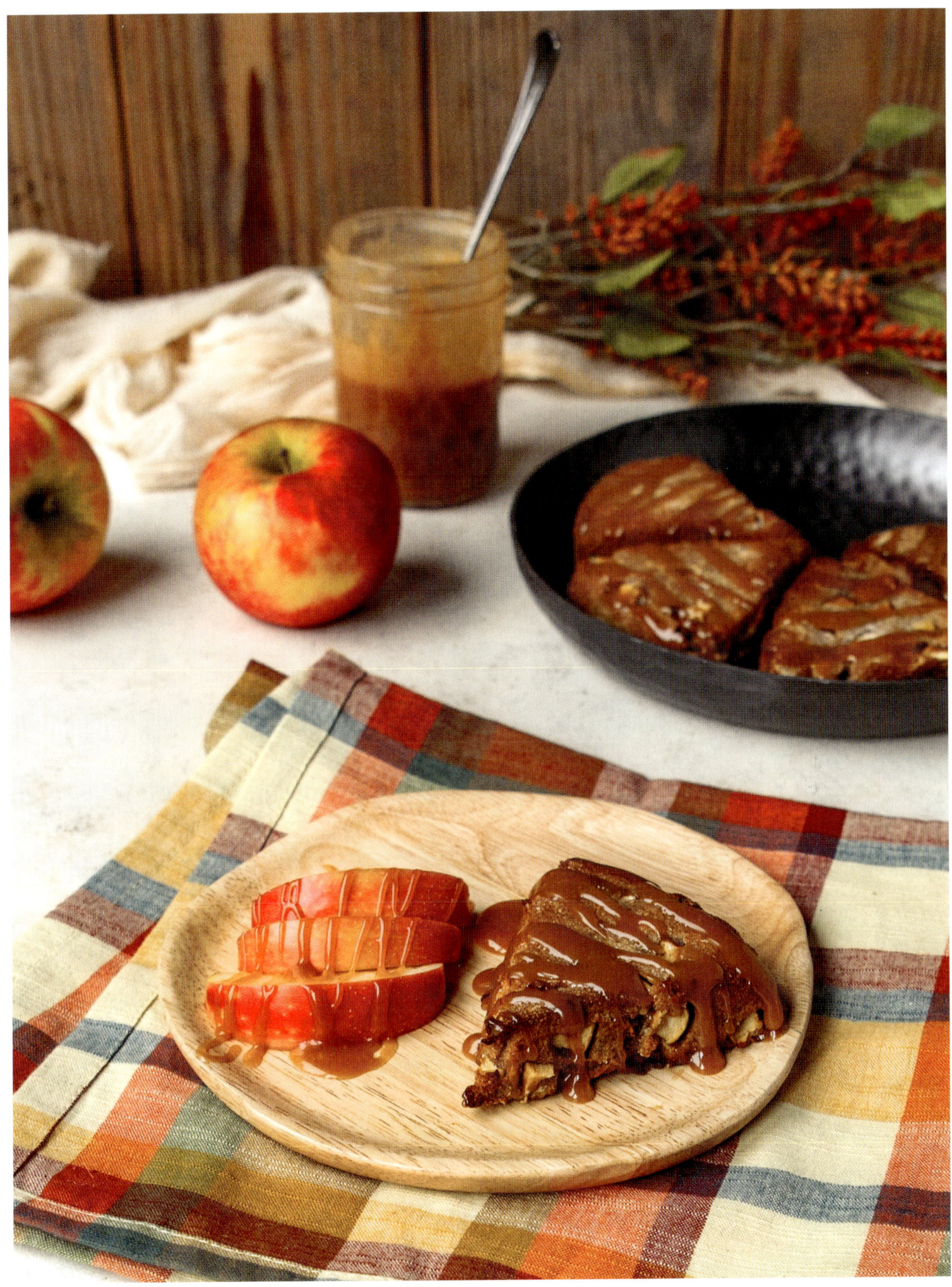

YIELD: 6 egg muffins (1 per serving)

PREP TIME: 10 to 15 minutes, depending on muffin variation

COOK TIME: 25 minutes

EGG MUFFINS—4 WAYS

 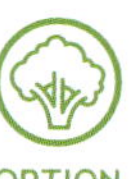 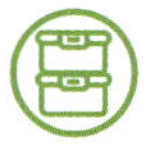

OPTION

You have the choice of making basic egg muffins—a fabulous recipe for meal prepping for the week ahead when you need a quick, wholesome breakfast option—or, when you have some extra time, making any of the three flavored varieties. Of course, you can always use the basic muffin recipe as a base for your own creative inventions, using your favorite add-ins!

FOR BASIC EGG MUFFINS:

12 large eggs

1/3 cup heavy cream or milk of choice

1/2 teaspoon fine sea salt

1/4 teaspoon ground black pepper

FOR MUSHROOM AND BELL PEPPER EGG MUFFINS:

3 ounces mushrooms of choice, sliced

2 ounces bell peppers (any color), diced

FOR HAM AND CHEDDAR EGG MUFFINS:

1 cup shredded cheddar cheese

3 ounces Canadian bacon, diced

FOR SPINACH AND MOZZARELLA EGG MUFFINS:

1 cup shredded mozzarella cheese (part skim)

3 ounces spinach leaves

3 ounces cherry tomatoes, sliced

Special equipment: 6-well silicone hamburger bun mold (optional)

1. Preheat the oven to 350°F. Set the mold on a rimmed baking sheet. (If not using a silicone mold, grease 6 wells of a standard-size muffin pan with cooking spray.)
2. Put the ingredients for the basic egg muffins in a large bowl and whisk together until well combined. Pour into the wells of the silicone mold or muffin pan, filling each well about three-quarters full.
3. Top evenly with the ingredients for the flavor variation you're making.
4. Bake for 20 to 25 minutes, or until the muffins are puffed and set in the center.
5. Store in an airtight container in the refrigerator for up to 5 days or in the freezer for up to 3 months. Reheat leftovers for 1 to 2 minutes in the microwave.

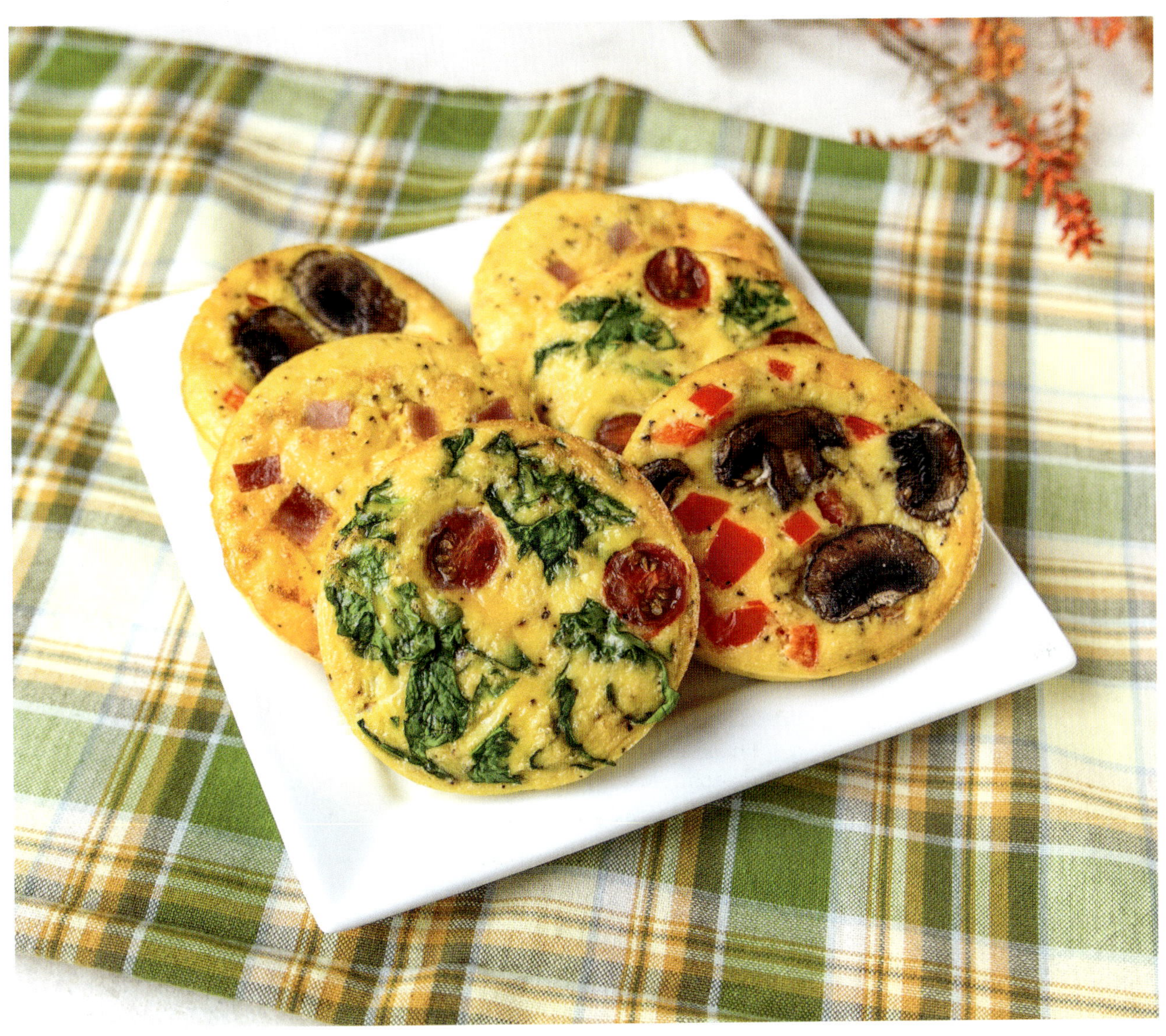

BASIC EGG MUFFINS

Calories	Fat	Protein	Total Carbs	Dietary Fiber	Net Carbs
187	14g	13g	1g	0.2g	0.8g

MUSHROOM AND BELL PEPPER EGG MUFFINS

Calories	Fat	Protein	Total Carbs	Dietary Fiber	Net Carbs
206	15.4g	13.5g	2.7g	.4g	2.3g

HAM AND CHEDDAR EGG MUFFINS

Calories	Fat	Protein	Total Carbs	Dietary Fiber	Net Carbs
267	20g	18g	1g	0.2g	0.8g

SPINACH AND MOZZARELLA EGG MUFFINS

Calories	Fat	Protein	Total Carbs	Dietary Fiber	Net Carbs
232	17g	16g	2g	1g	1g

YIELD: 9 muffins (1 per serving)
PREP TIME: 15 minutes
COOK TIME: 25 minutes

LEMON POPPYSEED MUFFINS

 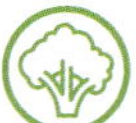

To instantly convert this breakfast muffin into an elegant brunch option or even dessert, serve them drizzled with my lemon curd (page 284).

- ½ cup (1 stick) butter, softened
- ⅓ cup cottage cheese (4% milkfat)
- 1 teaspoon grated lemon zest
- ⅓ cup fresh lemon juice
- ½ teaspoon lemon-flavored liquid stevia or liquid monk fruit
- 1 cup coconut flour
- ½ cup low-carb sweetener (granular or confectioners' style)
- 2 teaspoons baking powder
- ¼ teaspoon fine sea salt
- 1 teaspoon glucomannan or xanthan gum
- 1 teaspoon poppyseeds
- 6 large eggs

1. Preheat the oven to 425°F. Line 9 wells of a 12-well muffin pan with cupcake liners or grease the wells with cooking spray.
2. In the bowl of a stand mixer fitted with the paddle attachment, blend the butter, cottage cheese, lemon zest, lemon juice, and liquid sweetener on medium speed until smooth.
3. To the bowl with the wet ingredients, add the coconut flour, granular (or confectioners'-style) sweetener, baking powder, salt, glucomannan, and poppyseeds. Mix on low to combine. Taste the batter to check the sweetness level and add additional sweetener if desired.
4. Add one egg at a time to the bowl, mixing each one in before adding the next.
5. Pour the batter into the prepared muffin wells, filling each one about three-quarters full.
6. Bake the muffins for 5 minutes, then lower the temperature to 350°F and continue to bake for 20 to 25 minutes, until golden and a toothpick inserted in the center comes out clean.
7. Store in an airtight container in the fridge for up to 5 days. These can also be frozen for up to 3 months.

Calories	Fat	Protein	Total Carbs	Dietary Fiber	Net Carbs
199	15g	7g	7g	6g	1g

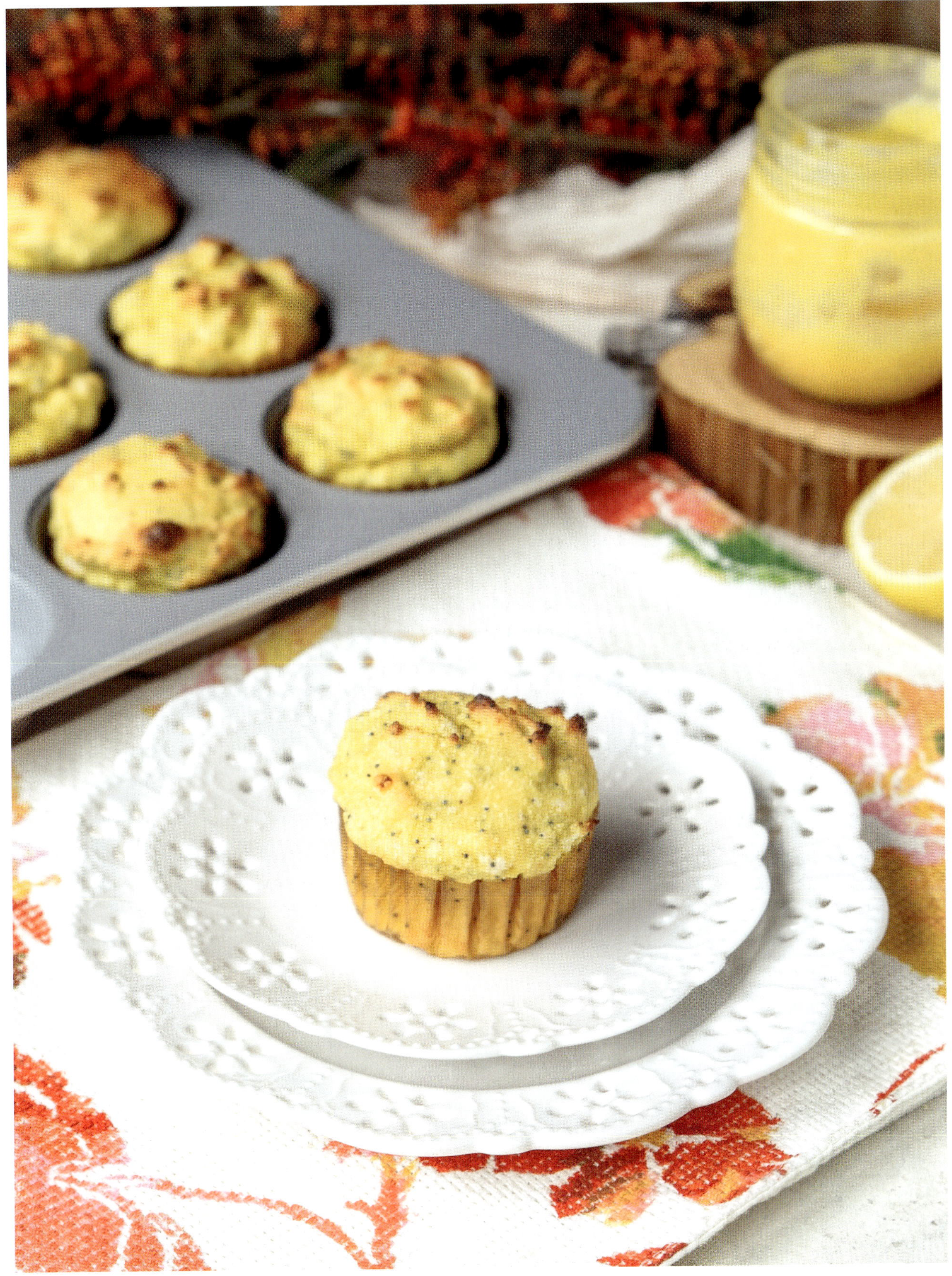

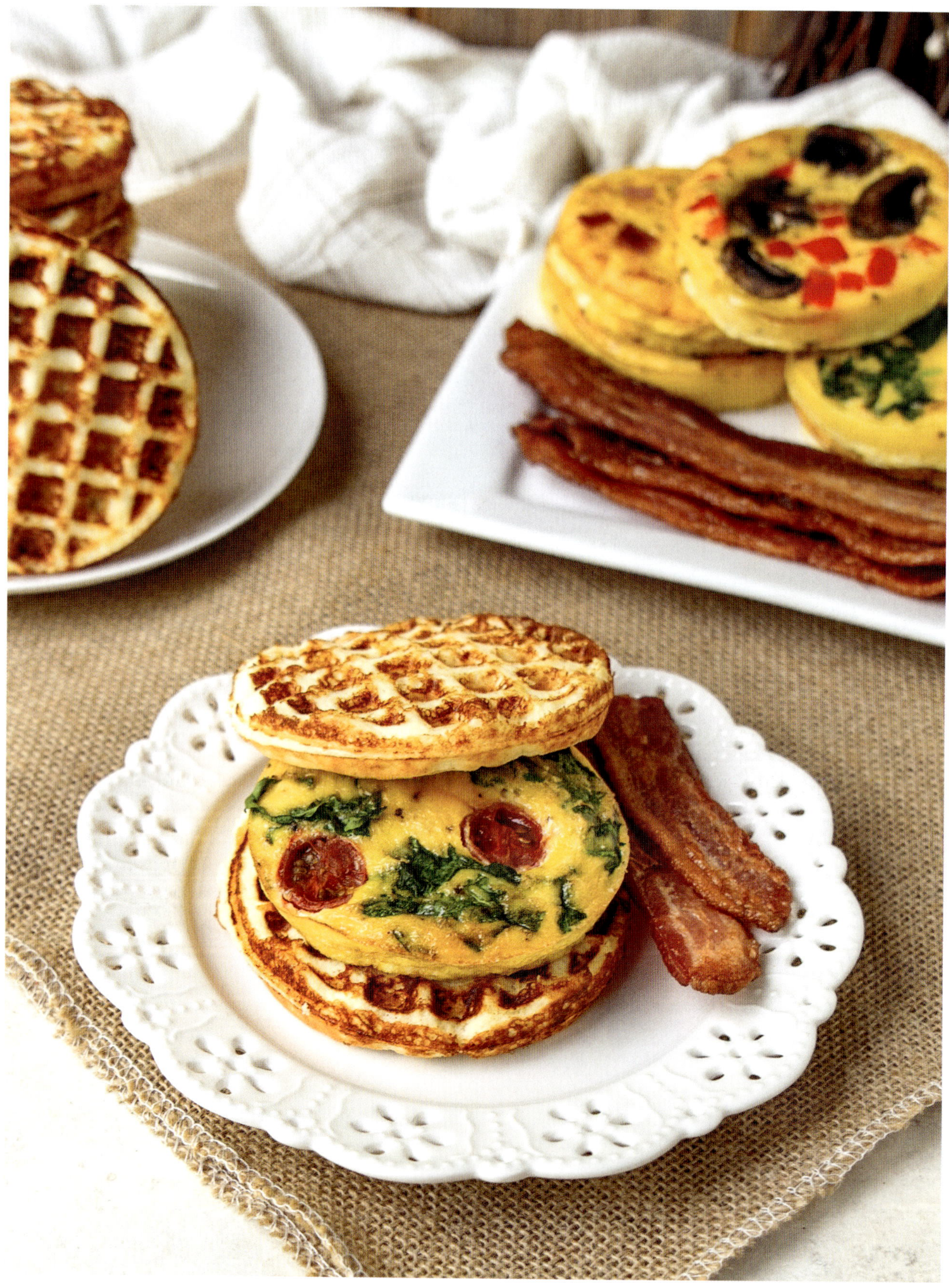

YIELD: 4 sandwiches (1 per serving)
PREP TIME: 15 minutes (not including time to cook waffles, egg muffins, or bacon)
REHEATING TIME: 10 minutes

PREP-AHEAD BREAKFAST SANDWICHES

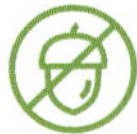 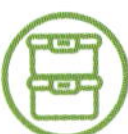 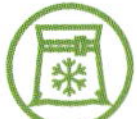

Meal prepped breakfast sandwiches make busy mornings easier—and delicious! To expedite the making of the three key components for these sandwiches, I suggest you get the egg muffins in the oven on one rack, with the bacon cooking away on another rack. While they're baking, you can make the waffles. Once the muffins, bacon, and waffles are cooled, you can assemble the sandwiches, wrap them up, and freeze them for later.

8 Cottage Cheese Protein Waffles (page 94)

4 Egg Muffins of choice (page 232)

8 slices thick-cut bacon, baked (see page 76)

4 cheddar cheese slices (optional)

1. Once the waffles, egg muffins, and bacon are cool enough to touch, assemble the sandwiches: Lay one waffle onto a piece of parchment paper. Lay one egg muffin on the waffle. Place 2 slices of bacon on top of the egg, and then top with a slice of cheese, if using. Lay the second waffle on top. Wrap in parchment paper and then foil and seal in a quart-size zip-top bag. Repeat with remaining ingredients to make a total of 4 sandwiches. Freeze for up to 3 months.
2. To reheat, remove a sandwich from the freezer to the refrigerator and allow to defrost overnight. Defrosted sandwiches will heat up more evenly and quickly. Preheat the oven to 350°F. Place the wrapped sandwich in the oven until heated through, about 10 minutes. If desired, open the wrapping and continue baking for a few minutes to brown the top of the sandwich.

MADE WITH THE BASIC EGG MUFFINS

Calories	Fat	Protein	Total Carbs	Dietary Fiber	Net Carbs
583	40g	50g	5g	0g	5g

YIELD: 3 servings

PREP TIME: 20 minutes (not including time to cook eggs and bacon)

COOK TIME: 50 minutes

ON-THE-GO COTTAGE CHEESE EGG SALAD WITH HOMEMADE WRAPS

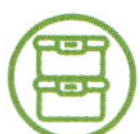

This cottage cheese egg salad is a great high-protein meal to take on the go. With a little bit more of your time, you can enjoy the salad with homemade ricotta wraps.

FOR THE WRAPS:

3/4 cup ricotta cheese (part skim)

3 large egg whites

1/4 teaspoon fine sea salt

1/4 teaspoon garlic powder

1/4 teaspoon onion powder

1 tablespoon ground flaxseed

1 tablespoon everything bagel seasoning, for garnish

FOR THE SALAD:

3 cups chopped romaine lettuce

1 1/2 cups cottage cheese (4% milkfat)

6 large hard-boiled eggs, peeled and chopped, or 1 batch Hard-Baked Eggs (page 166), chopped

3/4 cup sliced cucumbers

3/4 cup chopped tomatoes (or quartered if small)

3 tablespoons chopped red onions

6 slices regular-cut bacon, baked (see page 76)

Dressing of choice, for serving (optional)

Everything bagel seasoning, for garnish (optional)

1. To make the wraps, preheat the oven to 325°F. Line a rimmed baking sheet with parchment paper, then spray it with cooking spray. Set aside.
2. Put all the ingredients, except the everything bagel seasoning, in a large bowl and whisk together until combined into a thick batter.
3. Using a 1/3-cup measuring cup, scoop the batter onto the prepared pan and spread with the back of a spoon to create a 6-inch circle. Repeat to make a total of 3 rounds. Sprinkle with the everything bagel seasoning.
4. Bake for 45 to 50 minutes, until browned around the edges and the center is set. When the wraps are done, allow to cool for 15 minutes before removing from the pan and serving. While the wraps are baking, meal prep the salads.
5. To make the salads, evenly divide the chopped lettuce among 3 (4-cup) storage containers, putting 1 cup in each one.
6. In a medium bowl, gently mix the cottage cheese and chopped egg together, then evenly divide the mixture among the containers, scooping it into a mound for a pretty presentation, if desired.
7. Add 1/4 cup sliced cucumbers, 1/4 cup chopped tomatoes, and 1 tablespoon chopped onions to each container. Cover with the lid.
8. Place 2 slices of cooked bacon in each of 3 zip-top bags or wrap in parchment paper. Place 1 bag with each container.

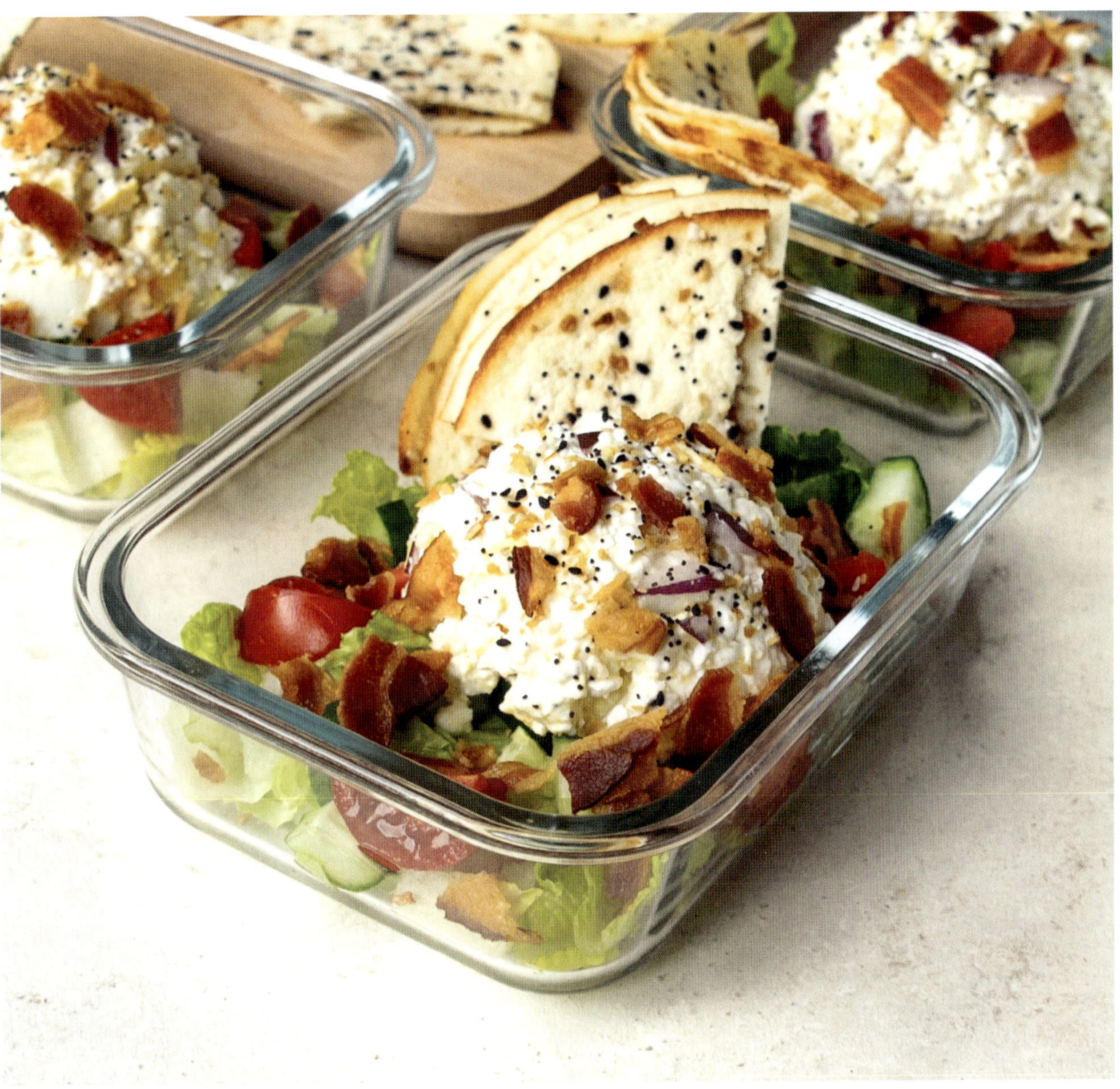

9. Refrigerate for up to 3 days. When you're ready to enjoy, crumble the bacon over the salad. Drizzle with your dressing of choice and garnish with everything bagel seasoning, if desired. Serve 1 wrap with each salad.
10. Store leftover wraps in the refrigerator in a zip-top bag for up to 5 days. To freeze, sandwich the wraps between parchment paper and store in a zip-top bag for up to 1 month. Thaw the night before using. Enjoy cold from the fridge or toast for 1 to 2 minutes to warm.

Calories	Fat	Protein	Total Carbs	Dietary Fiber	Net Carbs
455	23g	45g	11g	2g	9g

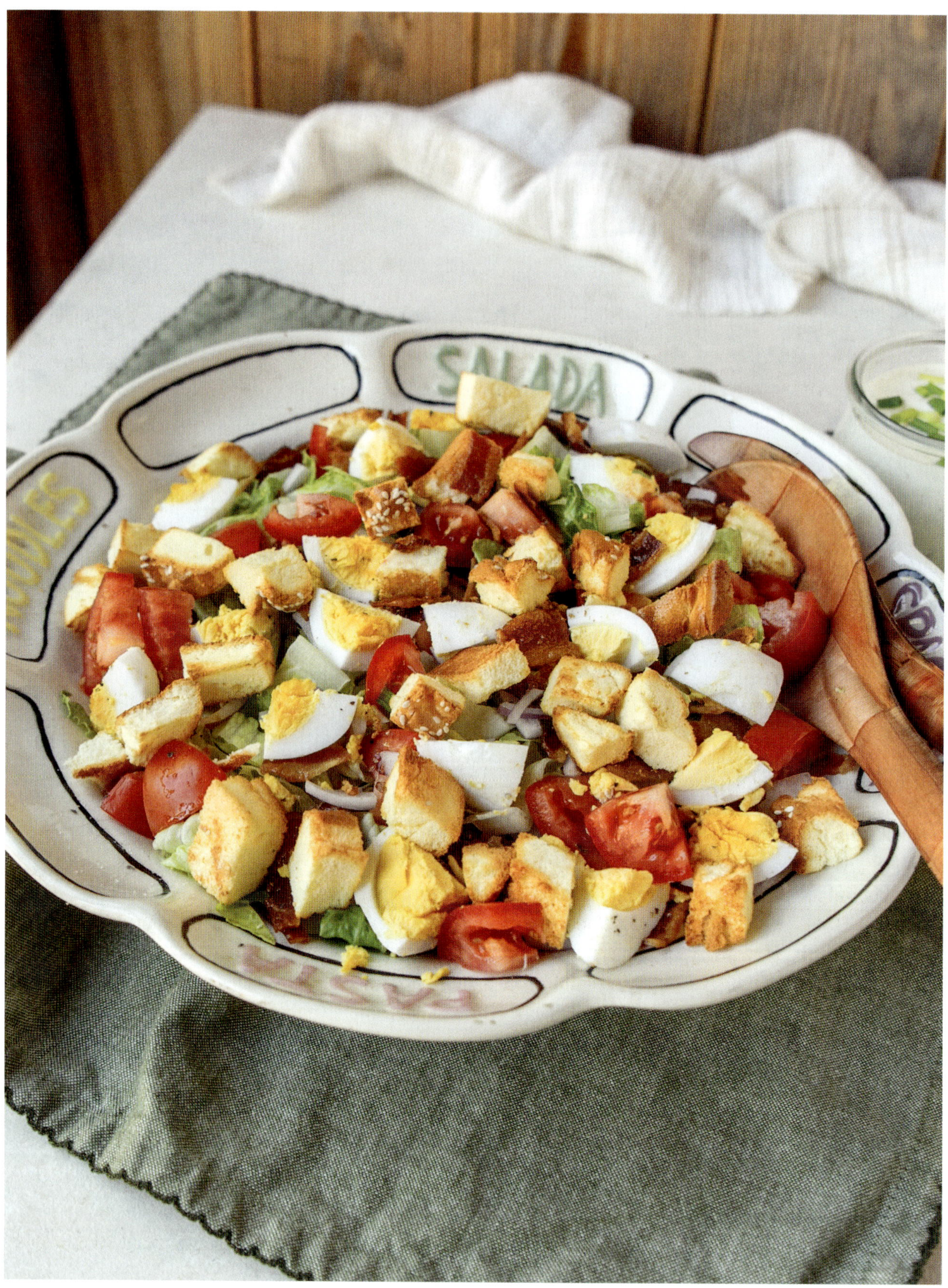
SALADA
NOODLES
PASTA

YIELD: 4 servings

PREP TIME: 10 minutes (not including time to cook bacon, eggs, or rolls)

COOK TIME: 5 minutes

BEST BLT SALAD

This recipe takes the BLT salad in the Better chapter and makes it more filling and elaborate with the addition of homemade low-carb croutons. To save time peeling the eggs, try my recipe for Hard-Baked Eggs on page 166. You can also trim off some time by using store-bought cloud bread rolls for the croutons.

2 romaine lettuce hearts (about 11 ounces)

8 ounces bacon, baked (see page 76)

2 large Roma tomatoes (about 6 ounces)

1 small red onion (about 1¾ ounces)

4 large hard-boiled eggs, peeled and chopped, or 1 cup chopped Hard-Baked Eggs (page 166)

FOR THE CROUTONS:

1 cloud bread roll, homemade (page 88) or store-bought

1 tablespoon salted butter, melted

FOR THE DRESSING:

¼ cup avocado oil mayonnaise

¼ cup sour cream

1 tablespoon extra-virgin olive oil

1 clove garlic, minced

¼ teaspoon fine sea salt

¼ teaspoon ground black pepper

2 tablespoons sliced scallions

1. Chop the lettuce and place in a large serving bowl or in 4 individual containers if meal prepping. Chop the bacon, tomato, and onion. Toss with the lettuce.
2. To make the croutons, preheat the oven to 350°F. Chop the roll into bite-sized pieces and place on a rimmed baking sheet. Drizzle the pieces with melted butter. Bake for 5 minutes, or until lightly browned.
3. Whisk together all the dressing ingredients in a small bowl.
4. When ready to serve, toss the salad with the dressing and croutons, or keep the 3 elements in separate containers for meal prepping. When stored separately, the salad, dressing, and croutons will keep for up to 2 days.

Calories	Fat	Protein	Total Carbs	Dietary Fiber	Net Carbs
290	25g	12g	8g	2g	6g

YIELD: 1 sandwich
PREP TIME: 12 minutes
COOK TIME: 30 minutes

RICOTTA FLATBREAD SANDWICH

When you have flatbread made ahead and some easy sandwich fixings on hand, you can put together a healthy low-carb lunch in no time. Deli ham is one of my go-to sandwich fillings, but use any fillings you prefer. The flatbread recipe makes enough for 4 sandwiches, so you'll have plenty for the week ahead.

FOR THE FLATBREAD:

(Makes 8 pieces)

4 large eggs

1 cup ricotta cheese (part skim)

⅓ cup unflavored whey protein powder

1 teaspoon Italian seasoning

½ teaspoon fine sea salt

SANDWICH FIXINGS (PER SANDWICH):

2 pieces flatbread (from above)

1 tablespoon avocado oil mayonnaise

2 ounces deli ham (see note)

2 tomato slices

1 piece lettuce

1. To make the flatbread, preheat the oven to 350°F. Line a rimmed baking sheet with parchment paper.
2. Place all the ingredients for the flatbread in a large bowl and mix to combine.
3. Scoop the dough onto the prepared pan and use the back of a spoon to spread into a 9 by 12-inch rectangle.
4. Bake for 30 minutes, or until slightly browned and set in the center. Let cool on the pan. Cut into 8 squares.
5. To make a sandwich, spread two pieces of flatbread with the mayonnaise, then fill with the ham, tomato, and lettuce.
6. Store leftover flatbread pieces in an airtight container in the fridge for up to 5 days. To freeze, place individual servings between pieces of parchment paper and then store in an airtight container in the freezer for up to 1 month. Thaw before using.

FOR SANDWICH

Calories	Fat	Protein	Total Carbs	Dietary Fiber	Net Carbs
248	15g	23g	5g	0.4g	4.6g

FOR 1 SERVING FLATBREAD (2 PIECES)

Calories	Fat	Protein	Total Carbs	Dietary Fiber	Net Carbs
186	10g	20g	5g	0.2g	0.9g

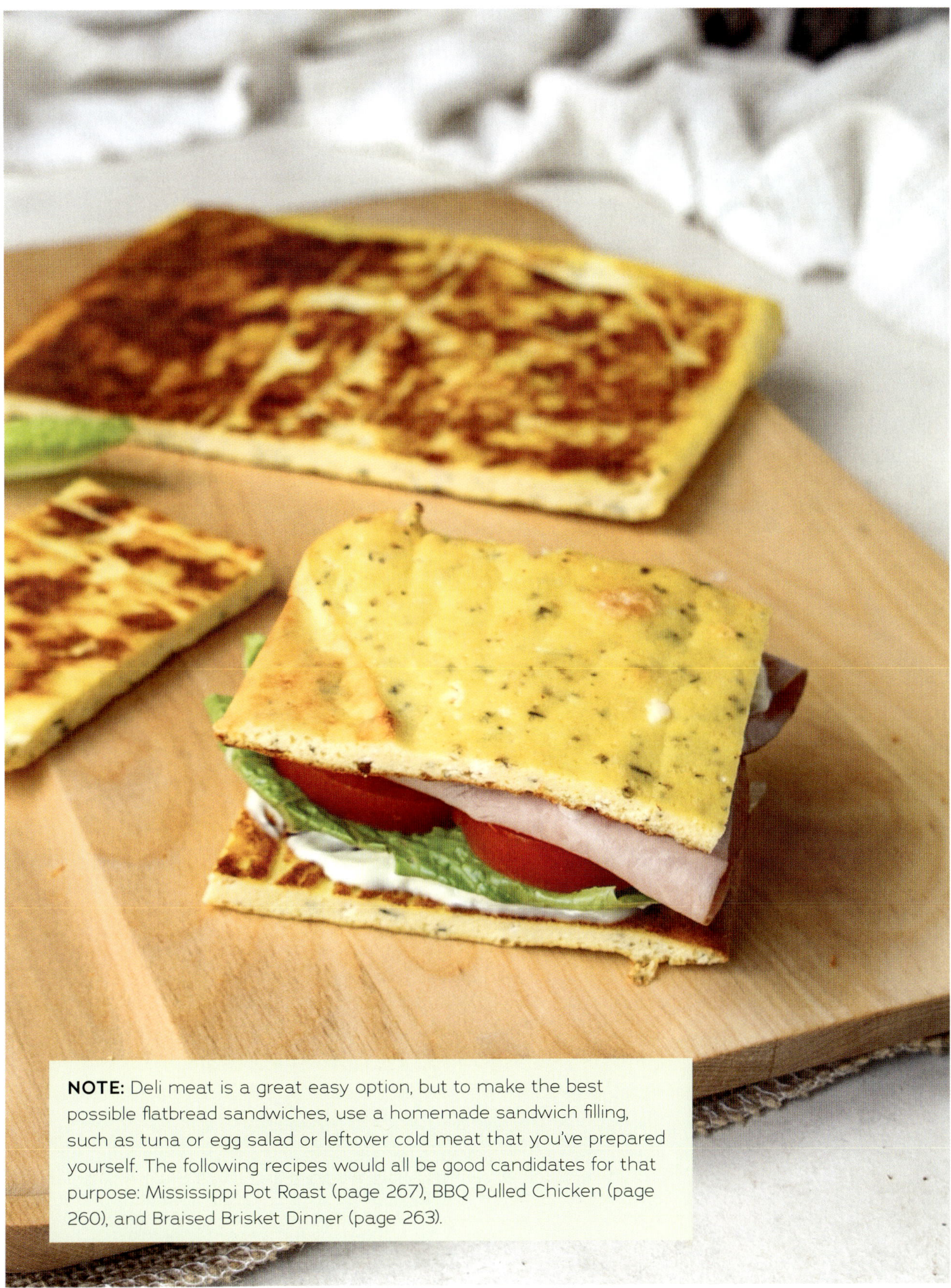

NOTE: Deli meat is a great easy option, but to make the best possible flatbread sandwiches, use a homemade sandwich filling, such as tuna or egg salad or leftover cold meat that you've prepared yourself. The following recipes would all be good candidates for that purpose: Mississippi Pot Roast (page 267), BBQ Pulled Chicken (page 260), and Braised Brisket Dinner (page 263).

YIELD: 6 servings (8 gnudi per serving)
PREP TIME: 25 minutes
COOK TIME: 3 to 15 minutes, depending on method

GNUDI (RICOTTA GNOCCHI)

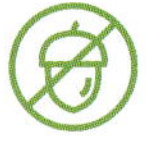
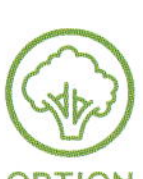
OPTION
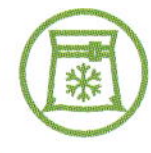

These soft and pillowy ricotta gnocchi, traditionally called gnudi, are simple to whip up and pretty quick to cook too! It's great to have these premade for a quick pastalike meal choice. And you have three options for cooking them: bake in the oven, fry in a pan, or simmer in marinara sauce. Unlike true gnocchi, they do not include potato, making them a good low-carb replacement. I like to make these ahead, freeze them, and then pull out the quantity I need. No need to defrost before cooking! To treat myself to a hot lunch, I grab eight gnudi from the freezer. In fifteen minutes or less, lunch is ready. I've written the cooking instructions for a single portion, but you can cook any quantity you like (see the note after the last step). To make these part of a heartier meal, try serving with my ricotta meatballs on page 206!

1 cup ricotta cheese (part skim)

1 cup grated Parmesan cheese, plus more for garnish if desired

1/2 cup coconut flour

2 large eggs

1 teaspoon garlic powder

1/2 teaspoon fine sea salt

1/4 teaspoon ground black pepper

1/2 teaspoon glucomannan or xanthan gum

FOR COOKING (STOVETOP METHODS ONLY):

2 tablespoons extra-virgin olive oil, or 2 cups low-carb marinara sauce

FOR GARNISH (OPTIONAL):

Extra-virgin olive oil, for drizzling

2 tablespoons chopped fresh basil

2 tablespoons chopped fresh parsley

1. Put all the ingredients in a food processor. Pulse until the mixture is pulling away from the sides of the bowl and has formed into a smooth and tacky dough.
2. Lay a piece of parchment paper on a work surface. Dump the dough out onto the parchment and, with wet fingers, form it into a 15-inch-long log. Cut the log in half lengthwise to make 2 thin ropes about 1/2 inch in diameter.
3. Cutting crosswise, slice 1-inch pieces from the thin ropes; you should get a total of 48 gnudi, each weighing 1/2 ounce (10 grams). Optionally, to form the classic ridges found on gnocchi, gently roll each piece of dough against the back of the tines of a fork. (If you're new to this process, turn the page for more detailed instructions.) You can cook the gnudi now or freeze for easy lunches later.

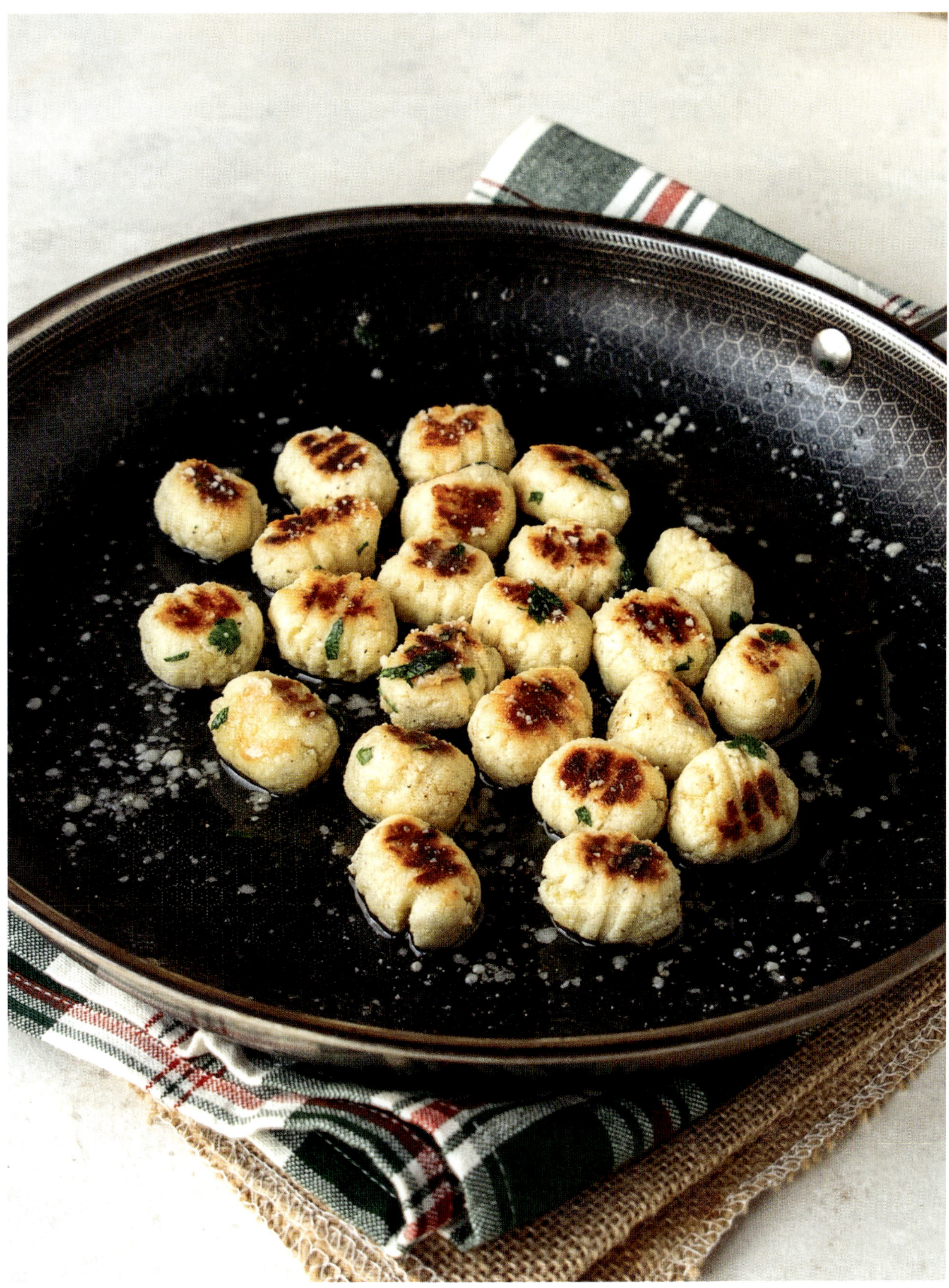

4. For freezer prep, arrange the gnudi in a single layer on a rimmed baking sheet lined with parchment paper, ensuring they don't touch. Cover the pan with plastic wrap and freeze for 1 hour, then transfer the gnudi to an airtight container, layering with parchment paper for easy removal later. They can be frozen for up to 3 months.
5. *If baking the gnudi,* preheat the oven to 350°F and line a rimmed baking sheet with parchment paper. Place 8 gnudi on the prepared pan and place in the oven. If cooking freshly made gnudi, bake for 5 minutes, then flip and bake for another 3 to 5 minutes, until golden brown. If cooking frozen gnudi, bake for 10 minutes, flip, and then bake for another 5 minutes or until golden brown. If desired, drizzle with some olive oil and gently toss to coat.

   If cooking the gnudi in marinara sauce, heat the sauce in a medium saucepan over medium heat. Add 8 gnudi, cover the pan, and simmer until the gnudi are heated through. If cooking freshly made gnudi, this should take just 2 to 3 minutes; if cooking frozen gnudi, allow them to simmer for 5 minutes, then gently turn them over, return the lid to the pan, and simmer for another 5 minutes.

   If pan-frying the gnudi, heat the olive oil in a medium skillet over medium heat. Place 8 gnudi in the hot pan and fry until browned on all sides and heated through. If frying freshly made gnudi, this should take 2 to 3 minutes. If frying frozen gnudi, after putting them in the pan, reduce the heat to medium-low, cover, and cook for about 5 minutes, or until browned. Flip over and fry, uncovered, for another 5 minutes, or until browned on all sides.
6. Serve the cooked gnudi garnished with grated Parmesan and chopped basil and parsley, if desired.

NOTES: To form ridges on the gnudi, set a fork on a work surface with the underside facing up. Hold the handle of the fork to keep it still; with your other hand, place a piece of gnudi dough on top of the fork, at the base of the tines. Using your thumb, press down gently on the dough until slightly flattened, so that the dough is well marked by the tines. Then roll the dough off the fork, rolling the top of the dough back onto itself to re-form it into a cylindrical shape.

If you want to fry more than one serving of gnudi, you can cook up to 16 at once using a large skillet and ¼ cup of olive oil, frying additional gnudi in batches and using more oil as needed. If you want to cook more than one serving in marinara sauce, simply increase the size of saucepan used as well as the quantity of sauce, using an additional ½ cup of sauce for every additional serving of gnudi.

If you're a strict vegetarian, make sure to use a Parmesan cheese made without animal rennet.

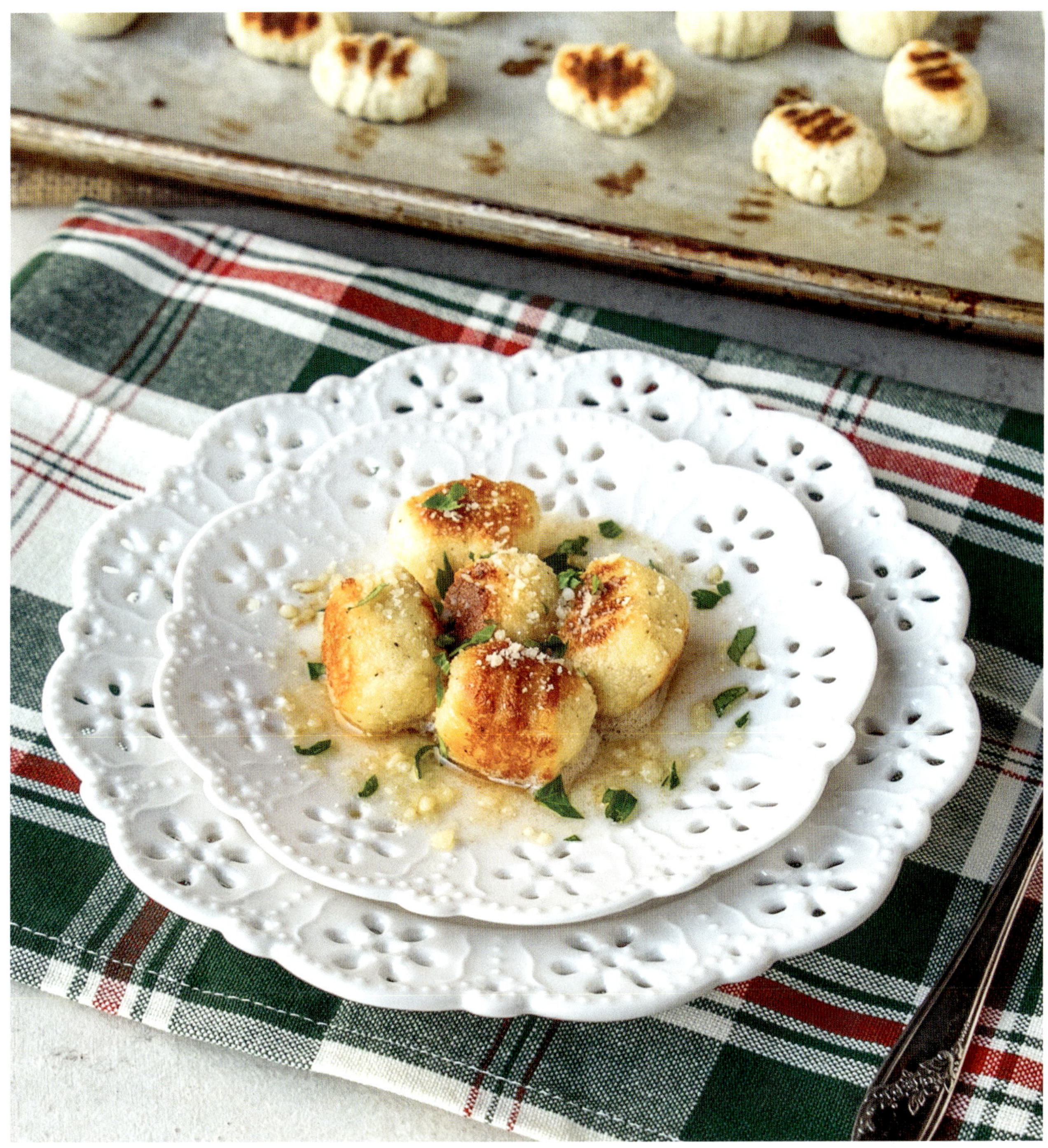

BAKED IN THE OVEN

Calories	Fat	Protein	Total Carbs	Dietary Fiber	Net Carbs
187	10g	14g	9g	4g	5g

COOKED IN MARINARA SAUCE

Calories	Fat	Protein	Total Carbs	Dietary Fiber	Net Carbs
200	11g	14g	10g	4g	6g

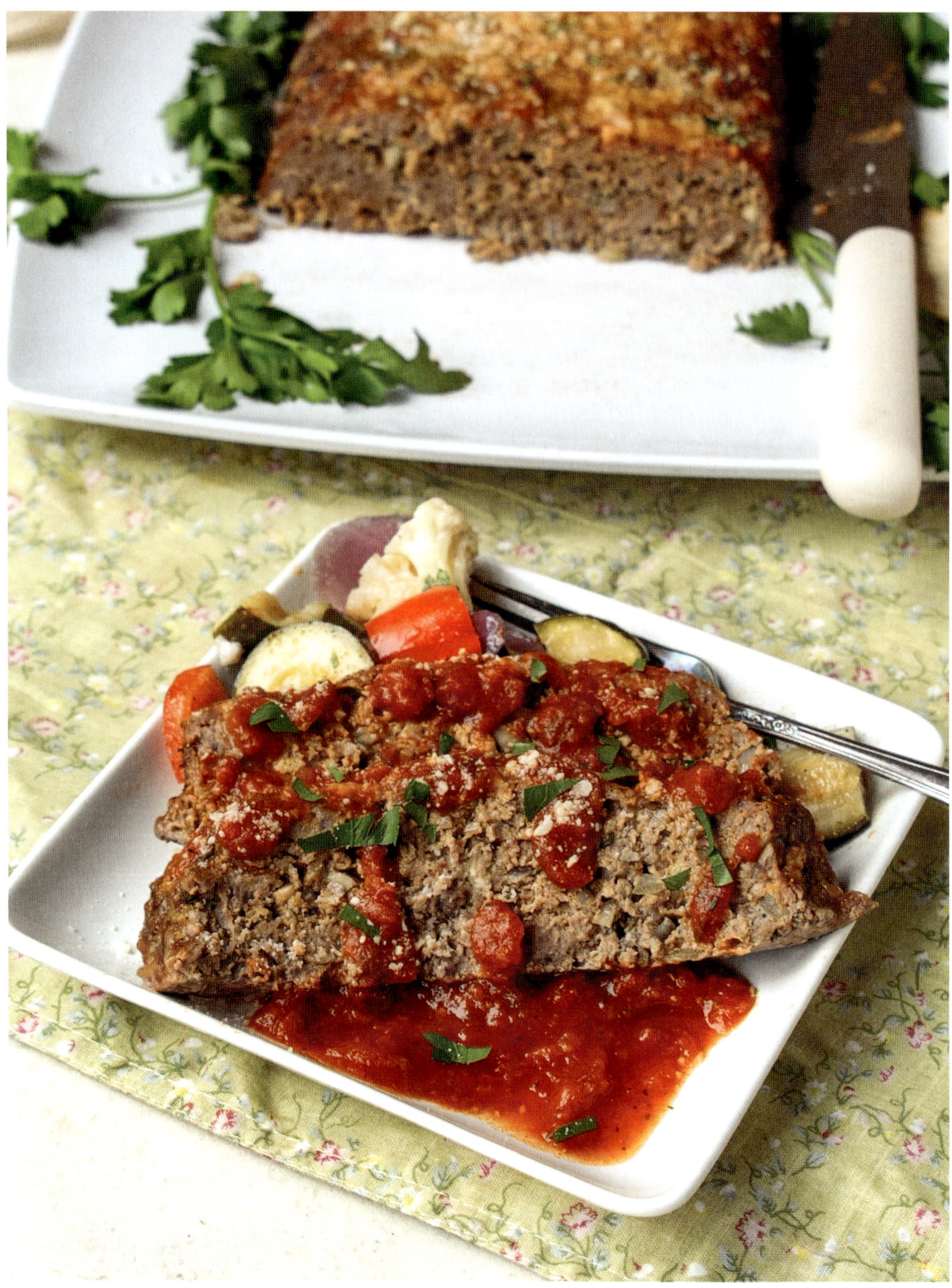

YIELD: 8 servings
PREP TIME: 15 minutes
COOK TIME: 1 hour

ITALIAN MEATLOAF

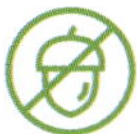 

My hubby loves a hearty meatloaf, and since I'm Italian, I had to create my own spin on the traditional meatloaf. My whole family loves how tender this meatloaf is and how delicious the leftovers are for lunches. I serve this with marinara sauce and roasted vegetables (page 264).

2 pounds 80/20 ground beef

2 large eggs, beaten

½ cup grated yellow onions

½ cup pork rind panko

⅓ cup heavy cream

½ cup low-carb marinara sauce, divided, plus more for serving if desired

⅓ cup shredded mozzarella cheese (part skim)

2 cloves garlic, minced

2 tablespoons chopped fresh parsley, plus more for garnish if desired

2 teaspoons Italian seasoning

½ teaspoon fine sea salt

¼ teaspoon ground black pepper

¼ cup grated Parmesan cheese, plus more for garnish if desired

1. Preheat the oven to 350°F. Line a rimmed baking sheet with parchment paper.
2. Place the ground beef, eggs, onion, pork panko, cream, and ¼ cup of the marinara sauce in a large bowl and mix gently with your hands to combine. Gently mix in the mozzarella, garlic, parsley, Italian seasoning, salt, and pepper; do not overmix. Overmixing will compact the meat too much and make it tough.
3. Scoop the meat mixture onto the prepared pan. Shape into a loaf that is 8 inches long by 4 inches wide and 2 inches thick.
4. Bake for 45 minutes, then remove and top with the remaining ¼ cup of marinara sauce and the Parmesan cheese. Bake for another 10 to 15 minutes, until a thermometer inserted in the center of the loaf registers 165°F.
5. Allow to rest for 10 minutes before slicing. If desired, serve with additional marinara sauce, Parmesan cheese, and fresh parsley.

Calories	Fat	Protein	Total Carbs	Dietary Fiber	Net Carbs
411	32g	27g	3g	1g	2g

YIELD: 9 servings
PREP TIME: 15 minutes
COOK TIME: 40 minutes

TACO CASSEROLE

 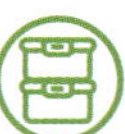 

Easy to prep and easy to make ahead! It's the perfect meal for a busy weeknight, and it can be frozen!

- 2 pounds 80/20 ground beef
- 1 tablespoon extra-virgin olive oil or avocado oil
- 3 cloves garlic, minced
- 1 teaspoon ground cumin
- 1 teaspoon smoked paprika
- ½ teaspoon ground dried oregano
- ½ teaspoon onion powder
- ½ teaspoon chili powder
- ½ teaspoon fine sea salt
- 1 (8-ounce) package cream cheese
- 1 cup salsa
- 2 large eggs
- ½ cup heavy cream
- 2 cups shredded cheddar cheese, divided

SUGGESTED TOPPINGS:

- Chopped tomatoes or salsa
- Sour cream
- Diced avocado
- Sliced black olives
- Chopped fresh cilantro
- Sliced jalapeños
- Sliced scallions

1. Preheat the oven to 400°F. Grease a 9 by 13-inch baking dish with cooking spray. Set aside.
2. Brown the meat in the olive oil in a 12-inch skillet over medium-high heat, 6 to 8 minutes, crumbling the meat as it cooks.
3. Once the ground beef is nicely browned, reduce the heat to low and add the garlic and seasonings. Stir together, then add the cream cheese and salsa and continue to stir until the cream cheese is well combined and there are no lumps. Spread this meat mixture evenly in the prepared baking dish.
4. In a large bowl, whisk the eggs, cream, and 1 cup of the shredded cheese. Pour over the meat mixture. Top with the remaining cup of cheese.
5. Cover with aluminum foil and bake for 20 minutes. Remove the foil and broil for 4 to 5 minutes, until the cheese is nicely browned.
6. Enjoy immediately with your favorite taco toppings.
7. Once cooled, cover the casserole with aluminum foil and refrigerate for up to 3 days or place in an airtight container and freeze for up to 3 months.

Calories	Fat	Protein	Total Carbs	Dietary Fiber	Net Carbs
519	43g	27g	5g	1g	4g

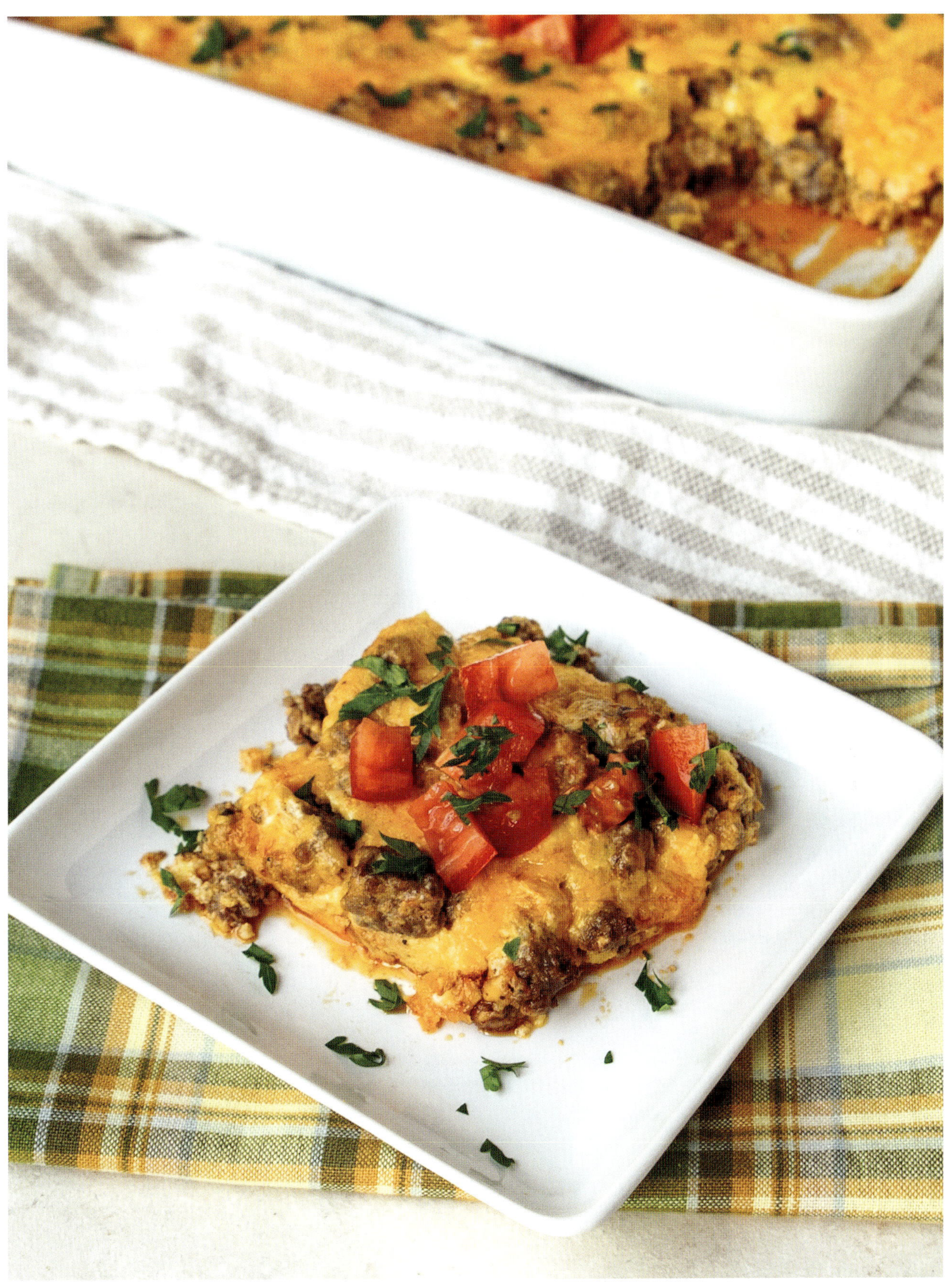

YIELD: 8 servings
PREP TIME: 25 minutes
COOK TIME: 45 minutes

SPAGHETTI SQUASH CASSEROLE

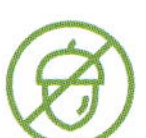 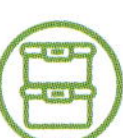 

This hearty casserole is made up of three delicious layers: Cooked spaghetti squash "noodles" form the base, a rich meat sauce forms the middle layer, and a creamy cheesy mixture is the top. It can also be cooked ahead, cooled, then frozen. Thaw the night before you need it, cover, and reheat in a preheated 350°F oven for 20 to 30 minutes or until heated through.

1 (1½-pound) spaghetti squash, sliced in half lengthwise

1 tablespoon extra-virgin olive oil

½ teaspoon fine sea salt

¼ teaspoon ground black pepper

2 pounds ground pork

2 cloves garlic, minced

16 ounces low-carb marinara sauce

2 large eggs

2 cups shredded mozzarella cheese (part skim), divided

1½ cups cottage cheese (4% milkfat) or ricotta cheese (part skim)

½ cup grated Parmesan cheese

1 teaspoon Italian seasoning

Chopped fresh parsley, for garnish (optional)

1. Preheat the oven to 400°F.
2. You need just 12 ounces of spaghetti squash for this recipe, which is one-half of the squash, so you can place the second half in the refrigerator for another use. (Alternatively, while you have the oven on, you could bake both halves and use the roasted squash from one of the halves for another recipe.) Scoop out the seeds and pulp of the squash and discard. Line a rimmed baking sheet with parchment paper. Place the squash on the prepared baking sheet, cut side up. Rub the cut surface of the squash with a drizzle of oil. Place cut side down on the prepared baking sheet. Roast for 25 minutes, until golden brown and easily pierced with a knife. Remove from the oven and allow to sit until cool enough to handle, then use a fork to scrape the inside to loosen the "spaghetti" threads. Season with the salt and pepper.
3. While the squash is in the oven, cook the pork. In a large skillet over medium-high heat, brown the pork until no longer pink, then add the garlic and sauce. Simmer for 15 minutes to allow the flavors to develop.
4. While the meat sauce is simmering, stir together the eggs, 1 cup of the mozzarella, the cottage cheese, Parmesan, and Italian seasoning in a large bowl until combined. Set aside.
5. To assemble the casserole, spread the spaghetti squash threads in a 9 by 13-inch baking pan. Spread the meat sauce over the spaghetti squash. Spread the egg and cheese mixture over the meat sauce. Sprinkle the remaining cup of mozzarella over the top.

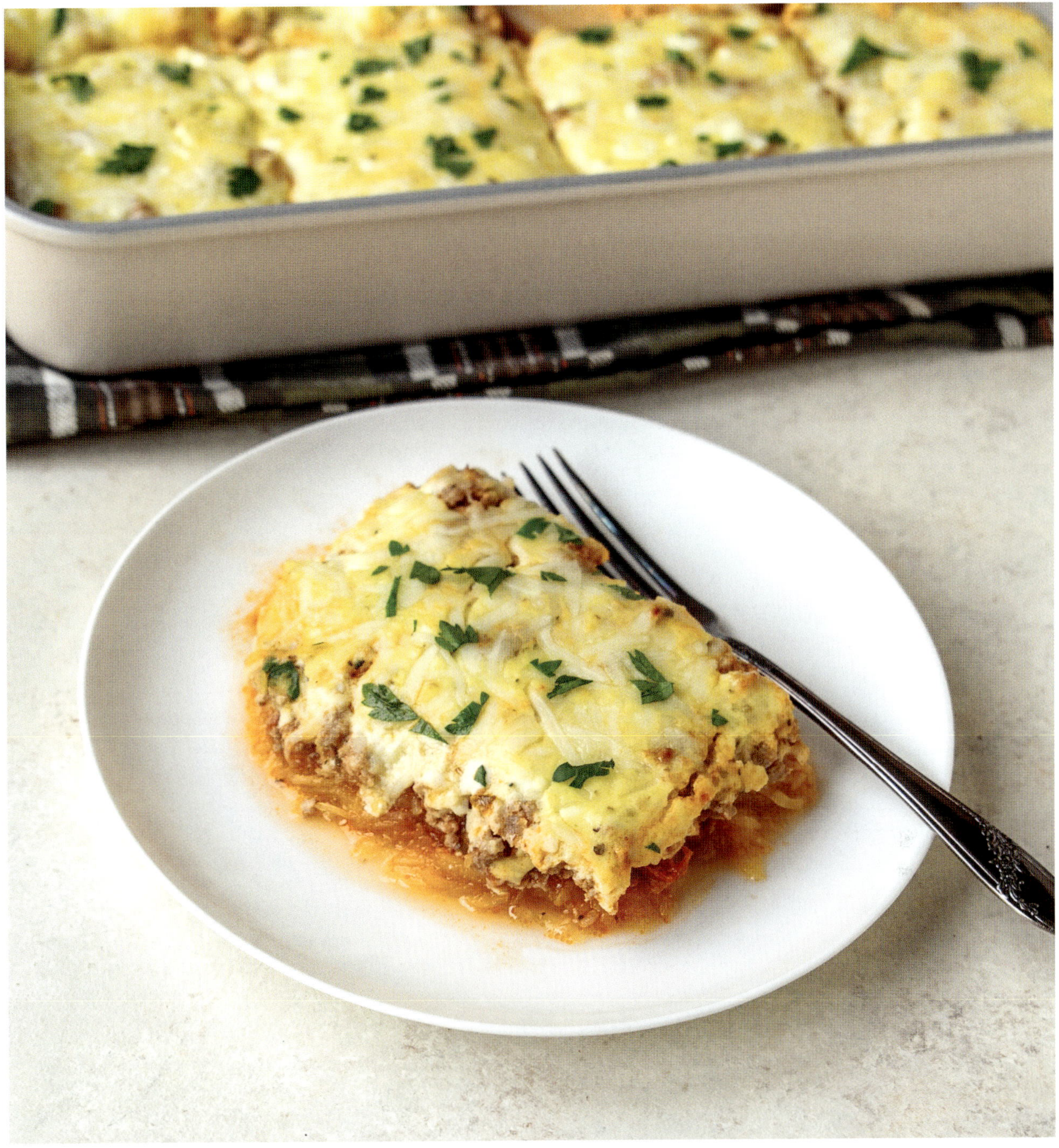

6. Bake for 20 minutes, or until the cheese is melted and the edges of the casserole are browned. Garnish with chopped parsley before serving, if desired.
7. Cover and store leftovers in the fridge for up to 3 days.

Calories	Fat	Protein	Total Carbs	Dietary Fiber	Net Carbs
518	38g	35g	7g	1g	6g

YIELD: 12 servings
PREP TIME: 20 minutes
COOK TIME: 1 hour 15 minutes

CHICKEN SPINACH ALFREDO CASSEROLE

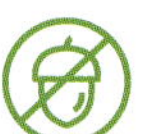

This hearty chicken casserole is full of protein and another great option for meal prep. This recipe makes a lot, but it freezes well. If you don't have time to make homemade Alfredo sauce, you can certainly purchase a low-carb prepared option from the brands Rao's and Primal Kitchen. If using store-bought sauce, you'll need 4 cups to make this recipe.

FOR THE ALFREDO SAUCE:

1/4 cup (1/2 stick) salted butter or bacon grease

2 cups heavy cream

1 large egg yolk

1/2 teaspoon onion powder

1/4 teaspoon fine sea salt

1/4 teaspoon ground white pepper

1/4 cup grated Parmesan cheese

1 teaspoon grated lemon zest

1/4 teaspoon ground nutmeg

8 cups chopped cooked chicken breast

10 ounces frozen spinach, thawed, squeezed of excess water

6 large eggs

1 cup cottage cheese (4% milkfat)

1 cup shredded mozzarella cheese (part skim)

1/4 teaspoon fine sea salt

1/4 teaspoon ground black pepper

6 slices thick-cut bacon, baked (see page 76) and chopped, for garnish (optional)

1. To make the Alfredo sauce, bring the butter and cream to a boil in a large saucepan over medium heat. Lower the heat to maintain a simmer and stir in the egg yolk until well incorporated.
2. Stir in the onion powder, salt, and white pepper. Continue to simmer, stirring constantly, until the sauce thickens, about 15 minutes. When sufficiently thickened, it will coat the back of a wooden spoon.
3. Remove the pan from the heat and stir in the Parmesan cheese, lemon zest, and nutmeg.
4. Preheat the oven to 350°F. Grease a 9 by 13-inch baking dish with cooking spray.
5. Put the chicken, thawed spinach, and Alfredo sauce in a large mixing bowl and stir to combine.
6. In another mixing bowl, mix together the eggs, cottage cheese, mozzarella, salt, and black pepper until well combined. Scoop this mixture into the bowl with the chicken and stir to combine.
7. Evenly spread in the prepared baking dish.

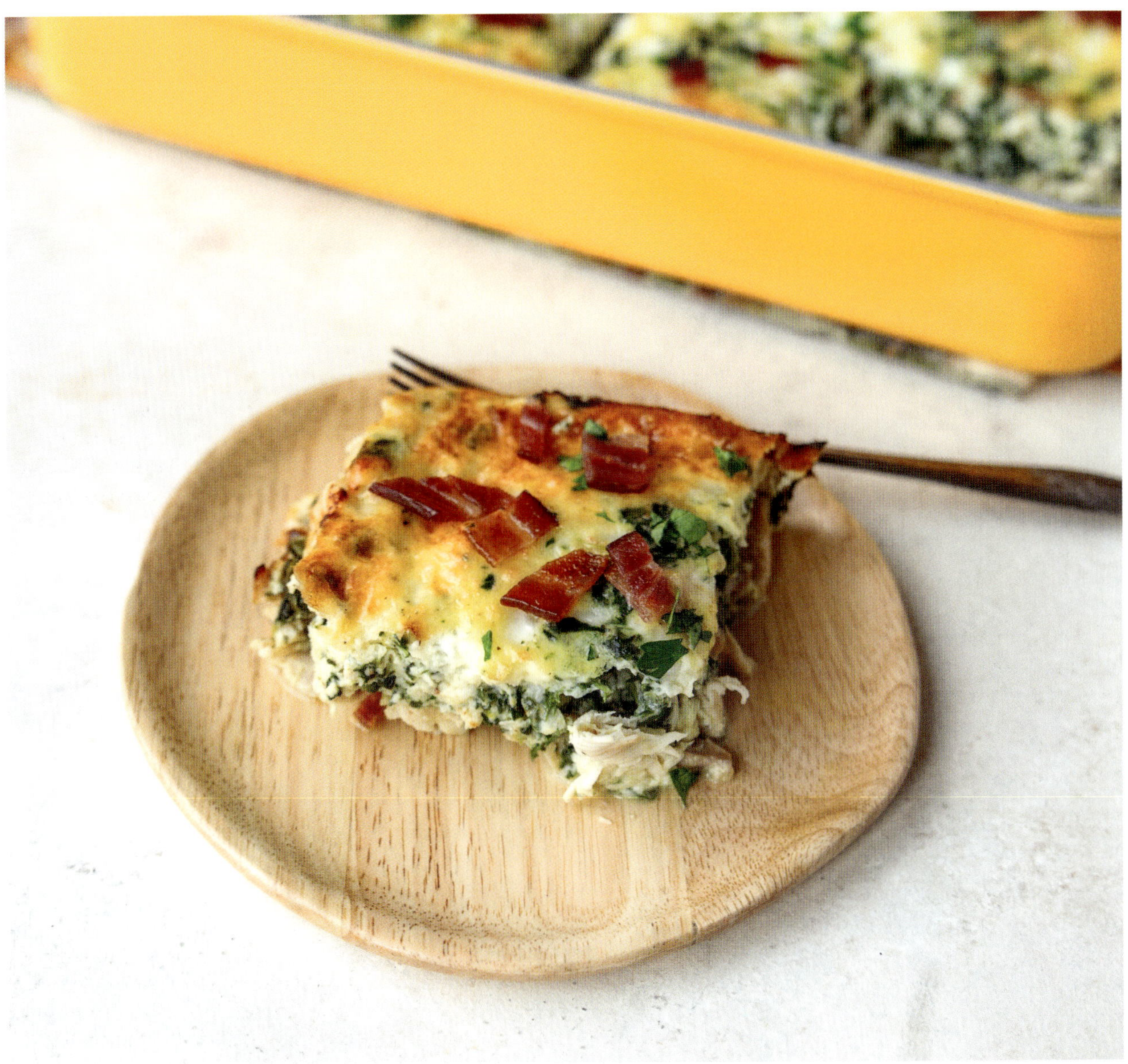

8. Bake for 45 minutes to 1 hour, until the mixture is set in the center and slightly browned around the edges of the pan.
9. Remove from the oven and allow to rest for 10 minutes before slicing and serving. Garnish with chopped bacon, if desired. Once cooled, portion the casserole as you like, place in airtight containers, and refrigerate for up to 5 days or freeze for up to 3 months. To reheat, transfer the container to the fridge to thaw overnight then bake in an air fryer or oven at 350°F for 5 minutes.

Calories	Fat	Protein	Total Carbs	Dietary Fiber	Net Carbs
432	30g	33g	3g	1g	2g

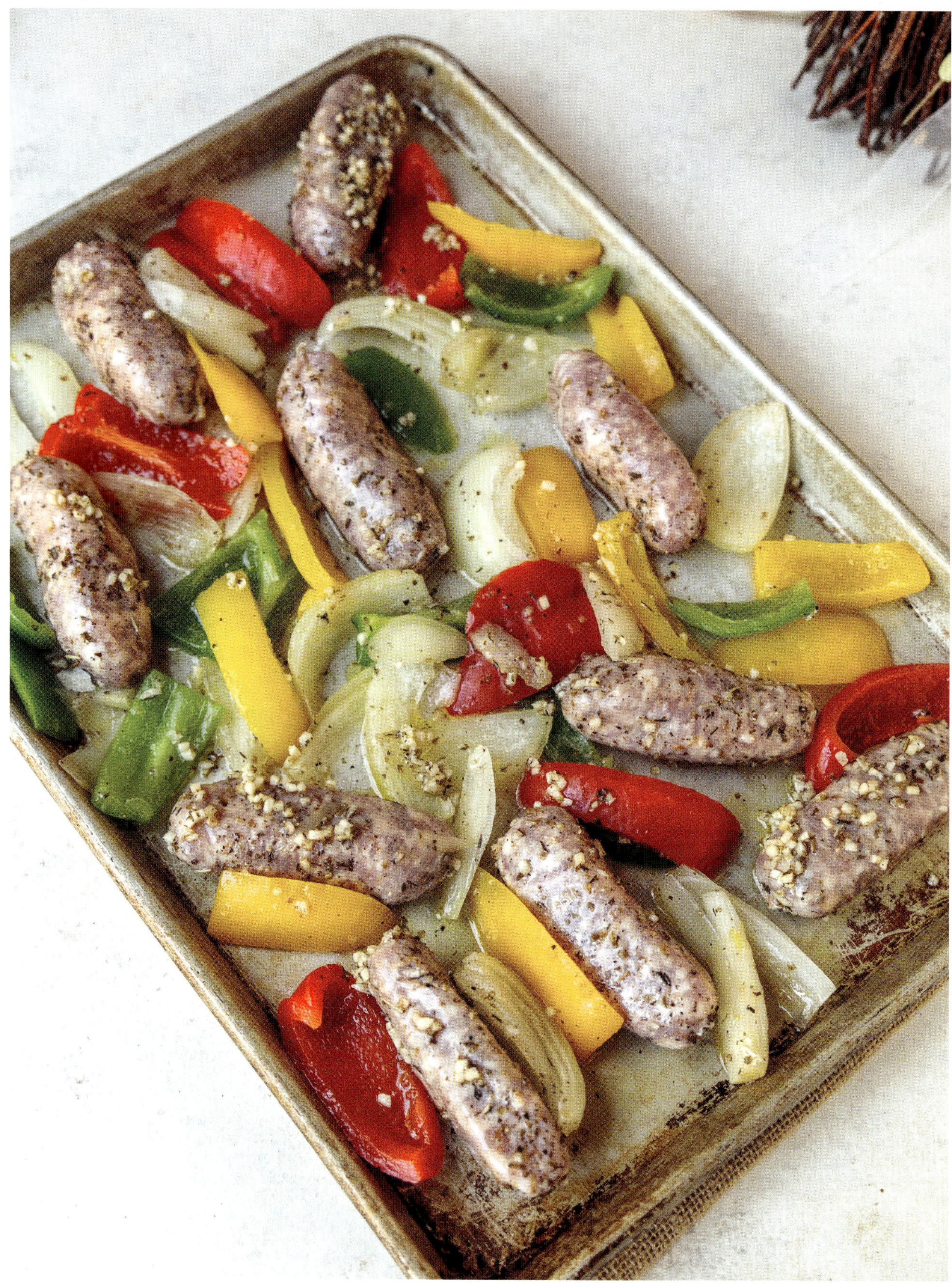

YIELD: 4 servings
PREP TIME: 15 minutes
COOK TIME: 30 minutes

ITALIAN SAUSAGE & PEPPERS

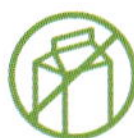  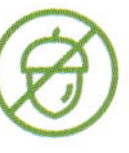 
  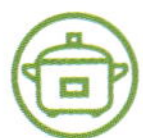

You have a few options to make this traditional Italian sausage and peppers dinner. Baking will give the sausage and peppers a nice browned color and more bite as opposed to using the Instant Pot or slow cooker.

- **1½ pounds Italian sausages**
- **3 cups sliced bell peppers (red, green, and/or yellow)**
- **1 cup yellow onion quarters**
- **4 cloves garlic, minced**
- **2 tablespoons extra-virgin olive oil**
- **2 teaspoons Italian seasoning**
- **½ teaspoon fine sea salt**
- **¼ teaspoon ground black pepper**

1. If freezer prepping, place all the ingredients in a gallon-size zip-top bag and freeze for up to 3 months. Thaw overnight before cooking in the oven, Instant Pot, or slow cooker.
2. Preheat the oven to 400°F. Put all the ingredients in a large mixing bowl and gently toss to coat in the oil and seasonings. Spread in a single layer on a rimmed baking sheet. (If freezer prepping, simply place the thawed contents of the freezer bag on a rimmed baking sheet and spread out.)
3. Bake for 30 minutes, or until the internal temperature of the sausages is 165°F and the vegetables are softened.

VARIATIONS:

Instant Pot Italian Sausage & Peppers. Pour ¼ cup of water into an Instant Pot. Then add all the ingredients (or, if freezer prepping, the thawed contents of the freezer bag) to the pot. Seal and cook on manual mode at high pressure for 25 minutes. Press cancel to end cooking and allow the pot to naturally release pressure.

Slow Cooker Italian Sausage & Peppers. Put all the ingredients (or the thawed contents of the freezer bag) in an 8-quart slow cooker. Cover and cook on low for 5 to 6 hours, until the internal temperature of the sausages is 165°F and the vegetables are softened.

Calories	Fat	Protein	Total Carbs	Dietary Fiber	Net Carbs
703	61g	26g	13g	4g	9g

YIELD: 8 servings (1 cup per serving)
PREP TIME: 30 minutes
COOK TIME: 35 minutes

BEEF STEW

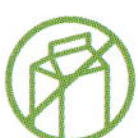

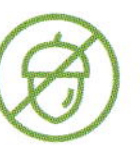
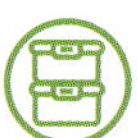

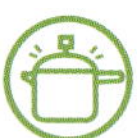
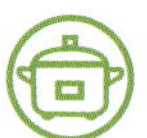

My hubby begs me for this beef stew on a weekly basis. Cooking up a big batch of it keeps everyone happy. Hubby is able to grab a serving from the freezer whenever he wants, which makes my life easier, especially when my kids want something else for dinner.

2 pounds boneless beef chuck roast or cubed beef stew meat

2 tablespoons extra-virgin olive oil, divided

1 teaspoon fine sea salt, divided

1/2 teaspoon ground black pepper, divided

4 cups beef bone broth

3 cloves garlic, minced

2 tablespoons tomato paste

1 teaspoon Italian seasoning

1 teaspoon ground thyme

1 cup chopped yellow onions

1 cup 1-inch-cubed carrots

2 cups peeled and 1-inch-cubed daikon radish

1 teaspoon glucomannan or xanthan gum (optional, to thicken)

1 tablespoon chopped fresh parsley, for garnish

1. If using chuck roast and not precut stew meat, cut the beef into 2-inch cubes.
2. Heat 1 tablespoon of the olive oil in the Instant Pot using the sauté mode. When the oil is hot, add half of the beef. Sprinkle with half of the salt and pepper.
3. Sear the beef cubes on the first side without moving them until browned and they easily release from the bottom of the pot, about 5 minutes. Flip over and brown the other side. Remove to a covered container to keep warm.
4. Repeat with the remaining oil, beef, salt, and pepper. When browned, return the first batch of seared beef to the pot.
5. Pour in the broth, then add the garlic, tomato paste, Italian seasoning, and thyme and stir to combine.
6. Add the onions, carrots, and radish. Turn off the sauté mode.
7. Seal the lid and cook on manual mode at high pressure for 35 minutes. Once the timer ends, allow the pressure to naturally release for 10 minutes. Then, using a long wooden spoon, push the steam valve to release the pressure quickly.
8. Carefully open the lid, stir the beef stew, and decide if you'd like a thicker broth. If so, sprinkle the glucomannan over the stew and stir to combine.
9. Serve with a sprinkle of fresh parsley and enjoy immediately!
10. For meal prepping, allow the stew to cool before placing individual servings in airtight containers. Store in the fridge for up to 3 days or freeze for up to 3 months.

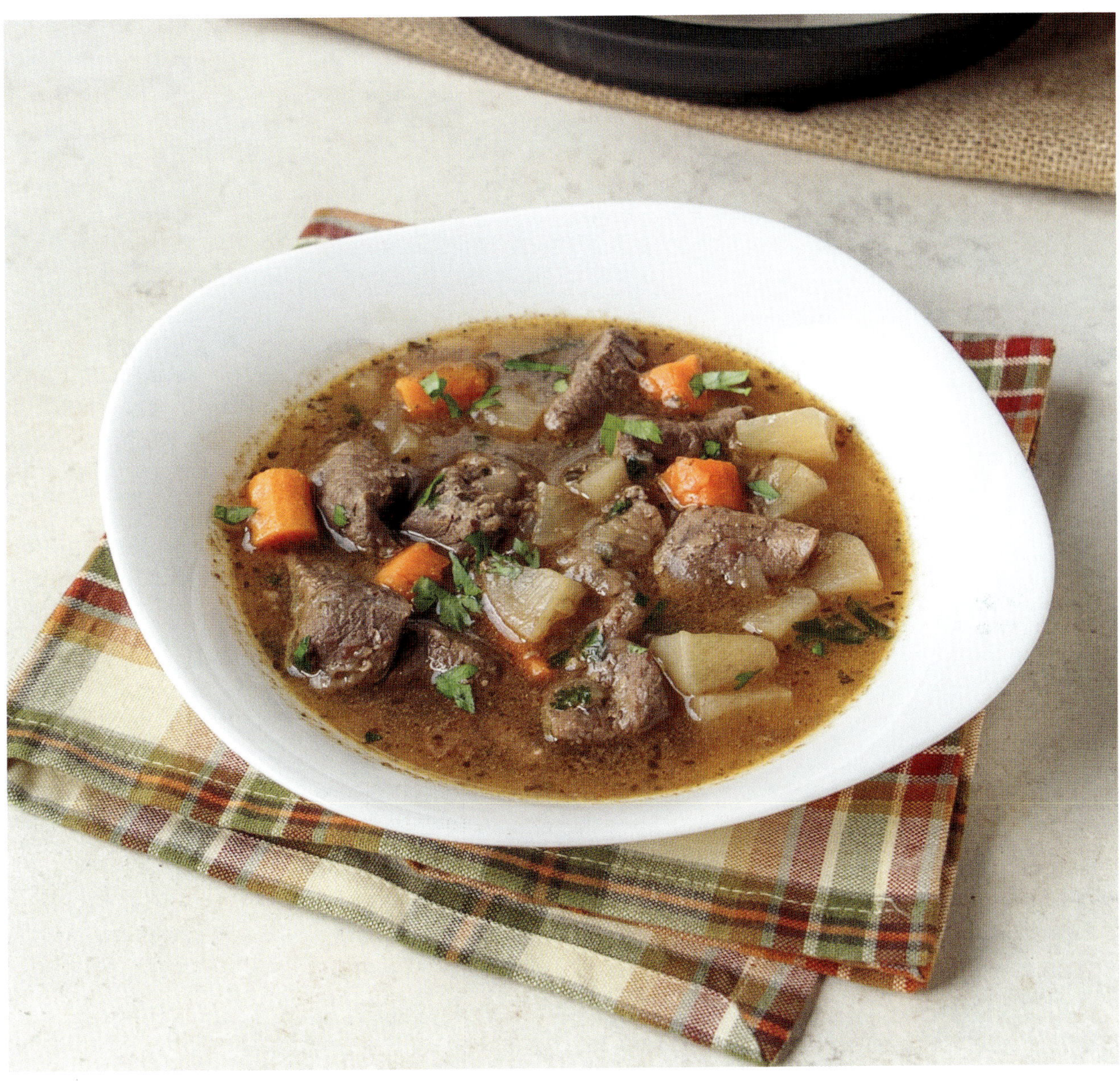

VARIATION: Slow Cooker Beef Stew. Complete Steps 1 through 4 as written, but use a large skillet for the searing step. You can sear all the meat at once, using 2 tablespoons of oil, if your skillet is large enough to sear the entire amount without crowding. Transfer the seared meat to a 7-quart slow cooker, then add the rest of the ingredients, except the glucomannan, and stir to combine. Cover and cook on low 8 to 10 hours or on high 4 to 6 hours, until the meat and vegetables are fork-tender. Complete Steps 8, 9, and 10 as written.

Calories	Fat	Protein	Total Carbs	Dietary Fiber	Net Carbs
278	17g	27g	6g	2g	4g

YIELD: 6 servings (1¼ cups per serving)
PREP TIME: 10 minutes
COOK TIME: 12 minutes

BBQ PULLED CHICKEN

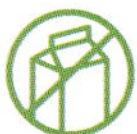  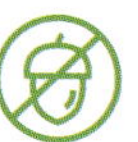 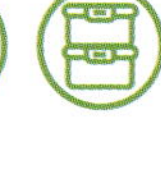
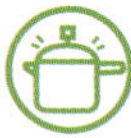 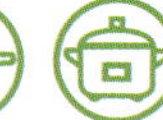

BBQ pulled chicken is a versatile recipe that can accommodate picky family members because you can serve it in a few different ways. If you want the keto option, serve the chicken in two or three butter lettuce leaves with keto toppings of choice. To make it low carb, enjoy it in a bowl served over cauliflower rice, or try it in low-carb tortillas. Thanks to the Instant Pot, this recipe cooks very quickly; however, if you don't have one, you can make the chicken in a slow cooker (see the variation below).

2 teaspoons dried minced onion

1 teaspoon garlic powder

1 teaspoon ground cumin

1 teaspoon fine sea salt

½ teaspoon ground black pepper

1 tablespoon smoked paprika

2 teaspoons chili powder (optional)

2 pounds boneless, skinless chicken thighs

½ cup chicken bone broth

½ cup sugar-free BBQ sauce, homemade (page 79) or store-bought

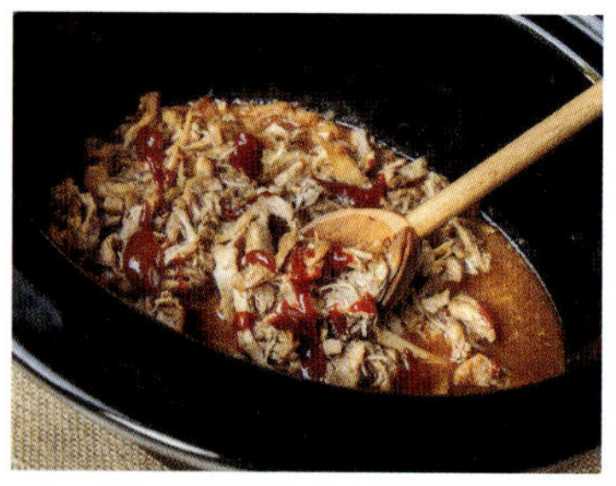

1. In a small bowl, whisk together the minced onion, garlic powder, cumin, salt, pepper, paprika, and chili powder, if using. Rub this all over both sides of each chicken thigh.
2. Pour the chicken broth and BBQ sauce into the Instant Pot. Add all the chicken thighs to the pot.
3. Seal the lid of the Instant Pot. Press the Poultry button and set the timer for 12 minutes. Once it beeps, use a long wooden spoon to prevent the steam from burning your finger and switch to "venting" to allow the Instant Pot to quick release.
4. Carefully open the lid and shred the chicken using two forks, stirring the meat in the sauce to coat. Serve right away or allow to cool before storing it.
5. For meal prepping, allow to cool, then divide into individual servings in airtight containers. Store in the fridge for up to 3 days or freeze for up to 3 months. Thaw before reheating in a microwave for 1 minute or in a skillet over medium heat for about 5 minutes.

VARIATION: Slow Cooker BBQ Pulled Chicken. Complete Step 1 as written. Pour the broth and BBQ sauce into an 8-quart slow cooker, then place the thighs in the slow cooker. Cover and cook on high for 3 hours or on low for 6 hours, until the chicken is cooked through. (When fully cooked, a thermometer should read 165°F when inserted in the thickest part of a thigh.) Complete Steps 4 and 5 as written.

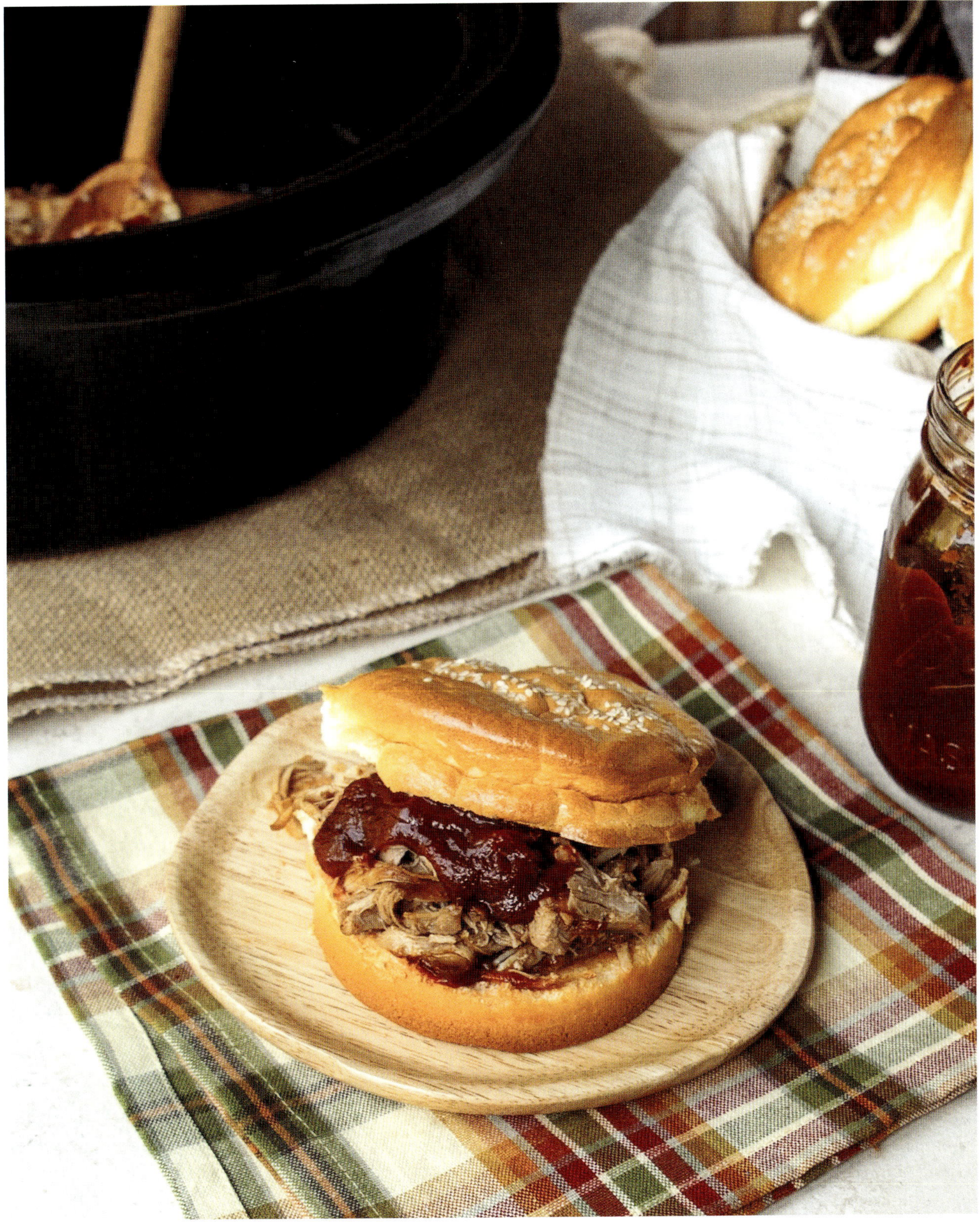

Calories	Fat	Protein	Total Carbs	Dietary Fiber	Net Carbs
203	6g	30g	5g	1g	4g

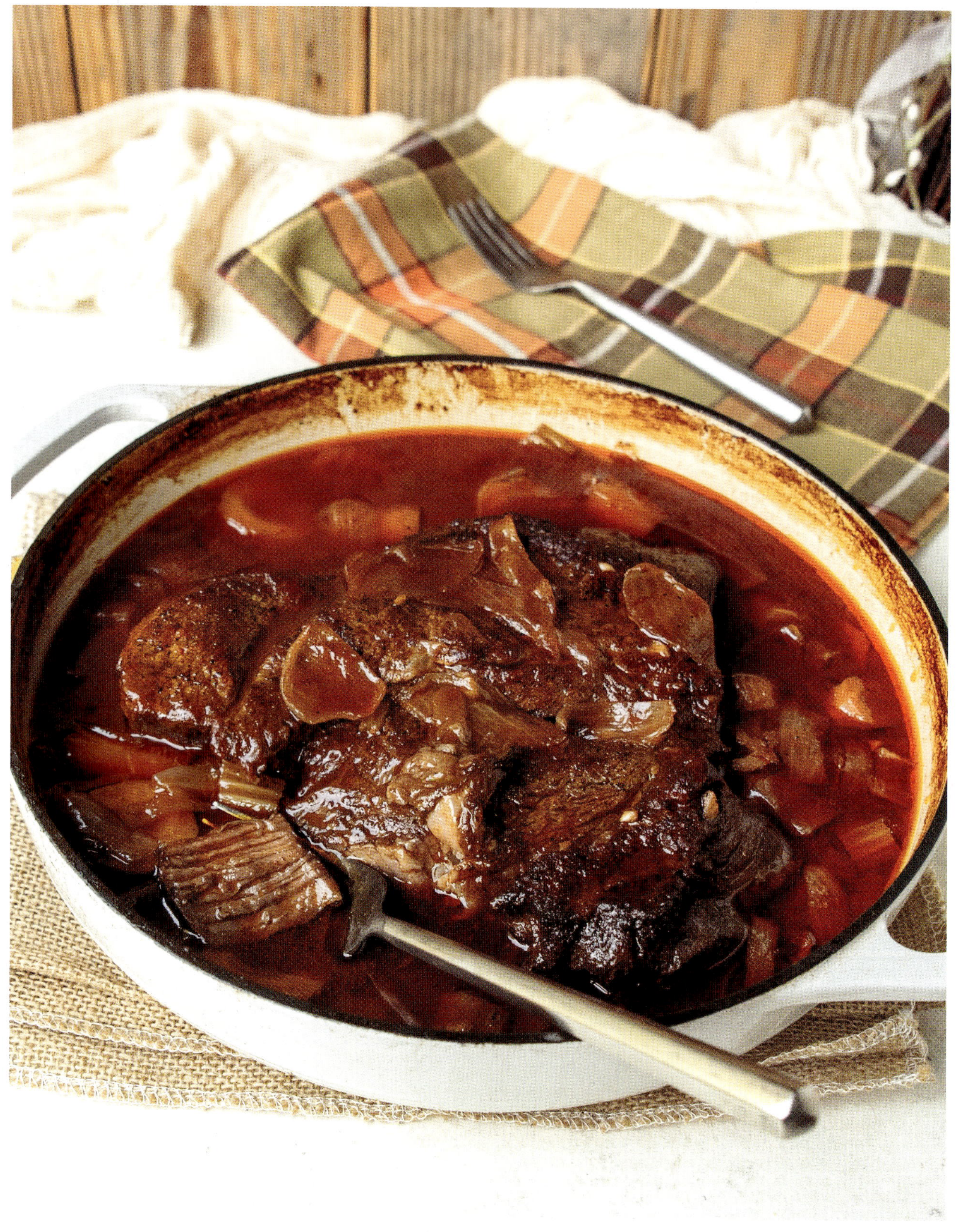

Calories	Fat	Protein	Total Carbs	Dietary Fiber	Net Carbs
488	26g	45g	10g	2g	8g

YIELD: 8 servings
PREP TIME: 15 minutes
COOK TIME: 3 hours

BRAISED BRISKET DINNER

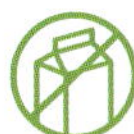

This makes for a scrumptious dinner when served with cauliflower rice or roasted vegetables. If you can't find brisket, you can use a boneless beef chuck roast instead.

3 pounds boneless beef brisket

1 teaspoon fine sea salt

1/2 teaspoon ground black pepper

2 cups beef bone broth, divided

1/2 cup sugar-free ketchup

2 teaspoons smoked paprika

2 tablespoons extra-virgin olive oil

1 cup chopped yellow onions

4 cloves garlic, minced

1 cup red wine

1 cup peeled and 1-inch cubed carrots

1 cup chopped celery

2 tablespoons chopped fresh parsley, for garnish

1. Preheat the oven to 325°F.
2. Season the meat with the salt and pepper on each side, then set aside.
3. In a small bowl, whisk together 1 cup of the broth with the ketchup and paprika. Set aside.
4. Heat the olive oil in a large braiser or a 6-quart Dutch oven over medium-high heat, then place the roast in the pot and sear on both sides until well browned and the meat easily releases from the bottom of the pot. Remove to a plate.
5. Add the onions to the pot and sauté until translucent, about 5 minutes. Stir in the garlic and cook about a minute, or until fragrant.
6. Pour in the wine and remaining cup of broth to deglaze the pan, stirring to scrape the meaty bits on the bottom of the pan.
7. Return the seared meat to the pot and bring to a boil.
8. Pour the broth and ketchup mixture over the top of the meat. Cover the pot with a lid.
9. Cook for 2 hours, then remove from the oven and add the carrots and celery. Cover and place back in the oven for another hour, or until the meat and vegetables are tender. Serve garnished with parsley and plenty of pot juices.
10. Once cooled, store leftovers covered in the refrigerator for up to 4 days or freeze for up to 2 months. Thaw overnight before reheating. To reheat, place in a preheated 325°F oven for 30 minutes to 1 hour, depending on the portion being reheated.

YIELD: 10 servings (1 cup per serving)
PREP TIME: 20 minutes
COOK TIME: 30 minutes

ROASTED VEGETABLES

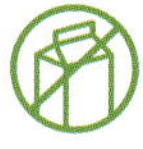 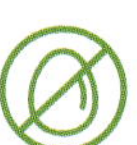 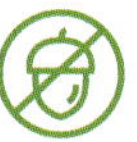 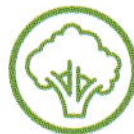

This is another great time-saving recipe, perfect for when you need a simple side that's precooked and stashed in the freezer. All you need do is defrost and reheat and serve with any protein you have on hand. A win-win!

- 2 cups chopped red and/or yellow bell peppers
- 4 cups sliced zucchini
- 6 cups cauliflower florets
- 2 cups chopped red onions
- 4 cloves garlic, sliced
- 2 tablespoons extra-virgin olive oil
- ½ teaspoon fine sea salt
- ¼ teaspoon ground black pepper
- ½ teaspoon onion powder
- ¼ teaspoon garlic powder
- 2 tablespoons chopped fresh parsley

1. Preheat the oven to 400°F.
2. Place all the vegetables on a 13 by 18-inch rimmed baking sheet.
3. Drizzle the vegetables with the olive oil, then sprinkle on the seasonings and fresh parsley. Toss to coat.
4. Bake for 30 minutes, or until the vegetables are fork-tender.
5. Store leftovers in an airtight container in the fridge for up to 5 days or freeze for up to 3 months.

Calories	Fat	Protein	Total Carbs	Dietary Fiber	Net Carbs
71	3g	3g	10g	3g	7g

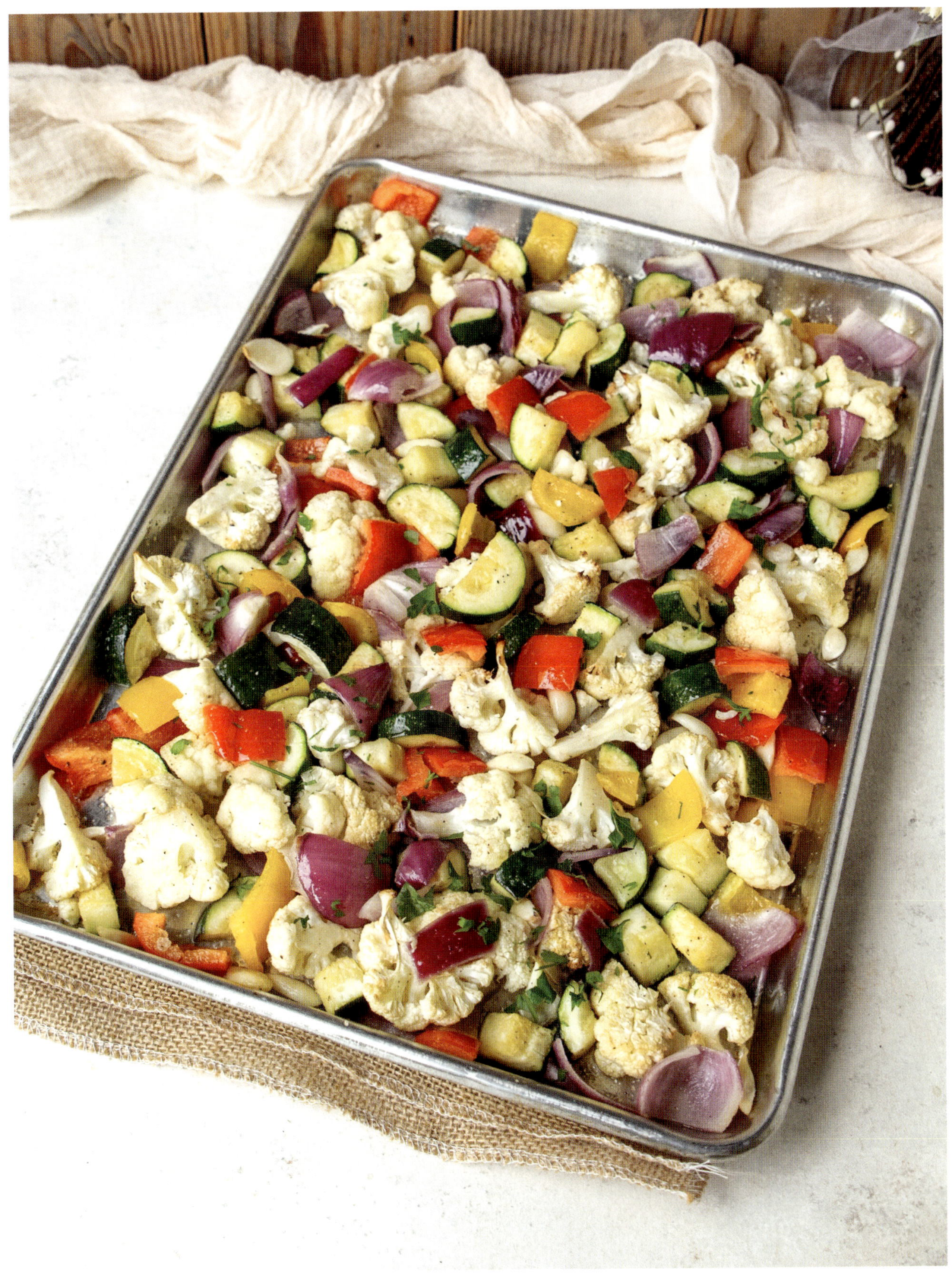

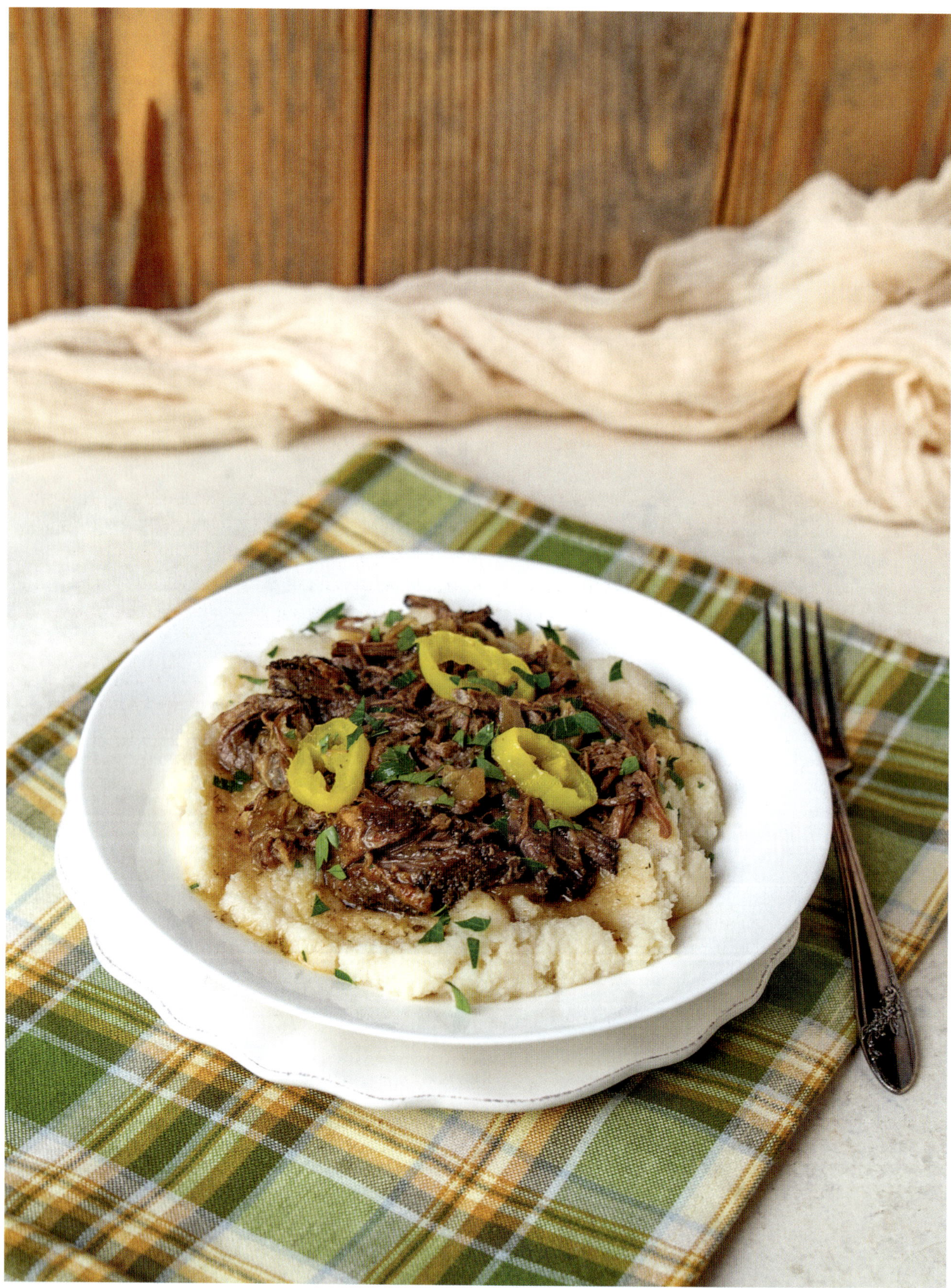

YIELD: 8 servings
PREP TIME: 5 minutes
COOK TIME: 1 hour or 4 to 8 hours, depending on method

MISSISSIPPI POT ROAST

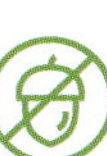
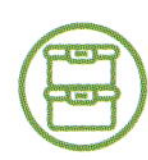
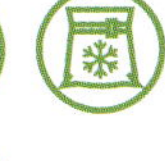

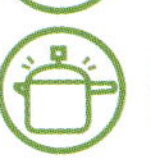
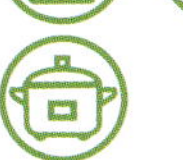

If you're new to batch cooking as I once was, once you try it, you will become addicted to doing it more often because it's truly a time-saver during the week.

2 tablespoons Italian seasoning

1 tablespoon onion powder

1 teaspoon garlic powder

1 teaspoon dried dill weed

½ teaspoon fine sea salt

½ teaspoon ground black pepper

4 pounds boneless beef chuck roast

1 cup sliced pepperoncini, plus more for garnish if desired

½ cup pepperoncini juice from the jar

½ cup (1 stick) salted butter, sliced

2 tablespoons coconut aminos

Chopped fresh parsley, for garnish (optional)

1. If not freezer prepping, skip ahead to Step 2. To freezer prep, put the seasonings in a gallon-size zip-top bag and shake vigorously. Add the roast, seal the bag, and shake to coat. Then add the remaining ingredients. Freeze for up to 3 months. Thaw overnight before putting the contents of the bag in an Instant Pot or an 8-quart slow cooker and cook following Step 3.
2. Mix the dry seasonings in a small bowl, then completely coat the chuck roast on all sides with the seasoning mixture. Place the roast and the rest of the ingredients in the Instant Pot or an 8-quart slow cooker.
3. *If using the Instant Pot,* seal the lid and cook on manual mode at high pressure for 60 minutes. Once the timer ends, allow the pressure to release naturally for 10 minutes. Then, using a long wooden spoon to prevent steam from burning your finger, push the steam valve to release the pressure quickly.

   If using the slow cooker, cover and cook on low for 6 to 8 hours or on high for 4 to 5 hours, until the meat is fork-tender.
4. Using two forks, shred the beef. Serve garnished with pepper rings and parsley, if desired.
5. Store leftovers in an airtight container in the refrigerator for up to 5 days or up to 3 months in the freezer.

Calories	Fat	Protein	Total Carbs	Dietary Fiber	Net Carbs
524	38g	44g	3g	1g	2g

YIELD: 8 servings
PREP TIME: 5 minutes
COOK TIME: 40 minutes or 4 to 6 hours, depending on method

GARLIC BUTTER CHICKEN THIGHS

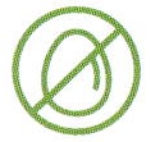
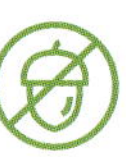
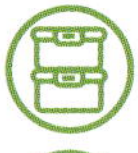
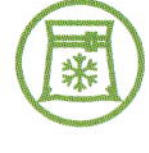

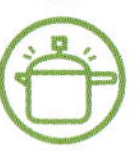
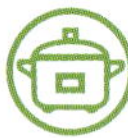

These buttery chicken thighs don't take long to prep, and you have the option to freezer prep them; then you can choose to cook them in a slow cooker or an Instant Pot, depending on the time you have. I serve this with my Garlic Parmesan Broccoli (page 137) for a complete meal.

8 (6-ounce) boneless, skinless chicken thighs

⅓ cup extra-virgin olive oil

2 tablespoons minced garlic

2 teaspoons fine sea salt

1 teaspoon ground black pepper

2 tablespoons salted butter

1 cup chicken bone broth

1. If not freezer prepping, skip ahead to Step 4.
2. *To freezer prep for the slow cooker,* place the chicken thighs in a gallon-size zip-top bag. In a small bowl, mix together the olive oil, garlic, salt, and pepper. Pour into the bag with the thighs, seal shut, and massage to coat the chicken. Add the butter and reseal. Freeze for up to 3 months. Thaw overnight before cooking in the slow cooker.

   To cook the freezer-prepped meal using the slow cooker, put the thawed contents of the bag in a 6-quart slow cooker. Pour in the chicken broth, then cover and cook on high for 4 to 6 hours, until a thermometer inserted in the thickest part of a thigh registers 165°F.
3. *To freezer prep for the Instant Pot,* follow the freezer prep instructions for the slow cooker, except do not add the butter to the zip-top bag. Thaw overnight before cooking in the Instant Pot.

   To cook the freezer-prepped meal using the Instant Pot, put the butter in the Instant Pot and press sauté. Once the butter is melted, add 4 of the seasoned chicken thighs. Brown on each side and remove to a plate. Add the rest of the seasoned chicken thighs and brown them on both sides. Turn off the sauté mode. Return the first set of chicken thighs to the pot, then pour in the chicken broth. Seal the lid and cook on manual mode at high pressure for 30 minutes. Once it beeps, use a long wooden spoon to prevent steam from burning your finger and switch to "venting" to allow the Instant Pot to quick release.

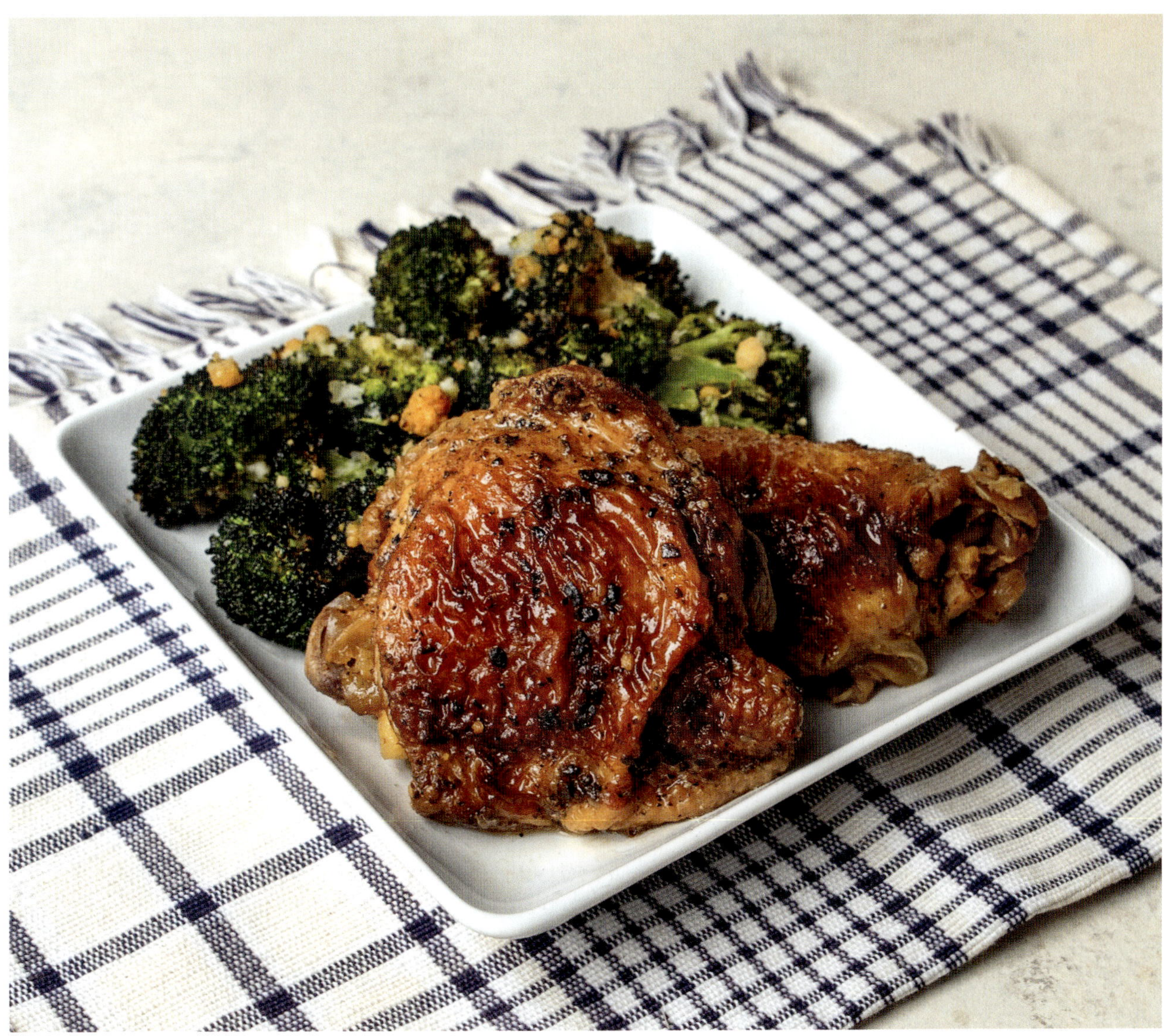

4. *To cook in a slow cooker,* put all the ingredients in a 6-quart slow cooker, cover, and cook on high for 4 to 6 hours, until a thermometer inserted in the thickest part of a thigh registers 165°F.

   To cook in an Instant Pot, place the chicken thighs in a large mixing bowl. In a small bowl, mix together the olive oil, garlic, salt, and pepper. Pour the seasoned oil over the thighs and massage the thighs with the oil. Cook in the Instant Pot following the directions in Step 3.

5. Store leftovers in the fridge for up to 4 days.

Calories	Fat	Protein	Total Carbs	Dietary Fiber	Net Carbs
312	19g	33g	1g	0.1g	0.9g

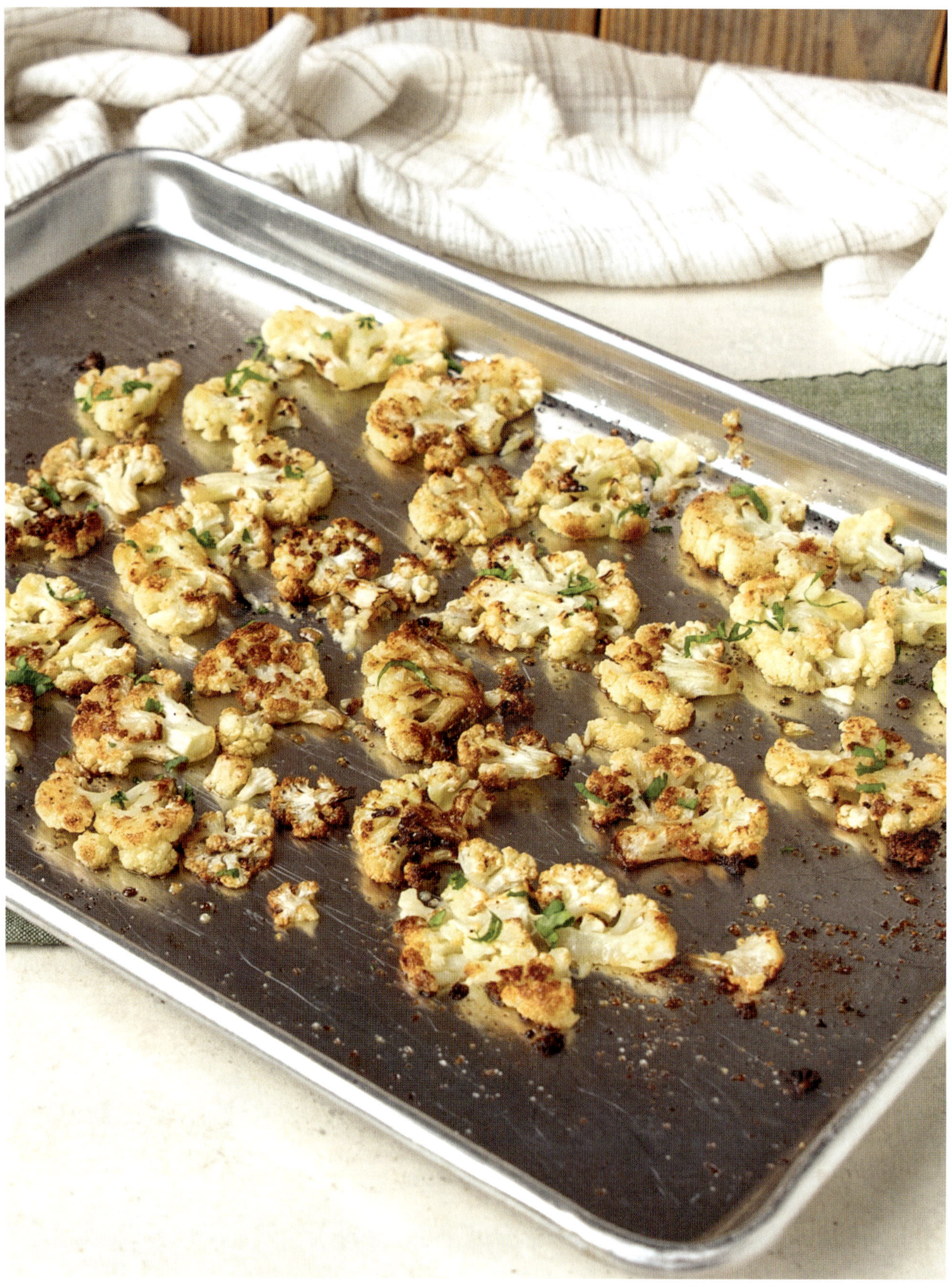

YIELD: 4 servings
PREP TIME: 10 minutes
COOK TIME: 30 minutes

CRISPY SMASHED CAULIFLOWER

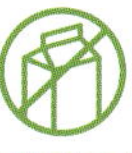

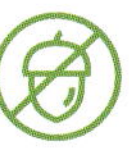
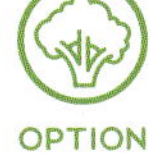

OPTION OPTION

Feel free to use precut cauliflower florets to save time in the kitchen. Just be sure to have a pound's worth for this recipe.

1 pound cauliflower florets (from 1 large head, about 2 pounds)

2 tablespoons extra-virgin olive oil

½ teaspoon fine sea salt

¼ teaspoon ground black pepper

¼ teaspoon garlic powder

¼ teaspoon onion powder

¼ cup grated Parmesan cheese (optional)

1. Preheat the oven to 400°F.
2. Place the cauliflower florets on a rimmed baking sheet. Drizzle with the olive oil and toss to coat. Sprinkle on the salt and spices and toss again. Arrange in a single layer.
3. Bake for 15 minutes, then remove and flip the florets over. Bake for another 10 minutes, or until golden brown.
4. Remove from the oven and increase the oven temperature to 450°F. Using a smooth meat mallet, smash the florets to about ½ inch thick. Sprinkle with the Parmesan cheese, if using. Return the pan to the oven and roast for 5 minutes, or until golden brown.

NOTE: If you're a strict vegetarian and you choose to use the Parmesan cheese, make sure to use a brand that doesn't include animal rennet.

Calories	Fat	Protein	Total Carbs	Dietary Fiber	Net Carbs
92	7g	2g	6g	2g	4g

YIELD: 3 servings
PREP TIME: 15 minutes
COOK TIME: 30 minutes

ROASTED ASPARAGUS WITH HOLLANDAISE

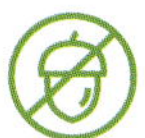 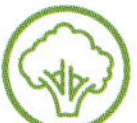

Roasted asparagus is great on its own, but when you have the extra time to make this delicious hollandaise sauce, you will feel like your dining room has turned into a fancy restaurant. This asparagus is perfect for a date night at home with my filet mignon recipe on page 213.

1 pound medium-thick asparagus, tough ends removed

2 tablespoons extra-virgin olive oil

½ teaspoon fine sea salt

½ teaspoon garlic powder

½ teaspoon onion powder

FOR THE HOLLANDAISE:

6 tablespoons (¾ stick) salted butter

2 large egg yolks

1 teaspoon fresh lemon juice

1 tablespoon heavy cream

Pinch of cayenne pepper (optional)

Pinch of fine sea salt

Pinch of ground black pepper

1. Preheat the oven to 400°F.
2. Place the trimmed asparagus on a rimmed baking sheet. Drizzle with the olive oil and toss to coat the spears. Sprinkle with the seasonings, toss to coat, and then arrange in a single layer. Roast for 30 minutes, or until tender.
3. While the asparagus is in the oven, make the hollandaise.
4. In a small saucepan over low heat, melt the butter.
5. Place the egg yolks in a small mixing bowl; set aside.
6. Once the butter is melted, add the lemon juice, cream, cayenne pepper (if using), salt, and black pepper. Stir to combine. To temper the yolks, pour a spoonful of the butter mixture at a time into the bowl with the yolks while whisking. Continue until most of the butter mixture is in the bowl with the yolks.
7. Once incorporated, pour the yolk mixture back into the saucepan and cook over low heat, stirring constantly, until it's thickened. Once the sauce coats the back of a wooden spoon, remove, cover, and keep warm at the back of the stove until the asparagus is tender.
8. Serve the roasted asparagus with the hollandaise.

BASED ON 4 OUNCES UNCOOKED TRIMMED ASPARAGUS BY WEIGHT AND ¼ CUP SAUCE

Calories	Fat	Protein	Total Carbs	Dietary Fiber	Net Carbs
362	37g	5g	6g	2g	4g

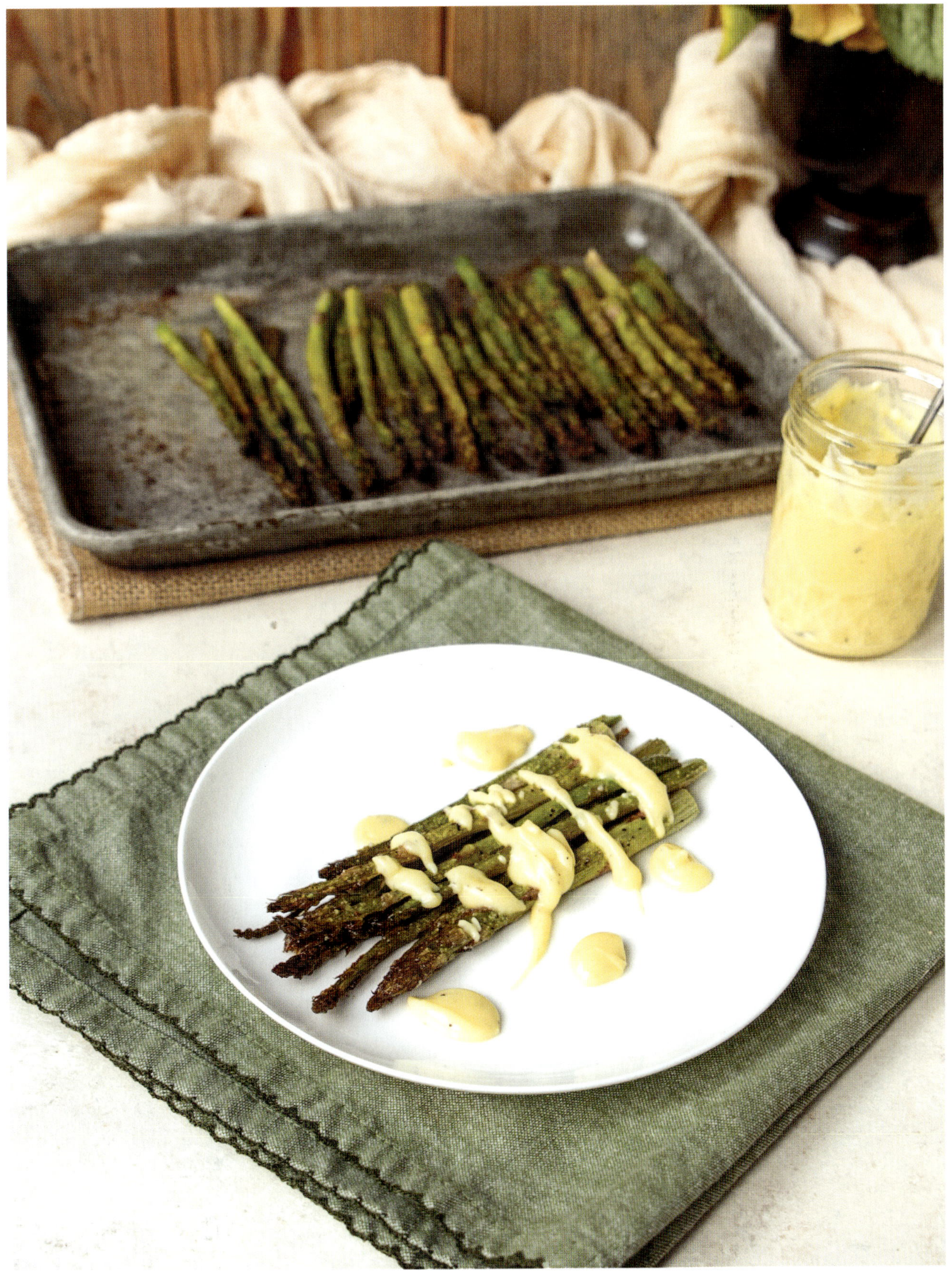

YIELD: 16 brookies (1 per serving)
PREP TIME: 20 minutes
COOK TIME: 35 minutes

BROOKIES

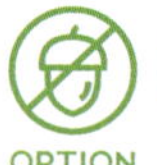
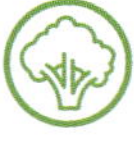

OPTION

Half cookie and half brownie, the brookie is an incredible combination that everyone loves. This recipe combines a half batch of my popular flourless brownies with a half batch of my popular bakery-style chocolate chip cookies, both found on SugarFreeMom.com.

FOR THE BROWNIE LAYER:

1 cup sugar-free chocolate chips

1/2 cup (1 stick) unsalted butter, coconut oil, or avocado oil

1/4 cup unsweetened sunflower seed butter, almond butter, or peanut butter

1/2 cup low-carb granular sweetener

1 teaspoon coffee extract (optional, enhances chocolate flavor)

2 teaspoons chocolate-flavored liquid monk fruit

1/2 teaspoon baking powder

3 large eggs

FOR THE CHOCOLATE CHIP COOKIE LAYER:

1/4 cup (1/2 stick) unsalted butter, softened

1/2 cup low-carb granular sweetener

1/2 teaspoon vanilla extract

1/2 teaspoon vanilla-flavored liquid stevia

1 cup hulled sunflower seeds

1/4 teaspoon baking powder

1/4 teaspoon glucomannan or xanthan gum

1 large egg

1/4 cup sugar-free chocolate chips

Pinch of fine sea salt

1. Preheat the oven to 350°F. Line an 8-inch square baking dish with parchment paper, allowing the paper to hang over the sides for easy removal. Set aside.
2. To make the brownie layer, set a tightly fitting heatproof bowl over a saucepan of simmering water. Make sure the water level is only an inch or two deep. Put the chocolate chips, butter, and sunflower butter in the bowl and heat until melted, stirring constantly. Continue to stir until smooth, with no lumps remaining. Remove the bowl from the pan. (You could also use a microwave-safe bowl and heat in the microwave in 30-second increments, stirring between, until melted and smooth.)
3. Pour the melted chocolate mixture into a large mixing bowl or the bowl of a stand mixer. Add the remaining brownie ingredients, except the eggs, and mix on medium speed using a hand mixer or the stand mixer until the batter is smooth. Taste the batter to decide if it's sweet enough. Add more sweetener if desired, then add the eggs, one egg at a time, mixing between each addition until combined.

(recipe continues)

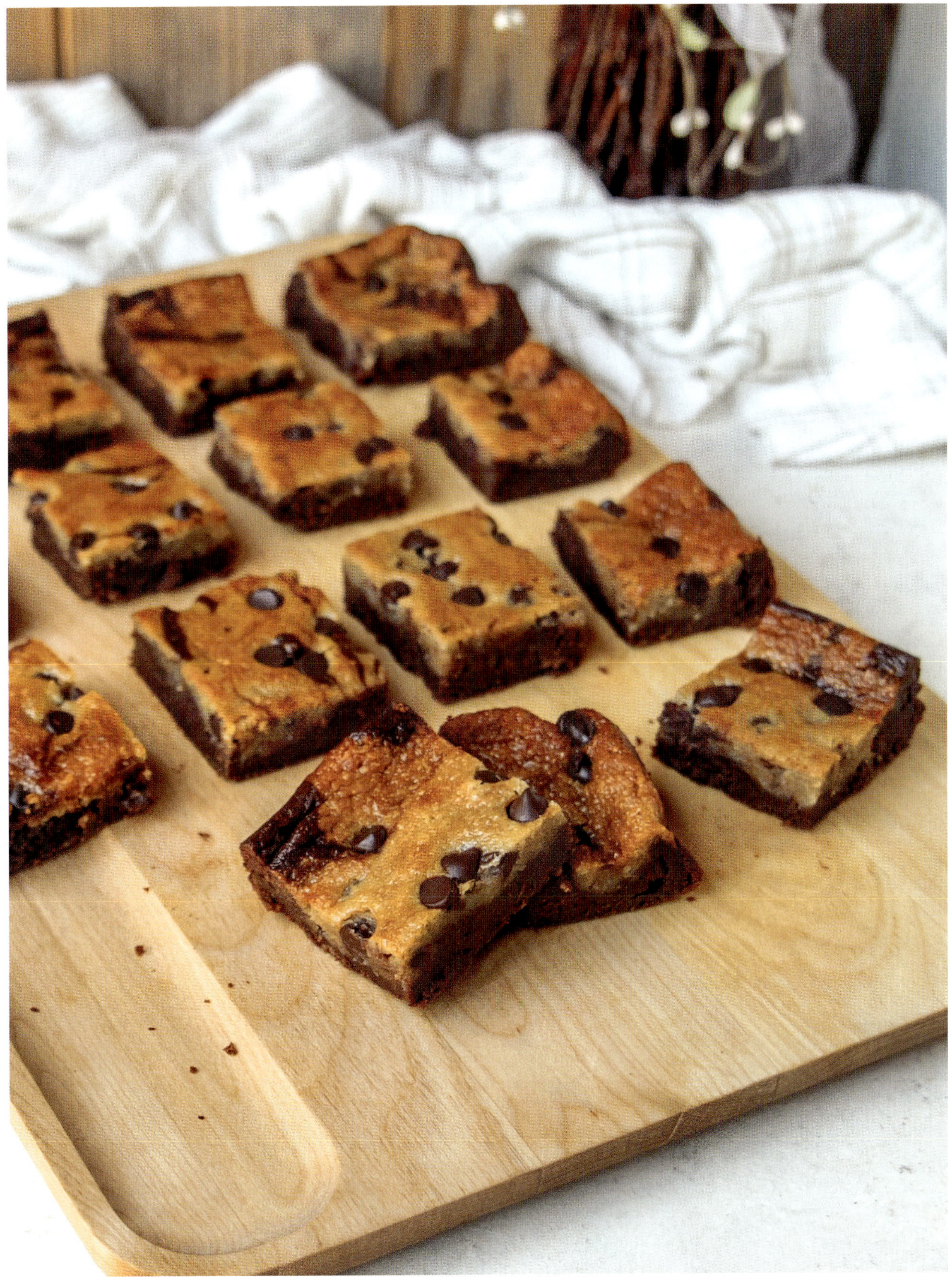

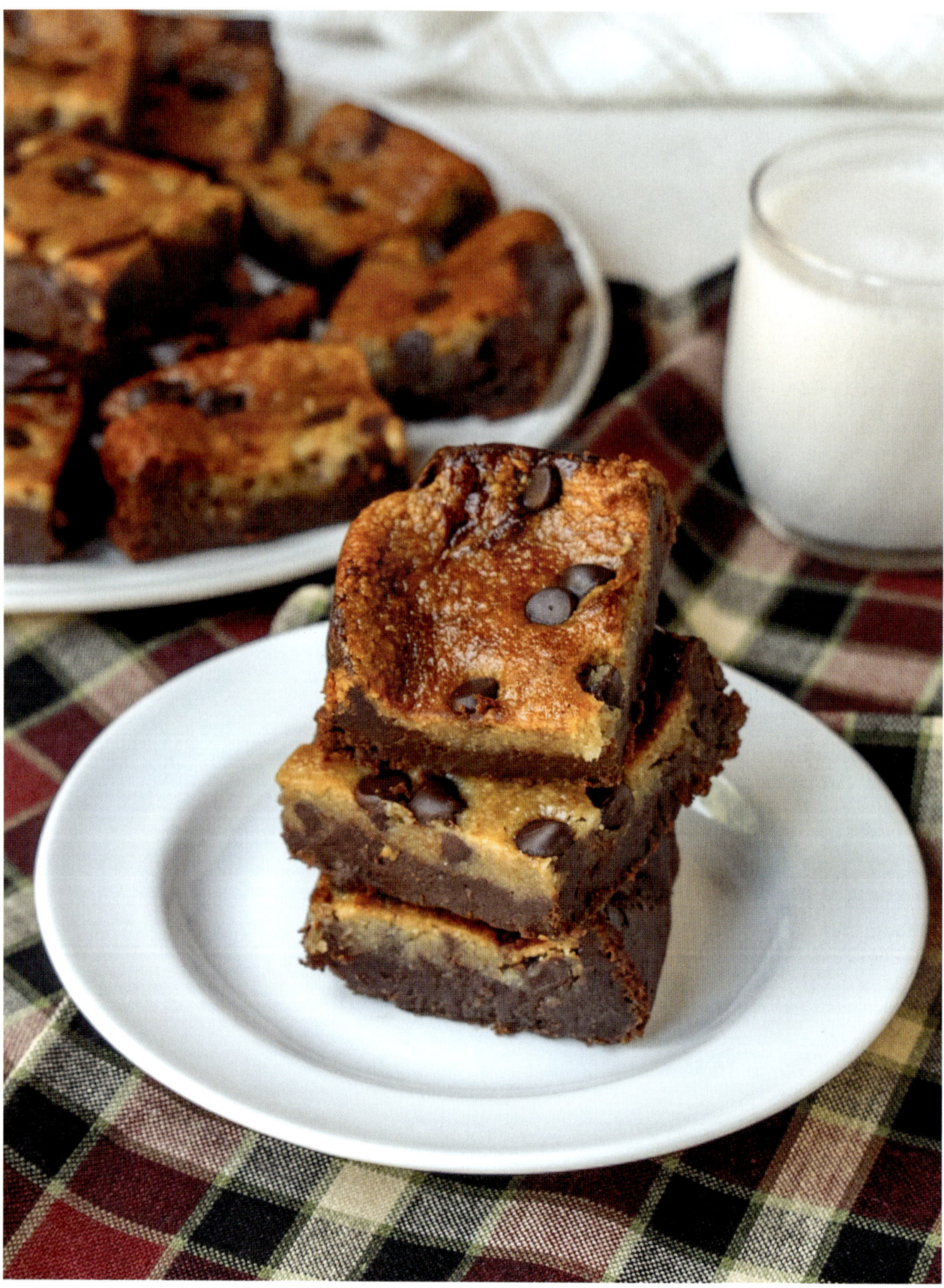

4. Pour the batter into the prepared baking dish and bake for 23 to 25 minutes, until the brownies are puffed up and a toothpick inserted in the center comes out clean. While the brownie layer is baking, make the cookie dough for the cookie layer.
5. To make the cookie dough, place all the ingredients, except the egg and chocolate chips, in a large mixing bowl or the bowl of a stand mixer fitted with the paddle attachment. Using a hand mixer or the stand mixer, mix on medium speed until combined. Taste and increase the sweetness if needed, then mix in the egg. Stir in the chocolate chips by hand. Refrigerate until the brownies are ready.
6. When the brownies are done, remove them from the oven and drop spoonfuls of the cookie dough over the top of brownies (the cookie dough will spread out as it bakes). Return to the oven and bake for another 10 to 12 minutes, until golden brown and the cookie layer is puffed up and a toothpick inserted in the center comes out clean.
7. Allow to cool for 15 minutes, then slice into 16 squares.
8. Store leftovers covered on the counter for up to 3 days. They will stay fudgy for days if you store them in an airtight container in the fridge for up to 1 week. You can also store them in the freezer for up to 3 months.

Calories	Fat	Protein	Total Carbs	Dietary Fiber	Net Carbs
218	21g	5g	5g	1g	4g

YIELD: 16 servings
PREP TIME: 25 minutes
COOK TIME: 25 minutes

BROWNIE COOKIES & CREAM TRIFLE

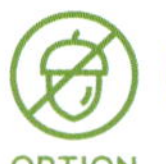
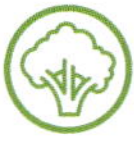
OPTION

Trifles always take a few more steps to prepare, but the layered effect is well worth the effort. You can prepare the brownies and the filling the day before you want to assemble the trifle. Perfect for a summer party!

FOR THE BROWNIE LAYER:

1 cup sugar-free chocolate chips

1/2 cup (1 stick) unsalted butter, coconut oil, or avocado oil

1/4 cup unsweetened sunflower seed butter, almond butter, or peanut butter

1/2 cup low-carb granular sweetener

1/2 teaspoon coffee extract (optional, enhances chocolate flavor)

2 teaspoons chocolate-flavored liquid monk fruit

1/2 teaspoon baking powder

3 large eggs

FOR THE COOKIES & CREAM FILLING:

1/2 cup hulled sunflower seeds or blanched almonds

1/4 cup unsweetened cocoa powder

1/4 cup confectioners'-style low-carb sweetener

1/4 cup (1/2 stick) unsalted butter, softened

2 (8-ounce) packages cream cheese, softened

1 cup heavy cream

1 teaspoon vanilla-flavored liquid stevia

FOR THE WHIPPED CREAM TOPPING:

2 cups heavy cream

1 teaspoon vanilla liquid stevia, plus more if needed

FOR GARNISH:

1 to 2 tablespoons cookie crumbs (reserved from above)

Special equipment: 3-quart trifle bowl or similarly sized clear glass bowl

1. Preheat the oven to 350°F. Line an 8-inch square baking dish with parchment paper, allowing the paper to hang over the sides for easy removal.
2. *To make the brownies,* set a tightly fitting heatproof bowl over a saucepan of simmering water. Make sure the water is only an inch or two deep. Put the chocolate chips, butter, and sunflower butter in the bowl and heat until melted, stirring constantly. Continue to stir until smooth, with no lumps remaining. Remove the bowl from the pan. (You could also use a microwave-safe bowl and heat in the microwave in 30-second increments, stirring between, until melted and smooth.)

(recipe continues)

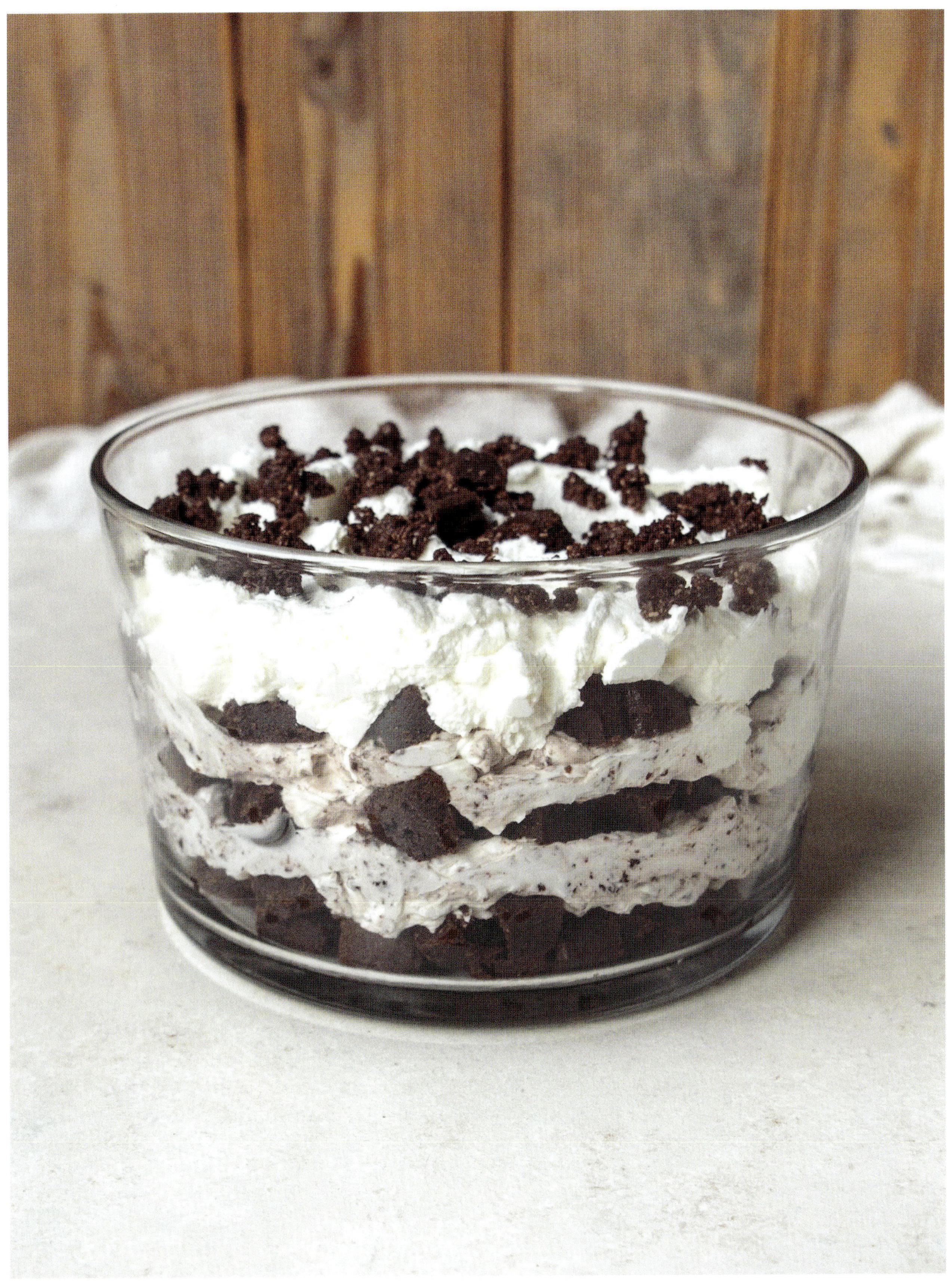

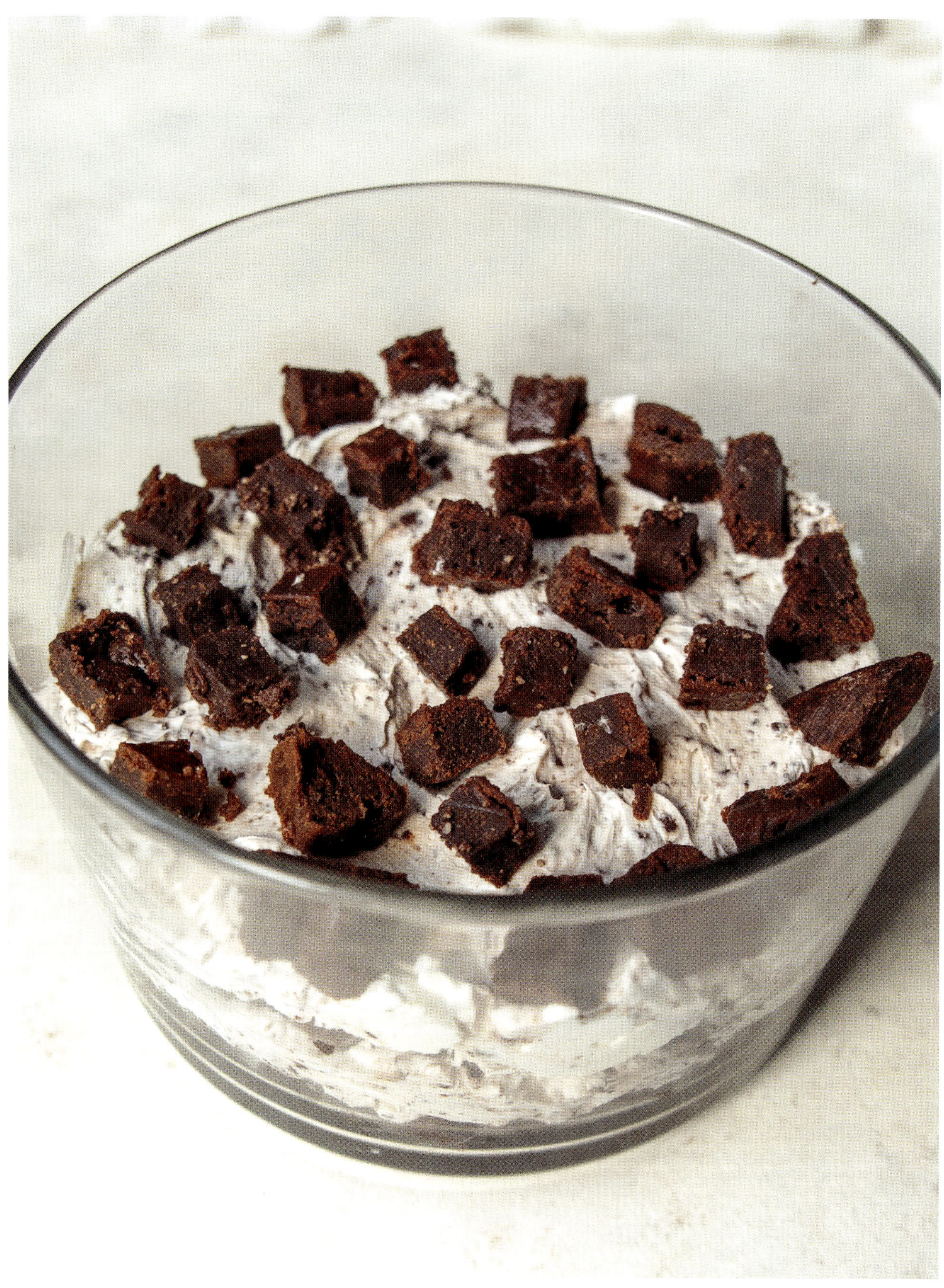

3. Pour the melted chocolate mixture into a large mixing bowl or the bowl of a stand mixer. Add the remaining ingredients, except the eggs, and mix on medium speed until the batter is smooth. Taste the batter to decide if it's sweet enough. Add more sweetener if desired, then add the eggs, one egg at a time, mixing between each addition until combined.
4. Pour the batter into the prepared baking dish and bake for 23 to 25 minutes, until the brownies are puffed up and a toothpick inserted in the center comes out clean. While the brownie layer is baking, make the filling.
5. To make the cookies and cream filling, put the sunflower seeds, cocoa powder, powdered sweetener, and butter in a small mixing bowl and mix until crumbs form. Set aside.
6. Put the cream cheese, cream, and liquid stevia in the bowl of a stand mixer (or use a large mixing bowl and a hand mixer) and mix on medium speed until smooth. Taste and adjust the sweetener if needed. Stir in the crumbs, reserving 1 to 2 tablespoons for the topping. Set aside in the refrigerator until ready to assemble the trifle.
7. When the brownie layer is done, remove it from the oven and allow to cool for 15 minutes.
8. To assemble, crumble or chop the brownies, then divide into thirds. Cover the bottom of a 3-quart trifle bowl with a third of the brownies. Spread half of the cookies and cream filling over the brownies. Add another third of the brownies, then spread the rest of the filling over the brownies. Top with the remaining brownies. You can keep this refrigerated for up to 2 days or until ready to serve.
9. When ready to serve, make the whipped cream topping by whipping the cream and sweetener with an electric mixer on high speed until stiff peaks form. Top the trifle with the whipped cream and reserved cookie crumbs. Serve immediately.
10. Leftover trifle can be covered and refrigerated for up to 3 days, but the whipped cream will likely flatten after a day or two.

Calories	Fat	Protein	Total Carbs	Dietary Fiber	Net Carbs
328	42g	5g	6g	1g	5g

YIELD: 12 slices (1 per serving)
PREP TIME: 30 minutes, plus 1 hour to chill
COOK TIME: 30 minutes

CHOCOLATE ÉCLAIR POKE CAKE

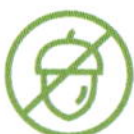 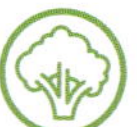

This recipe is popular with my kids because the éclair filling reminds them of a traditional éclair from the bakery. I love to serve this cake when family and friends gather for a holiday or birthday because it can be made ahead and left in the fridge until your guests arrive.

FOR THE CAKE:

- 8 large eggs
- 1 cup heavy cream
- 1 teaspoon vanilla extract
- 1 teaspoon vanilla-flavored liquid stevia
- ½ cup low-carb granular sweetener
- ½ cup coconut flour
- 2 teaspoons baking powder
- ½ teaspoon fine sea salt

FOR THE ÉCLAIR FILLING:

- 1½ cups heavy cream
- 4 large egg yolks
- ½ cup confectioners'-style low-carb sweetener
- 2 teaspoons vanilla extract
- ½ teaspoon glucomannan or xanthan gum

FOR THE CHOCOLATE TOPPING:

- 1 batch Ganache (page 84), freshly made

1. Preheat the oven to 350°F. Grease a 9 by 13-inch baking dish with cooking spray.
2. To make the cake, put the eggs, cream, vanilla, stevia, and low-carb granular sweetener in the bowl of a stand mixer (or use a large mixing bowl and a hand mixer) and mix on medium speed until combined. Alternatively, you can whisk the ingredients by hand.
3. In a small mixing bowl, whisk together the coconut flour, baking powder, and salt, then slowly pour the dry ingredients into the bowl with the wet ingredients while mixing on low speed. Once well combined, pour the batter into the prepared baking dish and smooth out the top with a spatula.
4. Bake for 30 minutes or until a toothpick inserted in the center comes out clean and the cake is just lightly golden brown around the edges. Once done, allow to cool for 10 minutes, then use a skewer to poke about 12 evenly spaced holes in the cake. While the cake is in the oven, prepare the filling.
5. To make the éclair filling, warm the cream in a medium saucepan over medium heat. While the cream is heating, whisk the egg yolks in a medium mixing bowl until they are light in color.
6. Once the cream is hot but not boiling, pour a small amount of the cream into the whisked yolks to temper them. Whisk to combine, then slowly add about half of the hot cream to the yolks while continuously whisking. Pour the tempered yolk mixture into the saucepan and reduce the heat to low while continuing to whisk the mixture.

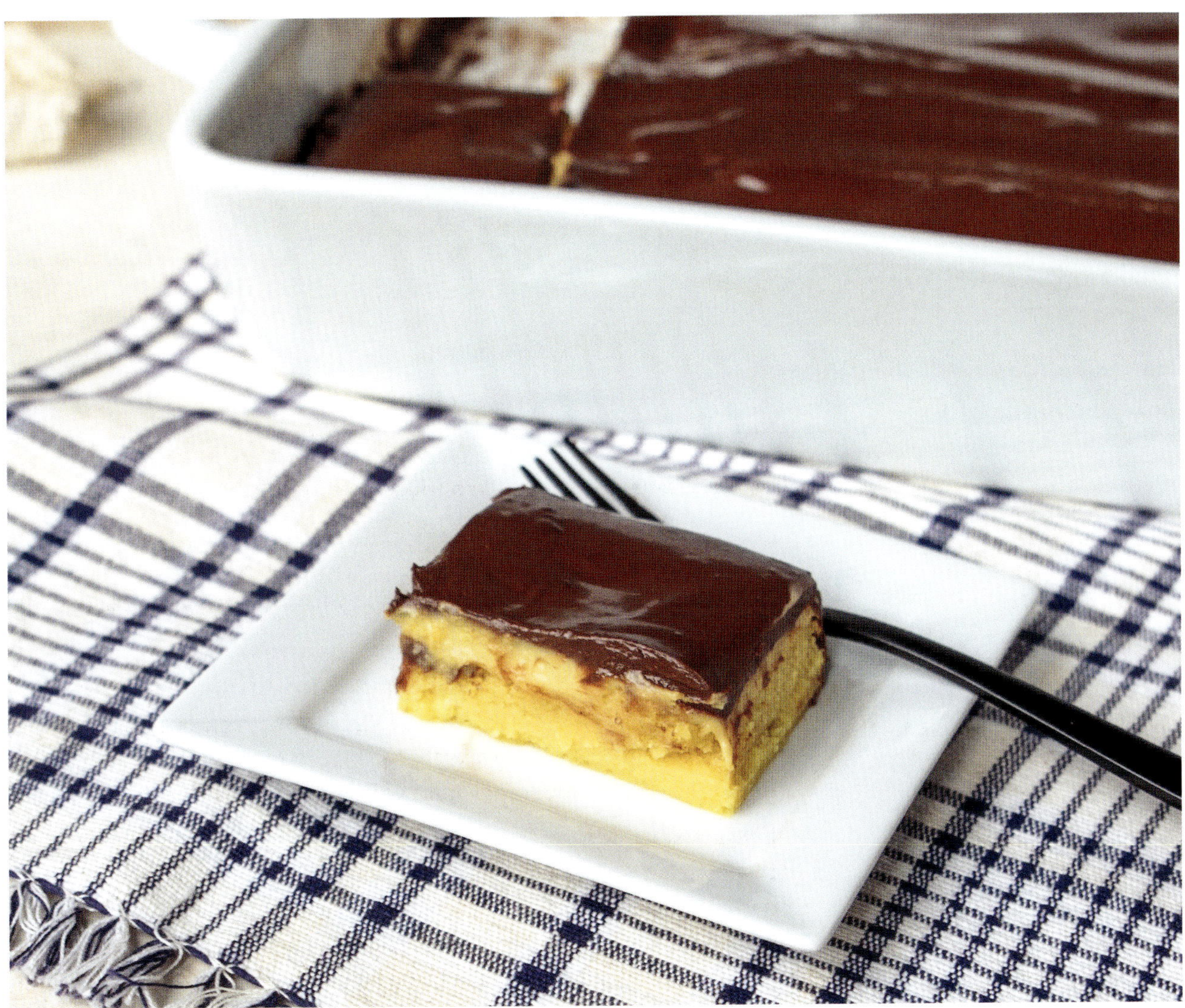

7. Add the sweetener and continue to whisk until the mixture is at a rolling boil. Remove the pan from the heat and whisk in the vanilla.
8. Sprinkle the glucomannan over the filling and whisk until it's all absorbed. Allow to cool for about 30 minutes, then spread over the cake and refrigerate for 1 hour.
9. When the cake and filling are almost done chilling, make the ganache. Pour the ganache evenly on the chilled cake and filling. Serve right away or, when the ganache layer is completely cooled, cover the cake with plastic wrap and refrigerate for later. You can store leftovers for up to 4 days in the refrigerator or freeze for up to 3 months.

Calories	Fat	Protein	Total Carbs	Dietary Fiber	Net Carbs
385	34g	7g	6g	2g	4g

YIELD: 1 cup (¼ cup per serving)
PREP TIME: 1 minute
COOK TIME: 5 minutes

LEMON CURD

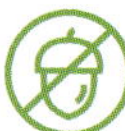
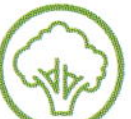

Using the juice from fresh lemons is always best for this recipe. Try this spooned over Lemon Poppyseed Muffins (page 234) or Lemon Ricotta Pie (page 287). Or simply enjoy a spoonful straight up to satisfy a sweet tooth.

2 large eggs

⅓ cup confectioners'-style low-carb sweetener

½ teaspoon lemon-flavored liquid stevia

1 teaspoon grated lemon zest

⅓ cup fresh lemon juice

¼ cup (½ stick) cold unsalted butter, diced

1. Whisk the eggs and confectioners'-style sweetener in a large saucepan over medium-low heat. Stir with a wooden spoon until the mixture thickens, 4 to 5 minutes.
2. Add the stevia, zest, and juice and whisk until combined. Drop pieces of butter on top and whisk until incorporated. Stir until smooth.
3. Remove and strain through a fine-mesh sieve into a heatproof bowl.
4. Cover the curd with plastic wrap, placing it directly on the surface to avoid forming a skin, and chill until you are ready to use. The curd will thicken more as it cools.
5. Store covered in the fridge for up to 1 week.

Calories	Fat	Protein	Total Carbs	Dietary Fiber	Net Carbs
141	14g	3g	2g	0.1g	1.9g

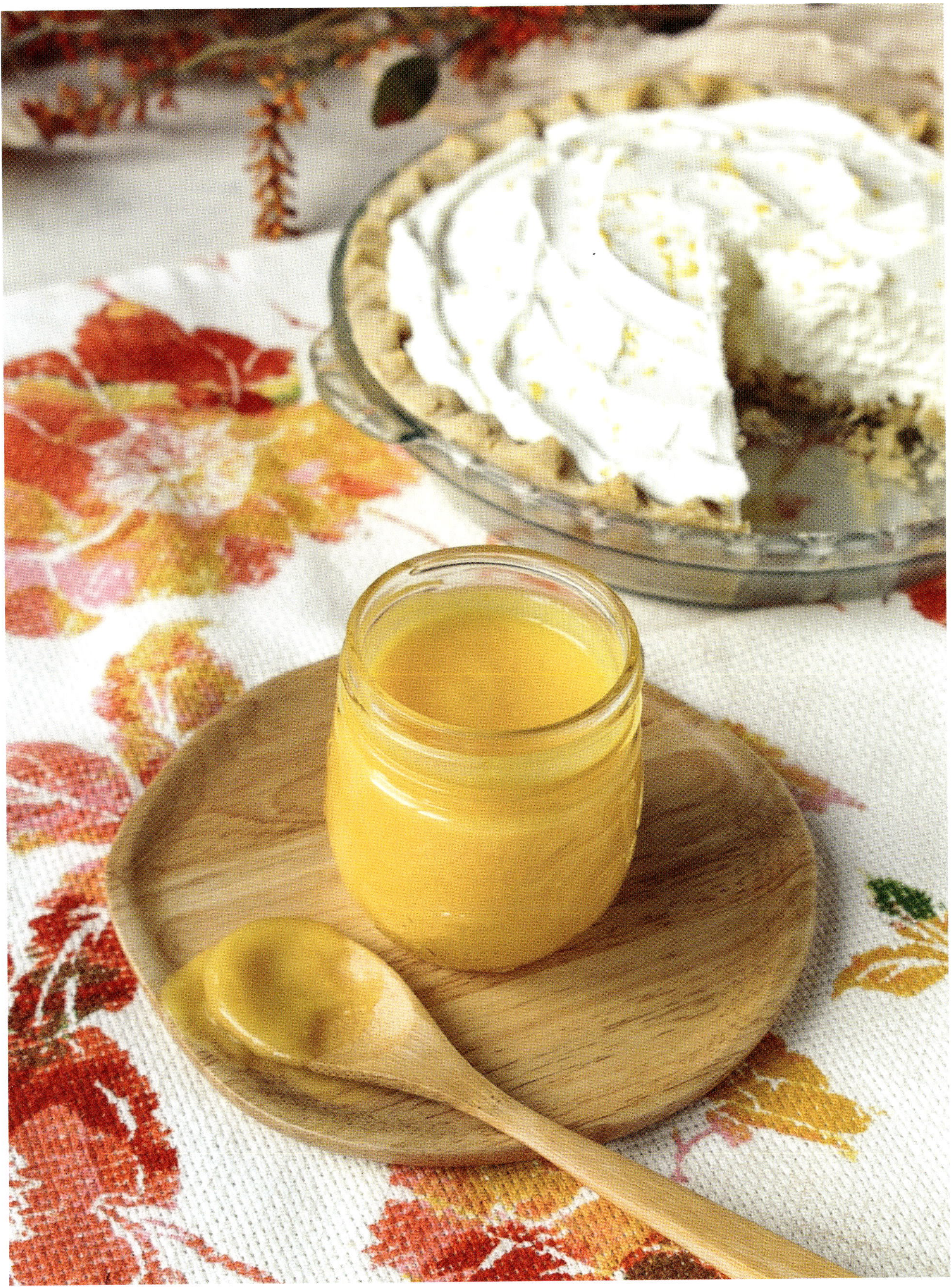

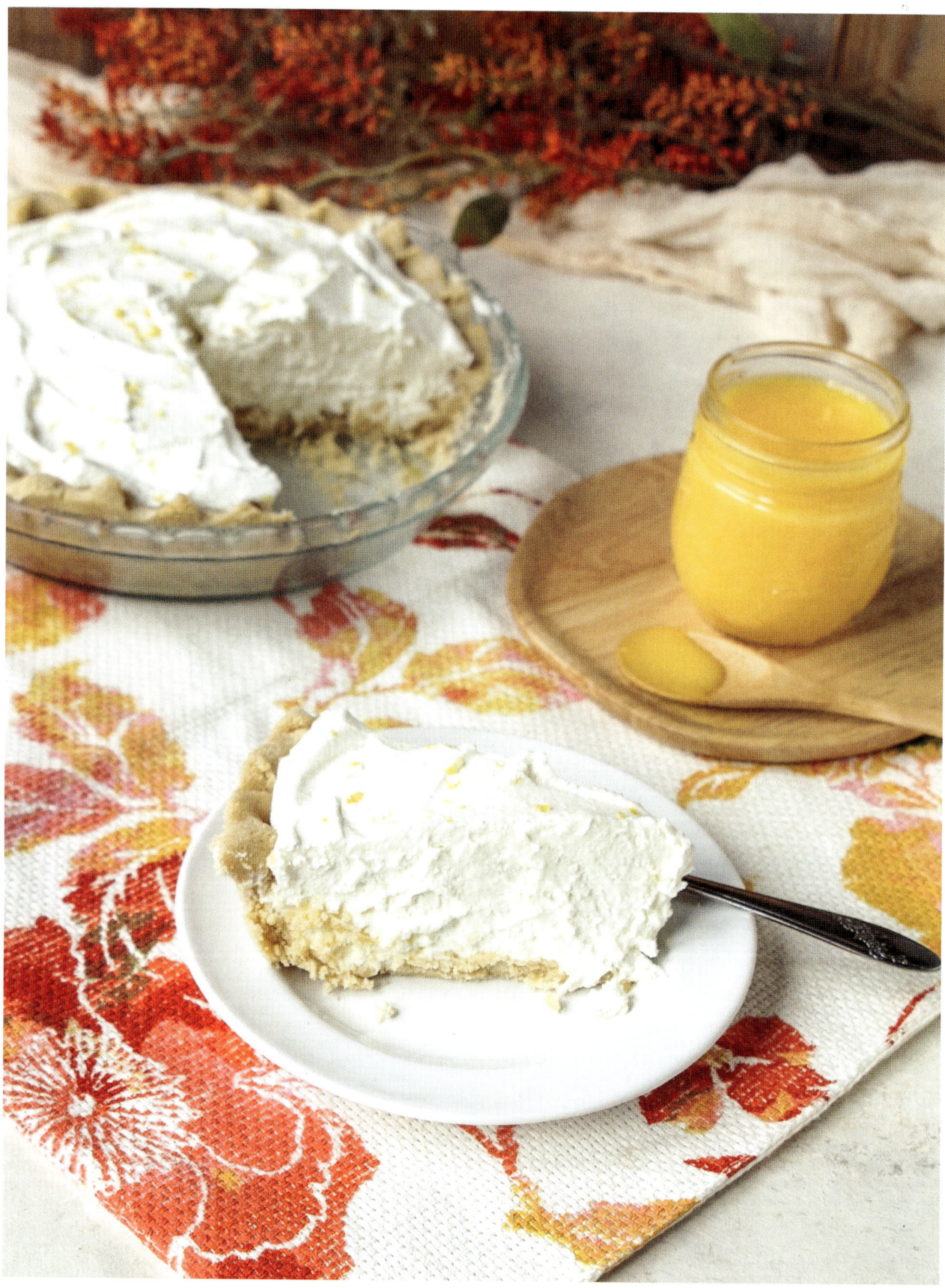

YIELD: 12 slices (1 per serving)
PREP TIME: 15 minutes, plus time to chill

LEMON RICOTTA PIE

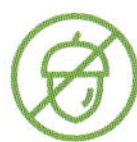

For an extra decadent treat, enjoy a slice of this pie drizzled with my lemon curd (page 284).

16 ounces ricotta cheese (part skim)

2 teaspoons lemon-flavored liquid stevia, divided

2 teaspoons grated lemon zest, divided

½ cup fresh lemon juice

4 teaspoons unflavored gelatin powder

1 pint heavy cream

1 batch Easy Keto Pie Crust (page 87), baked and cooled

1. Place the ricotta cheese, 1 teaspoon of the stevia, and 1 teaspoon of the lemon zest in the bowl of a stand mixer. Mix on medium speed until combined and smooth. (If you don't have a stand mixer, you can do this step in a food processor.) Set aside.
2. Pour the lemon juice into a small saucepan and heat over low heat until boiling, or place in a microwave-safe bowl and heat for 1 to 2 minutes, until boiling. Remove the pan from the heat, then slowly whisk in the gelatin a little at a time while continuing to whisk until it's completely dissolved and there are no lumps. Allow to cool before proceeding with the next step.
3. Pour the heavy cream into a medium mixing bowl and use an electric mixer to whip on high speed until stiff peaks form. Add the remaining teaspoon of stevia and whip just to combine.
4. Add the ricotta cheese mixture to the whipped cream and blend on medium speed until incorporated. With the mixer running on low speed, slowly drizzle in the cooled lemon juice gelatin mixture.
5. Spread the filling mixture in the cooled pie crust. Sprinkle the remaining lemon zest over the pie and chill before serving.
6. Store in an airtight container or tightly wrapped in the refrigerator for up to 3 days.

Calories	Fat	Protein	Total Carbs	Dietary Fiber	Net Carbs
335	28g	7g	7g	3g	4g

YIELD: 12 slices (1 per serving)
PREP TIME: 15 minutes
COOK TIME: 1 hour

CHOCOLATE BUNDT CAKE WITH PEANUT BUTTER CHEESECAKE FILLING

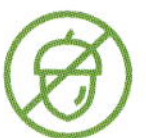 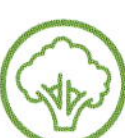 

Though I wouldn't consider myself a particularly skilled or artistic baker, I've had this recipe on my brain for a long time, waiting for the courage to attempt it. Once I did, I marveled at my accomplishment! Don't be intimated if you don't consider yourself a baker either; this isn't as hard as you think.

FOR THE CAKE:

2/3 cup sugar-free chocolate chips or chopped very dark chocolate (85% cacao)

10 tablespoons unsalted butter

1 cup espresso or strong brewed coffee

1/2 cup low-carb granular sweetener

2 teaspoons vanilla extract

4 large eggs

2/3 cup coconut flour

3 tablespoons unsweetened cocoa powder

2 teaspoons baking powder

1 teaspoon liquid monk fruit

FOR THE FILLING:

1/2 cup unsweetened peanut butter

4 ounces cream cheese (1/2 cup), softened

3 tablespoons confectioners'-style low-carb sweetener

FOR THE PEANUT BUTTER DRIZZLE (OPTIONAL):

2 tablespoons unsweetened peanut butter

1 1/2 teaspoons unsalted butter, melted

1 tablespoon confectioners'-style low-carb sweetener (optional)

FOR THE CHOCOLATE DRIZZLE (OPTIONAL):

3 tablespoons sugar-free chocolate chips

1 teaspoon unsalted butter

1 teaspoon chocolate-flavored liquid monk fruit (optional)

FOR GARNISH, IF USING ONE OR MORE DRIZZLES (OPTIONAL):

1 tablespoon roughly chopped roasted, salted peanuts

Special equipment: 9-inch silicone Bundt cake pan

1. To make the cake, set a tightly fitting heatproof bowl over a saucepan of simmering water. Make sure the water level is only an inch or two deep. Put the chocolate chips, butter, and espresso in the bowl. Heat, stirring continuously, until the butter and chocolate are melted and all the ingredients are combined.

(recipe continues)

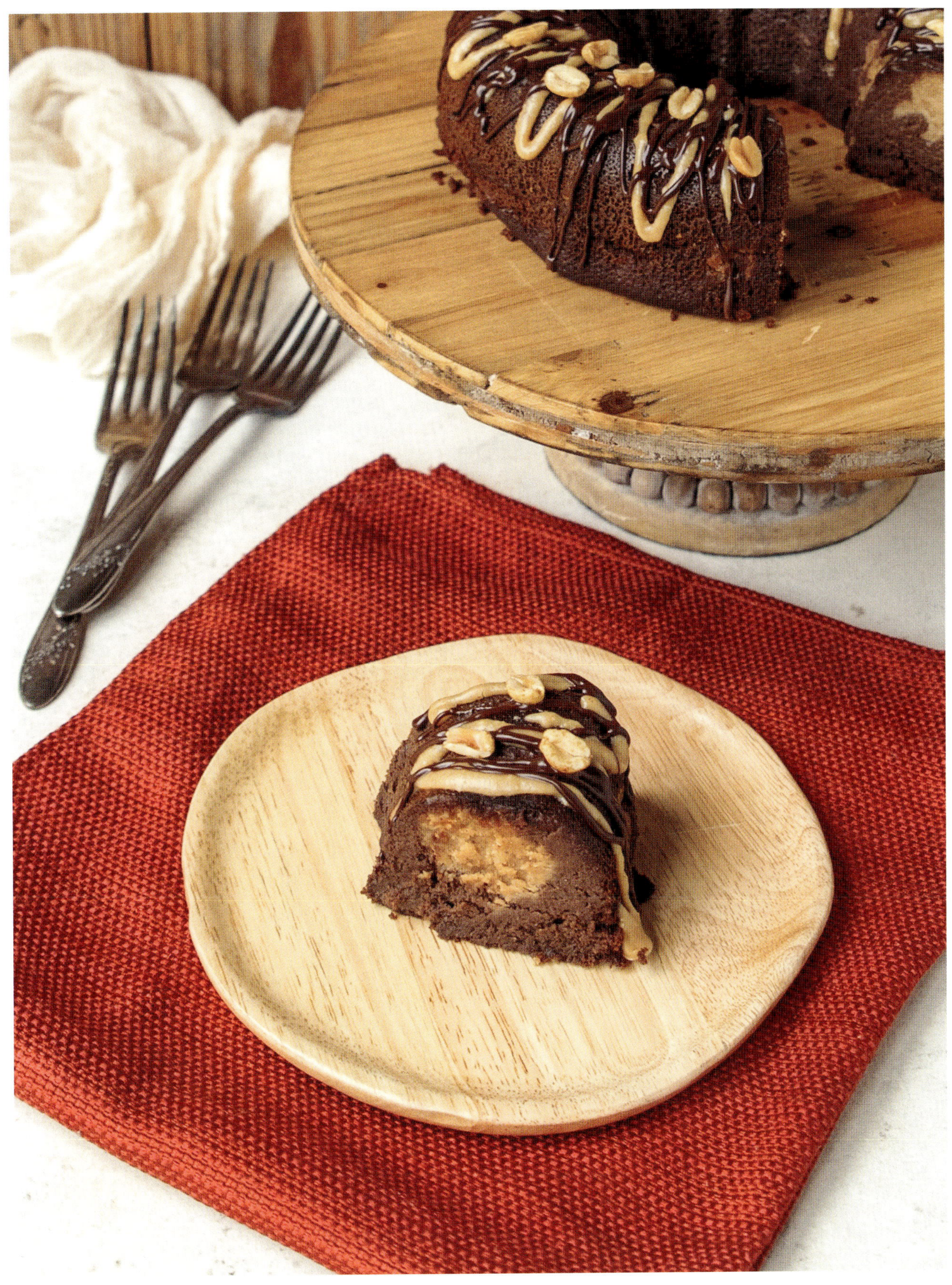

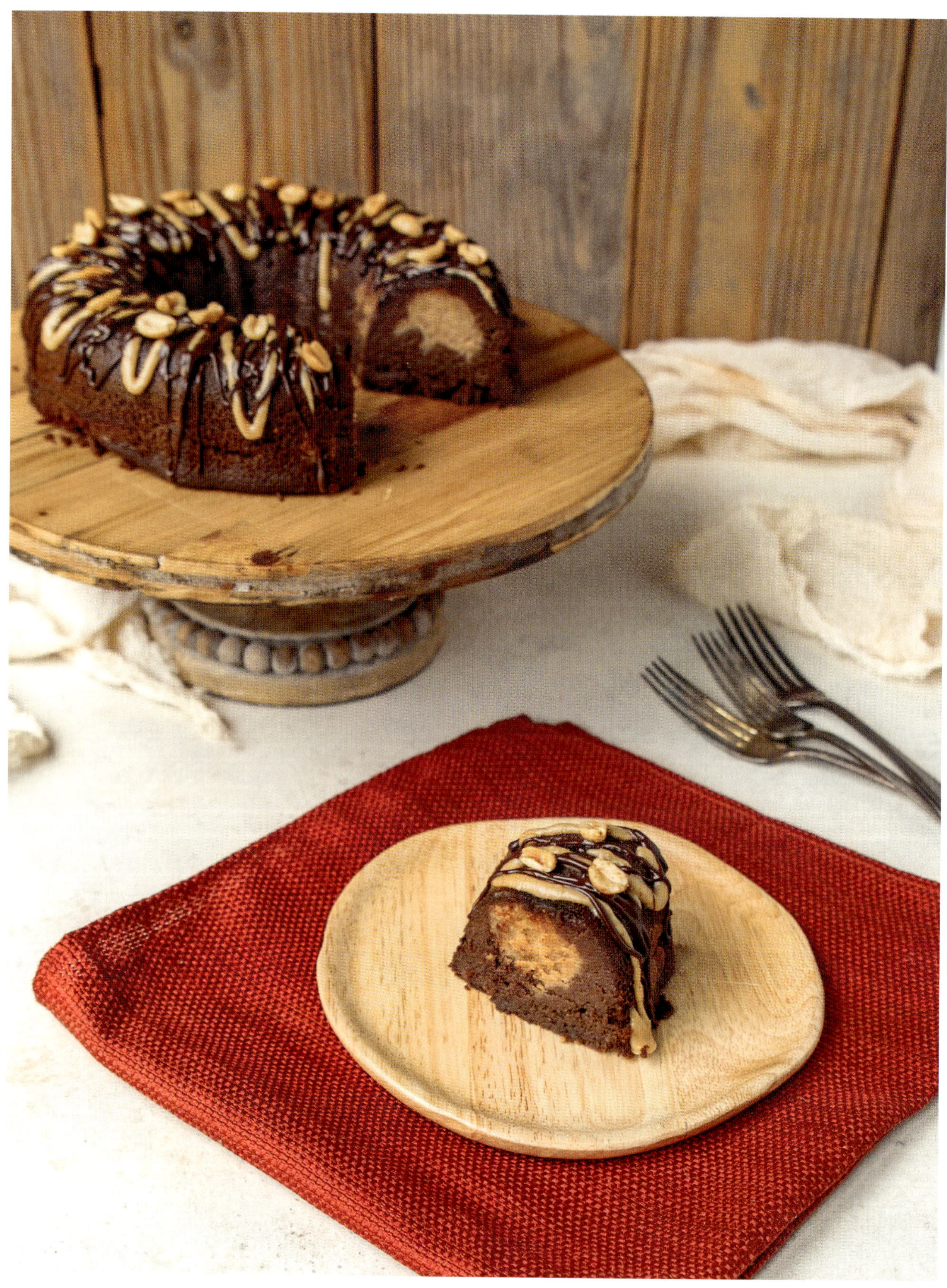

2. Add the sweetener and vanilla and stir until dissolved. Remove the bowl from the pan and beat in the eggs, one at a time.
3. Sift the coconut flour, cocoa, and baking powder together into a small bowl, then add to the chocolate mixture. Stir briskly until combined and smooth, with no lumps remaining.
4. The batter will look quite runny, but don't panic. Allow to sit for 15 minutes, and it will thicken.
5. Preheat the oven to 300°F. Grease a silicone 9-inch Bundt cake pan and place it on a rimmed baking pan. While the cake batter is sitting and the oven is preheating, make the filling.
6. To make the filling, place all the ingredients in a stand mixer fitted with the paddle attachment and mix on medium speed until smooth, no lumps. (Or mix in a bowl and use a hand mixer.) Taste and adjust the sweetness if needed.
7. Pour half of the thickened batter into the Bundt pan. Then drop spoonfuls of the filling evenly onto the cake batter in the Bundt pan. Pour the rest of the cake batter over the filling and gently smooth it out.
8. Bake for 1 hour, or until just set in the center. Remove and allow to cool in the pan before turning out onto a cake rack and serving. Store in the refrigerator for up to 3 days.
9. Optionally, once the cake has cooled, you can drizzle it with the peanut butter topping or the chocolate topping or both! To make the peanut butter topping, mix the ingredients in a small bowl and drizzle over the top of the cake before serving. To make the chocolate topping, put the chocolate chips and butter in a small microwave-safe bowl and microwave for 30 seconds, then stir until smooth. Stir in the chocolate-flavored sweetener, if using. Drizzle over the cake before serving. Garnish with peanuts, if desired.

Calories	Fat	Protein	Total Carbs	Dietary Fiber	Net Carbs
310	27g	8g	9g	4g	5g

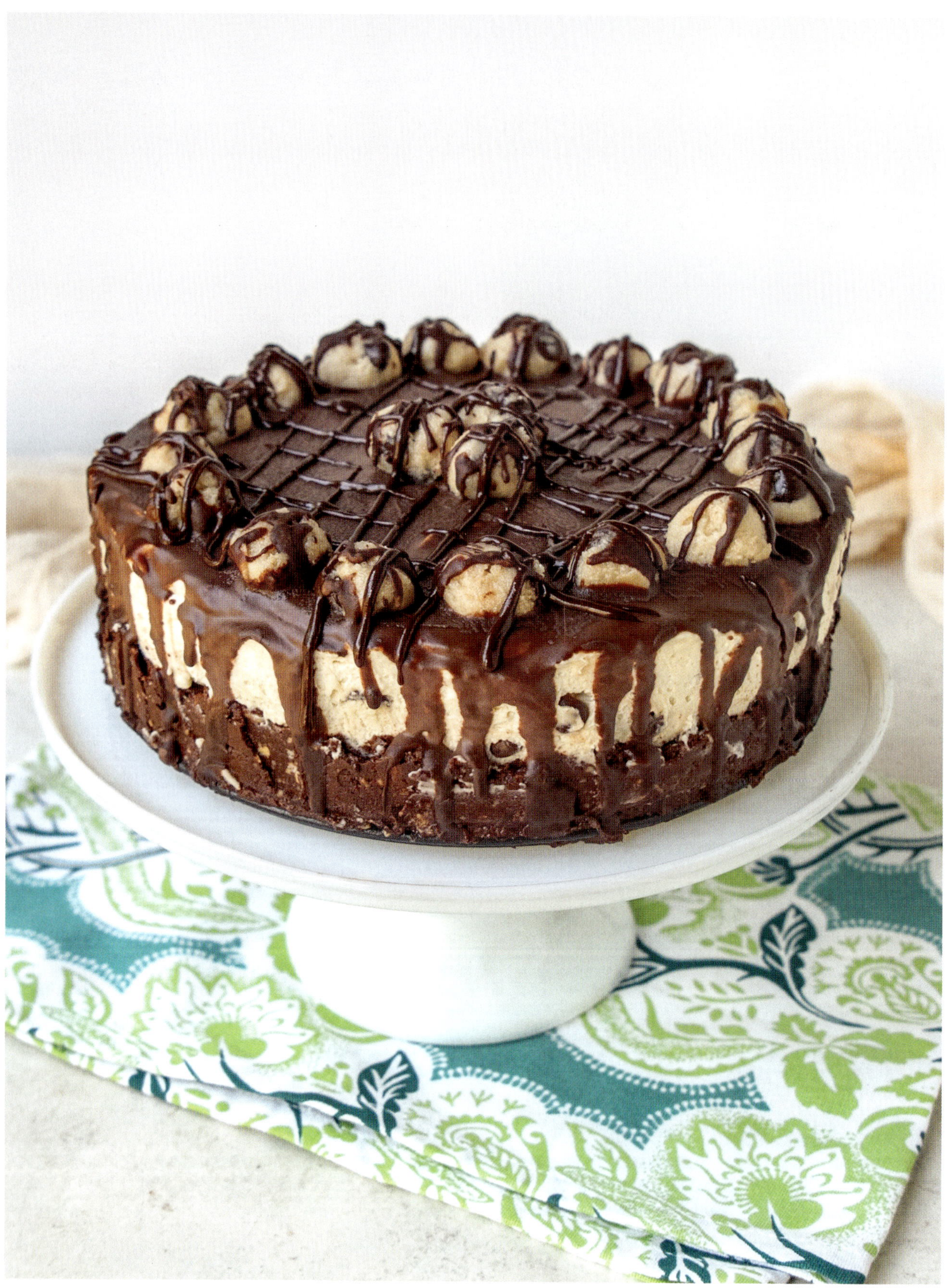

YIELD: 12 slices (1 per serving)
PREP TIME: 30 minutes, plus 3 hours to chill

NO-BAKE COOKIE DOUGH CHEESECAKE

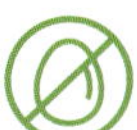
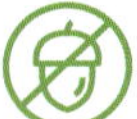

This is the dessert to make when you have family or friends coming over and want to impress them with your no-bake cheesecake skills. Those with food allergies will be grateful they can indulge like everyone else.

FOR THE CRUST:

1/3 cup sunflower seed meal or blanched almond flour

1/3 cup unsweetened cocoa powder

1/3 cup hulled sunflower seeds or blanched almonds

1/3 cup confectioners'-style low-carb sweetener

6 tablespoons (3/4 stick) unsalted butter, softened

FOR THE COOKIE DOUGH LAYER:

2 cups sunflower seed meal or blanched almond flour

1/2 cup (1 stick) unsalted butter

1/3 cup confectioners'-style low-carb sweetener

1/2 teaspoon vanilla extract

1/3 cup sugar-free chocolate chips

FOR THE FILLING:

2 teaspoons unflavored gelatin powder

1 1/2 cups heavy cream, divided

2 (8-ounce) packages cream cheese, softened

1/2 cup confectioners'-style low-carb sweetener

1 teaspoon vanilla extract

1/2 teaspoon vanilla-flavored liquid stevia

1/4 teaspoon fine sea salt

1/3 cup sugar-free chocolate chips

FOR THE GANACHE:

1/3 cup sugar-free chocolate chips

1/3 cup heavy cream

Special equipment: 8-inch springform pan

1. To make the crust, place all the ingredients in a food processor and process until moist and crumbly.
2. Using your hands, press the crust mixture into the bottom of an 8-inch springform pan. Set aside in the fridge while you make the cookie dough layer.
3. To make the cookie dough, place all the ingredients, except the chocolate chips, in a bowl and use a wooden spoon to mix until well combined. Stir in the chocolate chips.

(recipe continues)

4. Remove half of the cookie dough (about 1/2 cup), wrap tightly in plastic wrap, and place in the fridge until ready to decorate the cake. (You'll use the reserved dough to make 20 mini cookie dough balls.)
5. Take the remaining cookie dough and press it evenly over the crust in the springform pan. Place in the fridge to chill while you make the cheesecake filling.
6. To make the cheesecake filling, sprinkle the gelatin over 1/2 cup of the heavy cream in a microwave-safe bowl and allow to bloom for about a minute. Heat the cream mixture in the microwave for 2 minutes. Remove and stir until the gelatin is dissolved. Set aside to allow to come to room temperature.
7. Put the cream cheese in the bowl of a stand mixer fitted with the paddle attachment and mix on high until smooth. Add the cooled cream mixture, confectioners'-style sweetener, vanilla, stevia, and salt. Blend on high until incorporated.
8. Pour in the remaining cup of cream and whip on high until the mixture looks whipped and thickened, about 5 minutes. Gently stir in the chocolate chips.
9. Pour the filling onto the cookie layer in the pan. Refrigerate for at least 3 hours.
10. *When ready to decorate and serve,* form the mini cookie dough balls by scooping up a heaping teaspoon of the reserved dough and rolling it into a ball. Repeat with the rest of the dough until all is used. Remove the cake from the springform pan and set on a cake plate. Decorate the top with the cookie dough balls, placing a few balls to the center of the cake and the rest around the edge.
11. To make the ganache, put the chocolate chips in a medium heatproof bowl and heat the cream in a small saucepan over low heat until simmering.
12. Pour the hot cream over the chocolate chips and let stand for 5 minutes before stirring. After 5 minutes, stir until the ganache is completely smooth. Drizzle over the cheesecake.
13. Store covered or in an airtight container in the fridge for up to 1 week.

Calories	Fat	Protein	Total Carbs	Dietary Fiber	Net Carbs
505	49g	8g	10g	3g	7g

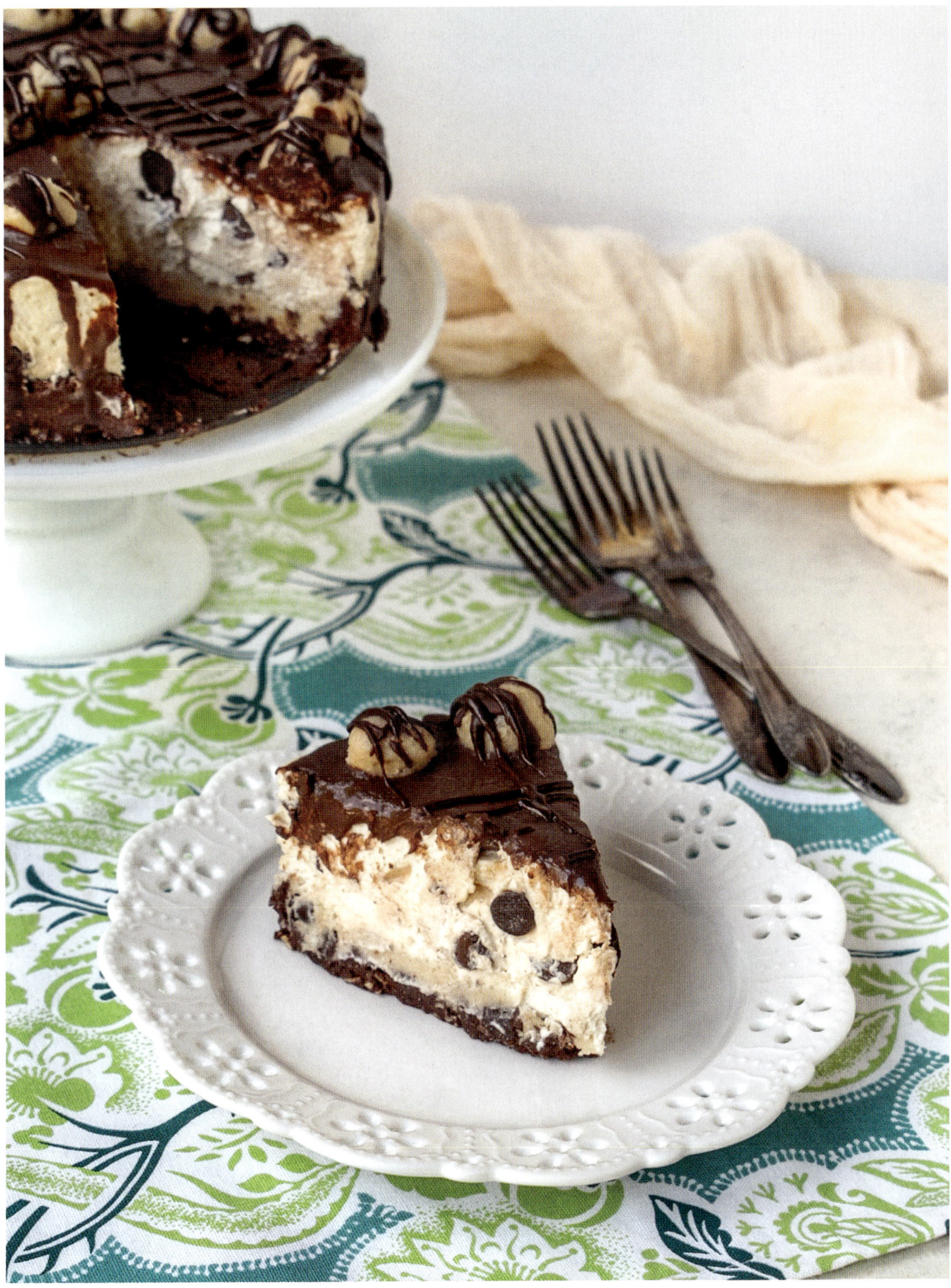

YIELD: 12 bites (1 per serving)
PREP TIME: 15 minutes
COOK TIME: 45 minutes

CHOCOLATE PECAN PIE BITES

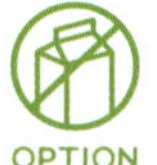
OPTION
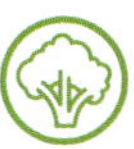
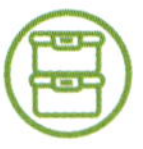

These little bites taste like the filling from the famous Kentucky Derby pie but without the crust!

- ¼ cup (½ stick) unsalted butter
- ¼ cup coconut flour
- ¼ teaspoon fine sea salt
- 1 cup chopped raw pecans
- ¾ cup sugar-free chocolate chips
- ¼ cup sugar-free maple syrup
- 1 teaspoon vanilla extract
- 1 cup low-carb brown sugar–style sweetener
- 4 large eggs, beaten
- Splash of bourbon (optional)

1. Preheat the oven to 350°F. Grease a 12-well muffin pan with cooking spray or use a 12-well silicone muffin pan (see note).
2. Melt the butter in a small saucepan over low heat. Set the pan aside.
3. In a large bowl, stir together the coconut flour, salt, pecans, chocolate chips, maple syrup, vanilla, brown sugar sweetener, and melted butter until combined. Taste the mixture and decide if it's sweet enough for you, adding more sweetener if desired.
4. Add the eggs and stir to combine. Then stir in the bourbon, if using.
5. Pour the mixture evenly into the muffin pan, filling each well about halfway full. Bake for 25 to 35 minutes, until the centers are no longer wet looking but are still jiggly. Allow to cool for about 15 minutes before removing from the pan and serving.
6. Store in an airtight container in the fridge for up to 1 week or freeze for up to 3 months.

NOTE: This recipe could be made dairy free by replacing the butter with coconut oil. If you prefer to bake the bites in paper liners for presentation reasons, as shown in the photo, be sure to spray the paper liners with cooking spray before filling them with the pie filling mixture; otherwise, the bites will stick to the paper.

Calories	Fat	Protein	Total Carbs	Dietary Fiber	Net Carbs
168	16g	4g	4g	2g	2g

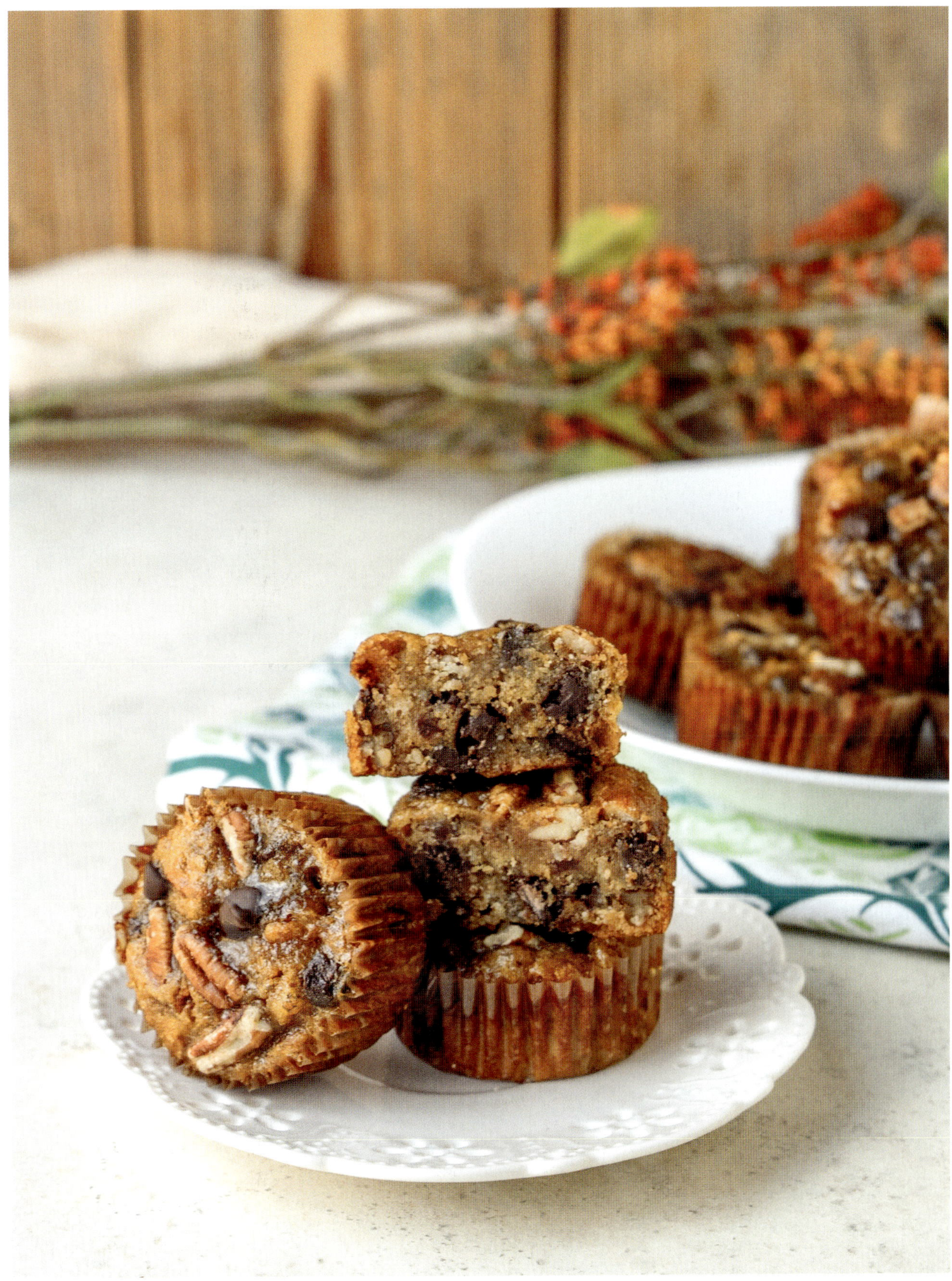

YIELD: 12 slices (1 per serving)

PREP TIME: 30 minutes, plus 2 hours to chill

STRAWBERRY SHORTCAKE PIE

I was thinking of my childhood in the summer, when the ice cream truck would come down the street ringing its bell, and all the children would run eagerly with money in hand to pick their favorite treat. Mine was always a strawberry shortcake on a stick! If you have those memories too, one bite will bring you right back to your childhood.

FOR THE FILLING:

2 cups heavy cream

1 teaspoon vanilla-flavored stevia

1 teaspoon unflavored gelatin powder

2 tablespoons water

1 (8-ounce) package cream cheese, softened

1 tablespoon fresh lemon juice

2 cups strawberries, fresh or frozen and thawed

1/2 cup confectioners'-style low-carb sweetener

1 recipe Easy Keto Pie Crust (page 87), baked and cooled

FOR THE CRUMBLE TOPPING:

1/2 cup (1 stick) cold unsalted butter, chopped

1/2 cup coconut flour

1/3 cup confectioners'-style low-carb sweetener

2 teaspoons fresh lemon juice

1 teaspoon natural red food coloring

1. To make the filling, place the cream and stevia in the bowl of a stand mixer fitted with the whisk attachment. (Or use a large mixing bowl and a hand mixer.) Mix on low speed for about 1 minute until the cream starts thickening. Then increase the mixer to high speed and whip until stiff peaks form. Set aside.
2. Sprinkle the gelatin over the water in a small microwave-safe bowl and allow to bloom for 1 minute. Microwave on high for 1 to 2 minutes. Stir until the gelatin dissolves completely. Set aside to cool.
3. In another bowl, beat the cream cheese and lemon juice with an electric mixer on high speed until no lumps remain.
4. Puree the strawberries and confectioners'-style sweetener in a blender or food processor. Pour this mixture into the cream cheese mixture and mix until combined. Gently fold this into the whipped cream in the stand mixer bowl. Drizzle the dissolved gelatin into the mixer bowl and mix on low speed until combined. Spread the filling onto the prepared pie crust.
5. Refrigerate for at least 2 hours before adding the topping.

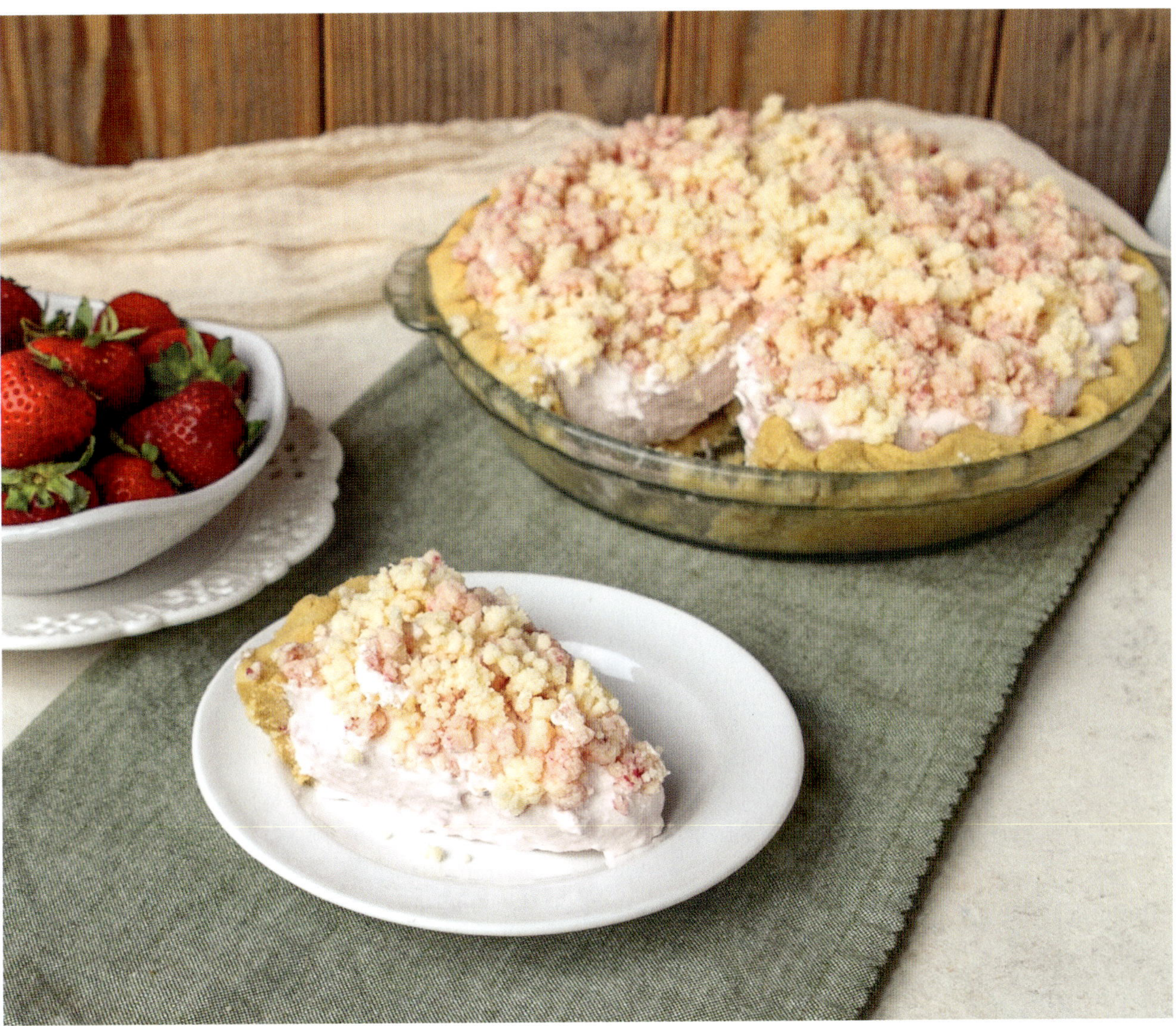

6. To make the crumble topping, place the topping ingredients, except the food coloring, in a food processor and pulse until crumbles form. Remove half to a bowl and place in the fridge.
7. To the remaining crumbles in the food processor, add the food coloring and pulse a few times to evenly incorporate it and the crumbles turn a light pink. Place in a separate bowl in the refrigerator until ready to decorate the pie.
8. When ready to serve, remove the pie from the refrigerator and sprinkle the pink and white crumb topping over the entire pie. Store covered in the refrigerator for up to 5 days.

Calories	Fat	Protein	Total Carbs	Dietary Fiber	Net Carbs
424	38g	4g	10g	5g	5g

YIELD: 12 cupcakes (1 per serving)
PREP TIME: 15 minutes
COOK TIME: 28 minutes

MOCHA CUPCAKES

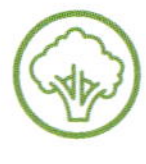

OPTION

Even if you're not a regular coffee drinker or really don't like the taste, I think you'll like these cupcakes. The espresso powder in the cupcakes and the ganache really enhances the chocolate flavor!

FOR THE CUPCAKES:

1 cup sugar-free chocolate chips

½ cup (1 stick) unsalted butter, coconut oil, or avocado oil

¼ cup unsweetened sunflower seed butter, almond butter, or peanut butter

½ cup low-carb granular sweetener

1 tablespoon instant espresso powder (optional)

2 teaspoons chocolate-flavored liquid monk fruit

½ teaspoon baking powder

3 large eggs

FOR THE MOCHA GANACHE:

½ cup heavy cream

½ cup sugar-free chocolate chips

1 tablespoon instant espresso powder

1. Preheat the oven to 350°F. Place cupcake liners in a 12-well muffin pan. Set aside.
2. In a heatproof bowl set over a saucepan with 1 to 2 inches of simmering water, heat the chocolate chips, butter, and sunflower seed butter over medium heat until melted, stirring constantly until smooth, with no lumps remaining. Remove from the heat. (You could also use a microwave-safe bowl and microwave in 30-second increments, stirring in-between, until melted and smooth.)
3. Pour the melted chocolate mixture into the bowl of a stand mixer fitted with the paddle attachment or a large mixing bowl. Add the remaining ingredients for the cupcakes, except the eggs, and mix on medium speed until combined and smooth. Taste the batter to check the sweetness, adding more sweetener if desired. Add the eggs one egg at a time, mixing to combine after each addition.
4. Pour the batter into the lined muffin wells, filling each halfway up, and bake for 20 to 22 minutes, until the cupcakes are puffed up and a toothpick inserted in the center comes out clean.
5. Remove from the oven and set aside to cool for 15 minutes before topping with ganache.
6. To make the mocha ganache, bring the cream to a simmer in a small saucepan over medium-low heat. Put the chocolate chips and espresso powder in a heatproof bowl. Stir to combine. Once the cream is simmering, pour it over the chocolate and let it sit for 5 minutes without stirring. After 5 minutes, stir until the ganache is completely smooth and there are no lumps. Spoon the warm ganache on top of the cupcakes. Serve right away or allow the ganache to harden.

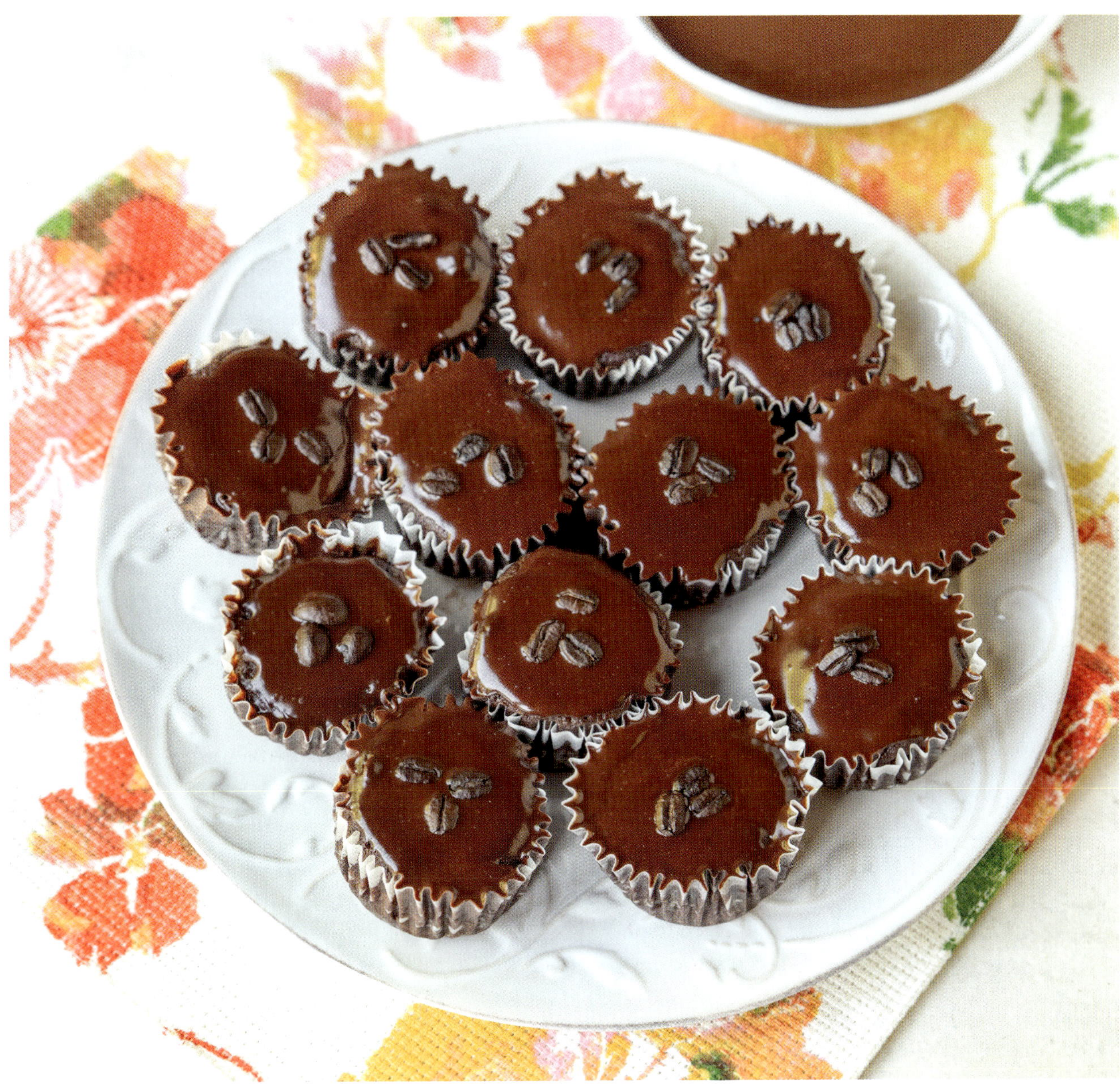

7. Store in an airtight container on the counter for up to 3 days or in the fridge for up to 1 week. (Storing them in the fridge will keep them fudgy.) Alternatively, freeze for up to 3 months.

Calories	Fat	Protein	Total Carbs	Dietary Fiber	Net Carbs
241	21g	5g	5g	0.3g	4.7g

ENDNOTES

1. Grant A. Pignatiello, Richard J. Martin, and Ronald L. Hickman, Jr., "Decision Fatigue: A Conceptual Analysis," *Journal of Health Psychology* 25, no. 1 (2018): 123–35, https://doi.org/10.1177/1359105318763510.

2. Goran Šimić et al., "Understanding Emotions: Origins and Roles of the Amygdala," *Biomolecules* 11, no. 6 (2021): 823, https://doi.org/10.3390/biom11060823.

3. Rupa Gupta et al., "The Amygdala and Decision-Making," *Neuropsychologia* 49, no. 4 (2011): 760–6, https://doi.org/10.1016/j.neuropsychologia.2010.09.029.

4. Michael Ascher and Lauren Ascher, "Overcoming Decision Fatigue in ADHD," *Psychology Today*, May 8, 2024, www.psychologytoday.com/us/blog/changing-the-narrative-on-adhd/202405/overcoming-decision-fatigue-in-adhd.

5. Daniela Jakubowicz et al., "Meal Timing and Composition Influence Ghrelin Levels, Appetite Scores and Weight Loss Maintenance in Overweight and Obese Adults," *Steroids* 77, no. 4 (2012): 323–31, https://doi.org/10.1016/j.steroids.2011.12.006.

6. David Raubenheimer and Stephen J. Simpson, "Protein Leverage: Theoretical Foundations and Ten Points of Clarification," *Obesity* (Silver Spring, MD) 27, no. 8 (2019): 1225–38, https://onlinelibrary.wiley.com/doi/10.1002/oby.22531.

7. Sarika Arora, "How to Stop Sugar Cravings," Women's Health Network, last updated April 27, 2025, www.womenshealthnetwork.com/blood-sugar/sugar-cravings/.

8. James J. DiNicolantonio, James H. O'Keefe, and William L. Wilson, "Sugar Addiction: Is It Real? A Narrative Review," *British Journal of Sports Medicine* 52, no. 14 (2018): 910–3, https://doi.org/10.1136/bjsports-2017-097971.

9. Jong-Woo Sohn, "Network of Hypothalamic Neurons That Control Appetite," *BMB Reports* 48, no. 4 (2015): 229–33, https://doi.org/10.5483/BMBRep.2015.48.4.272.

10. Anne-Marie Chang et al., "Evening Use of Light-Emitting eReaders Negatively Affects Sleep, Circadian Timing, and Next-Morning Alertness," *Proceedings of the National Academy of Sciences* 112, no. 4 (2015): 1232–7, https://doi.org/10.1073/pnas.1418490112.

11. Vennila Suriyagandhi and Vasanthi Nachiappan, "Protective Effects of Melatonin Against Obesity-Induced by Leptin Resistance," *Behavioural Brain Research* 417 (2022): 113598, https://doi.org/10.1016/j.bbr.2021.113598.

12. YongMin Cho et al., "Effects of Artificial Light at Night on Human Health: A Literature Review of Observational and Experimental Studies Applied to Exposure Assessment," *Chronobiology International* 32, no. 9 (2015): 1294–310, https://doi.org/10.3109/07420528.2015.1073158.

13. Gaétan Chevalier et al., "Earthing: Health Implications of Reconnecting the Human Body to the Earth's Surface Electrons," *Journal of Environmental and Public Health* (2012): 291541, https://www.ncbi.nlm.nih.gov/pmc/articles/PMC3265077/.

14. Clinton Ober, Stephen T. Sinatra, and Martin Zucker, *Earthing: The Most Important Health Discovery Ever!* (Basic Health Publications, 2014).

15. Maurice Ghaly and Dale Teplit, "The Biologic Effects of Grounding the Human Body During Sleep as Measured by Cortisol Levels and Subjective Reporting of Sleep, Pain, and Stress," *Journal of Alternative and Complementary Medicine* 10, no. 5 (2004): 767–76, https://pubmed.ncbi.nlm.nih.gov/15650465/.

16. Hans-Peter Landolt, "'No Thanks, Coffee Keeps Me Awake': Individual Caffeine Sensitivity Depends on *ADORA2A* Genotype," *Sleep* 35, no. 7 (2012): 899–900, www.ncbi.nlm.nih.gov/pmc/articles/PMC3368971/.

17. Oura Team, "How Caffeine Impacts Your Sleep," *The Pulse* (blog), August 31, 2023, https://ouraring.com/blog/how-caffeine-impacts-sleep/.

18. Ann F. Walker et al., "Mg Citrate Found More Bioavailable Than Other MG Preparations in a Randomised, Double-Blind Study," *Magnesium Research* 16, no. 3 (2003): 183–91, https://pubmed.ncbi.nlm.nih.gov/14596323/.

19. Ortho Molecular Products, "Reacted-Magnesium Powder," accessed September 30, 2024, www.orthomolecularproducts.ca/docs/canadalibraries/pdn/reacted-magnesium---information-sheet.pdf?sfvrsn=b34ea6c_5.

20. Neil Bernard Boyle, Clare Lawton, and Louise Dye, "The Effects of Magnesium Supplementation on Subjective Anxiety and Stress—A Systematic Review," *Nutrients* 9, no. 5 (2017): 429, www.ncbi.nlm.nih.gov/pmc/articles/PMC5452159/.

21. Joseph Levine, "Controlled Trials of Inositol in Psychiatry," *European Neuropsychopharmacology : the Journal of the European College of Neuropsychopharmacology* 7, no. 2 (1997): 147–55, https://pubmed.ncbi.nlm.nih.gov/9169302/.

22. V. Soldat-Stanković et al., "The Effect of Metformin and Myoinositol on Metabolic Outcomes in Women with Polycystic Ovary Syndrome: Role of Body Mass and Adiponectin in a Randomized Controlled Trial," *Journal of Endocrinological Investigation* 45, no. 3 (2022): 583–95, https://pubmed.ncbi.nlm.nih.gov/34665453/.

23. Meysam Zarezadeh et al., "Inositol Supplementation and Body Mass Index: A Systematic Review and Meta-Analysis of Randomized Clinical Trials," *Obesity Science & Practice* 8, no. 3 (2021): 387–97, www.ncbi.nlm.nih.gov/pmc/articles/PMC9159559/.

24. Tomohiko Mukai et al., "A Meta-Analysis of Inositol for Depression and Anxiety Disorders," *Human Psychopharmacology* 29, no. 1 (2014): 55–63, https://pubmed.ncbi.nlm.nih.gov/24424706/.

25. Benjamin E. Jewett and Sandeep Sharma, "Physiology, GABA," *StatPearls* [Internet], last updated July 24, 2023, www.ncbi.nlm.nih.gov/books/NBK513311/.

26. Gregor Hasler et al., "Effect of Acute Psychological Stress on Prefrontal GABA Concentration Determined by Proton Magnetic Resonance Spectroscopy," *The American Journal of Psychiatry* 167, no. 10 (2010): 1226–31, https://www.ncbi.nlm.nih.gov/pmc/articles/PMC3107037/.

27. YongMin Cho et al., "Effects of Artificial Light at Night on Human Health: A Literature Review of Observational and Experimental Studies Applied to Exposure Assessment," *Chronobiology International* 32, no. 9 (2015): 1294–1310, https://doi.org/10.3109/07420528.2015.1073158; Vera Popovic and Leonidas H. Duntas, "Brain Somatic Cross-Talk: Ghrelin, Leptin and Ultimate Challengers of Obesity," *Nutritional Neuroscience* 8, no. 1 (2005): 1–5, www.tandfonline.com/doi/abs/10.1080/10284150400027107; see note 11 above.

28. Jason Fanning et al., "Intervening on Exercise and Daylong Movement for Weight Loss Maintenance in Older Adults: A Randomized, Clinical Trial," *Obesity* (Silver Spring, MD) 30, no. 1 (2022): 85–95, https://www.ncbi.nlm.nih.gov/pmc/articles/PMC8711609/.

29. Nicola König et al., "How Therapeutic Tapping Can Alter Neural Correlates of Emotional Prosody Processing in Anxiety," *Brain Sciences* 9, no. 8 (2019): 206, https://pmc.ncbi.nlm.nih.gov/articles/PMC6721443.

30. Rachel A. Heckenberg et al., "Do Workplace-Based Mindfulness Meditation Programs Improve Physiological Indices of Stress? A Systematic Review and Meta-Analysis," *ScienceDirect* 114 (2018): 62–71, https://www.sciencedirect.com/science/article/abs/pii/S0022399918305749; Katey Davidson and Heather Hobbs, "11 Natural Ways to Lower Your Cortisol Levels," *Healthline*, updated January 29, 2024, www.healthline.com/nutrition/ways-to-lower-cortisol; Quinn A Conklin et al., "Meditation, Stress Processes, and Telomere Biology," *Current Opinion in Psychology* 28 (2019): 92–101, https://doi.org/10.1016/j.copsyc.2018.11.009.

31. Paola Helena Ponte Márquez et al., "Benefits of Mindfulness Meditation in Reducing Blood Pressure and Stress in Patients with Arterial Hypertension," *Journal of Human Hypertension* 33 (2019): 237–47, https://doi.org/10.1038/s41371-018-0130-6.

32. Dharma Singh Khalsa, "Stress, Meditation, and Alzheimer's Disease Prevention: Where the Evidence Stands," *Journal of Alzheimer's Disease* 48, no. 1: 1–12 (2015), https://doi.org/10.3233/JAD-142766; Hye Gyeong Son and Eun-Ok Choi, "The Effects of Mindfulness Meditation-Based Complex Exercise Program on Motor and Nonmotor Symptoms and Quality of Life in Patients with Parkinson's Disease," *Asian Nursing Research* 12, no. 2 (2018): 145–53, https://doi.org/10.1016/j.anr.2018.06.001.

33. Jason C. Ong et al., "A Randomized Controlled Trial of Mindfulness Meditation for Chronic Insomnia: Effects on Daytime Symptoms and Cognitive-

Emotional Arousal," *Mindfulness* 9 (2018): 1702–12, https://doi.org/10.1007/s12671-018-0911-6.

34. John T. Mitchell et al., "A Pilot Trial of Mindfulness Meditation Training for ADHD in Adulthood: Impact on Core Symptoms, Executive Functioning, and Emotion Dysregulation," *Journal of Attention Disorders* 21, no. 13 (2013), https://journals.sagepub.com/doi/abs/10.1177/1087054713513328.

35. Brenda Bennett, *The 30-Day Sugar Elimination Diet: A Whole-Food Detox to Conquer Cravings & Reclaim Health, Customizable for Keto or Low-Carb* (Victory Belt Publishing Inc, 2023).

36. Ju Young Kim, "Optimal Diet Strategies for Weight Loss and Weight Loss Maintenance," *Journal of Obesity & Metabolic Syndrome* 30, no. 1 (2020): 20–31, www.ncbi.nlm.nih.gov/pmc/articles/PMC8017325/.

37. Jamie I. Baum, Il-Young Kim, and Robert R. Wolfe, "Protein Consumption and the Elderly: What Is the Optimal Level of Intake?," *Nutrients* 8, no. 6 (2016): 359, www.ncbi.nlm.nih.gov/pmc/articles/PMC4924200/.

38. Jorn Trommelen et al., "The Anabolic Response to Protein Ingestion During Recovery from Exercise Has No Upper Limit in Magnitude and Duration *in vivo* in Humans," *Cell Reports Medicine* 4, no. 12 (2023): 101324, www.ncbi.nlm.nih.gov/pmc/articles/PMC10772463/.

39. See note 36 above.

40. Daniela Jakubowicz et al., "High Caloric Intake at Breakfast vs. Dinner Differentially Influences Weight Loss of Overweight and Obese Women," *Obesity* (Silver Spring, MD) 21, no 12 (2013): 2504–12, https://pubmed.ncbi.nlm.nih.gov/23512957/.

41. Lidia Satarpia, Franco Contaldo, and Fabrizio Pasanini, "Body Composition Changes After Weight-Loss Interventions for Overweight and Obesity," *Clinical Nutrition* 32, no. 2 (2013); 157–61, https://doi.org/10.1016/j.clnu.2012.08.016; Thais R. Silva, Karen Oppermann, Fernando M. Reis, and Poli Mara Spritzer, "Nutrition in Menopausal Women: A Narrative Review," *Nutrients* 13, no. 7 (2021): 2149, https://doi.org/10.3390/nu13072149; Gordon I. Smith et al., "Effect of a High-Protein Diet on Preservation of Muscle Mass and Metabolic Rate During Weight Loss in Postmenopausal Women," *Obesity* 23, no. 8 (2015): 1462–70, https://doi.org/10.1002/oby.21134.

42. Institute of Medicine (US) Subcommittee on Military Weight Management, "Weight-Loss and Maintenance Strategies," *Weight Management: State of the Science and Opportunities for Military Programs* (National Academies Press, 2004), https://www.ncbi.nlm.nih.gov/books/NBK221839/.

43. Kyung Jung Han, Mansoo Yu, and Omoshola Kehinde, "Effectiveness of Different Online Intervention Modalities for Middle-Aged Adults with Overweight and Obesity: A 20-Year Systematic Review and Meta-Analysis," *Journal of Prevention* 45 (2024): 123–57, https://link.springer.com/article/10.1007/s10935-023-00761-z.

RECIPE INDEX

BASICS

GOOD (ENOUGH)

BREAKFAST

LUNCH

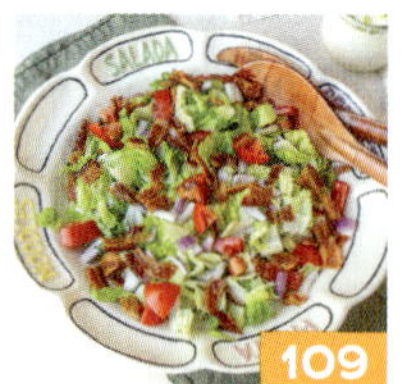

Good Enough BLT Salad

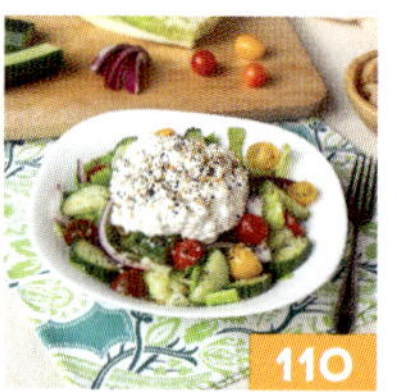

Cottage Cheese Lunch Bowl

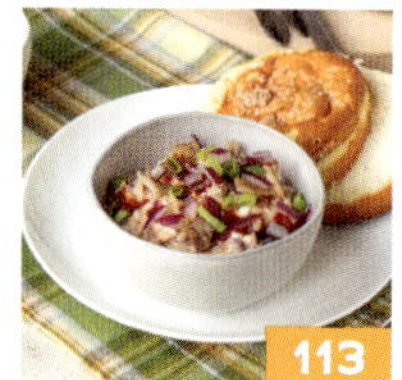

Hot BBQ Chicken Cottage Cheese Bowl

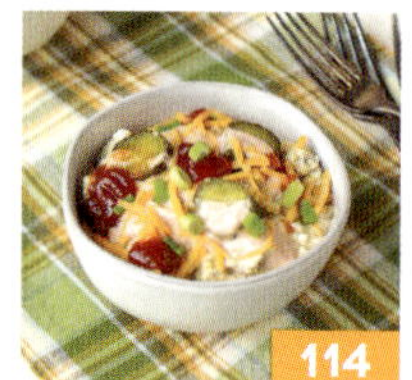

Hot Cheeseburger Cottage Cheese Bowl

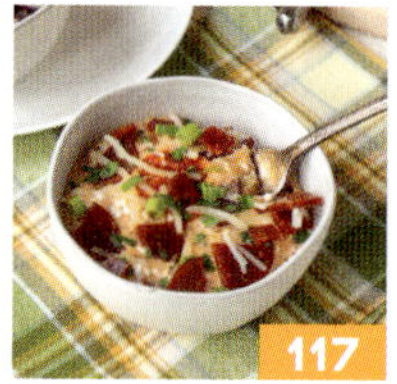

Hot Cottage Cheese Pizza Bowl

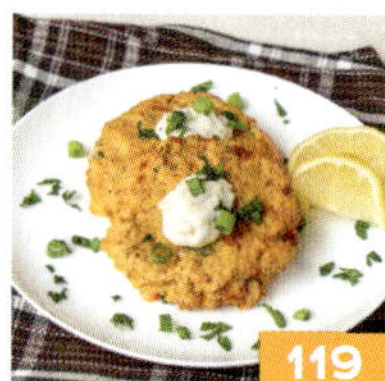

Salmon Patties

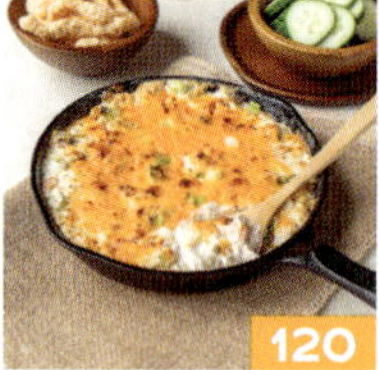

Hot Shrimp Dip

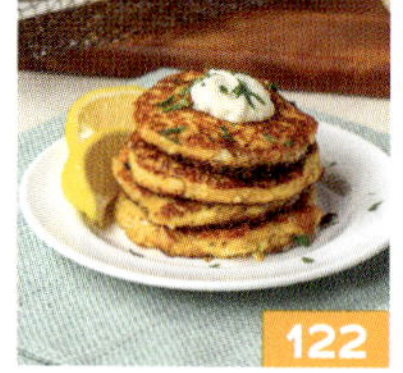

Tuna Cabbage Patties

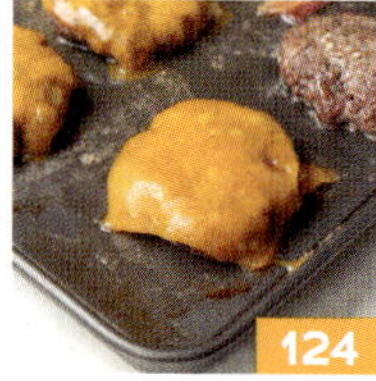

Sheet Pan Ranch Burgers

DINNER & SIDES

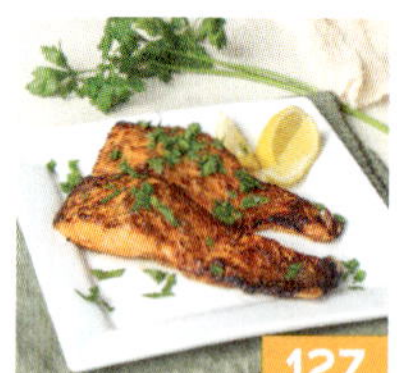

Air Fryer Salmon

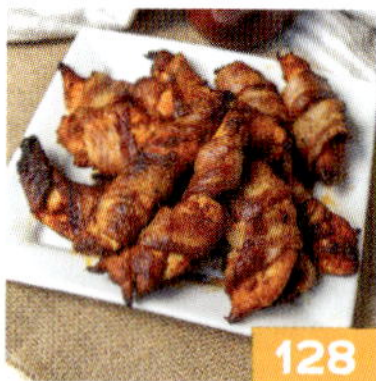

Bacon-Wrapped Chicken Tenders

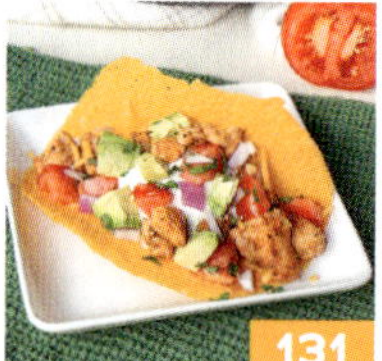

Chicken Tacos

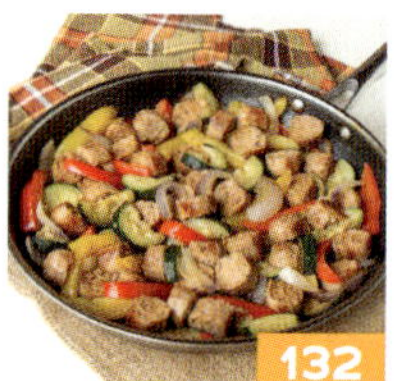

Turkey Sausage Pepper Zucchini Skillet

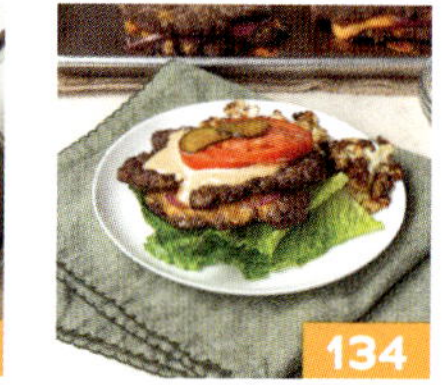

Sheet Pan Double Smash Cheeseburgers with Secret Sauce

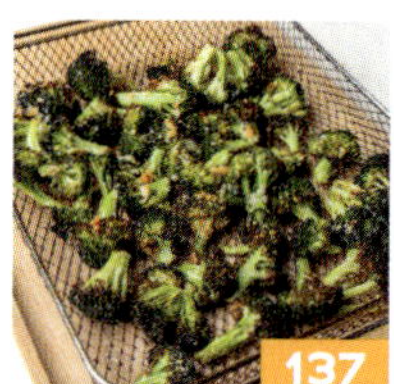

Garlic Parmesan Broccoli

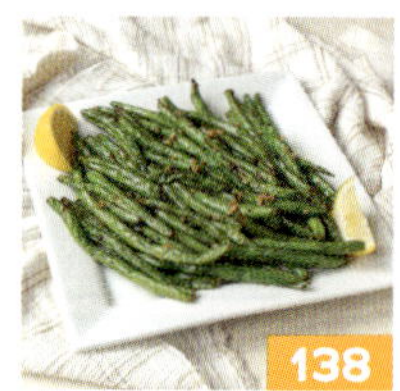

Garlic Green Beans

DESSERTS

BETTER

BREAKFAST

LUNCH

DINNER & SIDES

DESSERTS

BEST

BREAKFAST

LUNCH

DINNER & SIDES

DINNER & SIDES (continued)

DESSERTS

GENERAL INDEX

C

D

E

N

O

P

Q

R

T

V

W

Y–Z